A Practical Approach to Radiology

A Practical Approach to Radiology

Nancy M. Major, MD

Associate Professor
Radiology, Surgery, Biological Anthropology and Anatomy
Musculoskeletal Division
Duke University Medical Center
Durham, North Carolina

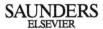

SAUNDERS
ELSEVIER

1600 John F. Kennedy Blvd.
Suite 1800
Philadelphia, PA 19103-2899

A Practical Approach to Radiology

ISBN-13: 978-1-4160-2341-8
ISBN-10: 1-4160-2341-0

Library of Congress Cataloging-in-Publication Data
Major, Nancy M.
    A practical approach to radiology/Nancy M. Major.
      p.; cm.
    ISBN-13: 978-1-4160-2341-8
    ISBN-10: 1-4160-2341-0
    1. Diagnosis, Radioscopic. 2. Diagnostic imaging. 3. Radiography, Medical. I. Title.
      [DNLM: 1. Radiology–methods. 2. Diagnostic Imaging–Methods. WN 180 M234p 2007]
    RC78.M35 2007
    616.07'57–dc22

                                                                                        2006041809

Acquisitions Editor: Meghan McAteer
Developmental Editor: Kim Davis
Project Manager: David Saltzberg
Design Direction: Karen O'Keefe Owens

To my son, Austin Michael Helms: Everyday you remind me of what a joy it is to teach. Your innate curiosity and quest for knowledge is a great source of pleasure for me. I am grateful to you for your patience during the creation of this book.

To my parents, Kathy and Paul: You spent more time at my house than your own during the writing of this book! Without your support and the care you provided for Austin this book clearly couldn't have happened. You gave me the gift of time and the incentive to make this happen. I am grateful to you for all you do and for the wonderful example you have provided.

To the greatest teacher I know, and the love of my life, Clyde Helms, this book is dedicated to you.

N. M. M.

Contents

Acknowledgments

It is misleading to think that I could have prepared this book on my own. While I am responsible for the content, I acquired it from a variety of sources. I must acknowledge my colleagues who helped by contributing images for your viewing pleasure. I am forever grateful to Mike Gotway, M.D., Elizabeth Mc Graw, M.D., Don Frush, M.D., Charles Gooding, M.D., Mike Hanson, M.D., Dave Williams, M.D., William Thompson, M.D., Carl Ravin, M.D., Jay Baker, M.D., Mary Scott Soo, M.D., Ralph Heinz, Tony Smith, M.D., Barbara Hertzberg, M.D., Srini Mukundan M.D., Susan Kealey M.D., and Clyde A. Helms, M.D. In addition to contributing numerous examples of pathology, William E. Brant, M.D. provided encouragement and mentorship. Those who have trained with him know he is an outstanding teacher, and I have the great fortune of calling him my dearest friend.

I'd like to acknowledge the secretarial support of Mirjana Cudic whose efficiency is unparalleled, and whose spell check seems to work better than mine!

I'd like to thank Dr. Carl Ravin, my Chairman, for being understanding during the time that I was preparing this book. His support and encouragement was especially helpful and unexpected. It is a privilege and pleasure to be a part of Duke Radiology, and to work with a Chairman who has created a marvelous atmosphere for me to maximize my interests and potential.

My section chief, Clyde Helms, was wonderfully supportive, and was patient while I missed weekends with him and our son in order to complete this project on time.

To the publisher, Elsevier, I'd like to acknowledge the support from Allan Ross and Meghan McAteer. Their enthusiasm for this project and guidance throughout will lead to the success of this book. Kim Davis and the art department were delightful to work with and have the same standard of excellence as I had for this book.

I must acknowledge the unending and tireless work of Glen Toomayan, MD. During the preparation of this book, Glen was involved in every step. He proofread every chapter for clarity as well as organization and detail. He edited the tables and key points for clarity and consistency. Glen also communicated with many of the radiologists mentioned previously in getting good examples for the textbook. His insight was invaluable and his computer skills far exceed anything I could aspire to. Glen is a radiology resident at Duke, and I believe he will make great academic contributions to the specialty of radiology. His friendship, support and desire for perfection made this book much better than it would have been without his involvement. I valued his suggestions and input and am grateful to him for identifying when changes needed to be made. I am indebted to him for spending countless hours listening to me pontificate about one topic or another. Never have I worked with a more kind, patient man who was one of the smartest medical students I have had the pleasure to teach. He also taught me a great deal during the creation of this book.

I have had the great pleasure to work with and teach many students that have come through Duke radiology. I thank every last one of them who have enriched my life.

Foreword

In the summer of 1999, in what has proven to be one of my best administrative decisions, I asked Dr. Nancy M. Major to become Director of our very popular medical student elective in diagnostic radiology. She agreed and, with her characteristic high energy and enthusiasm, set about energizing this already popular elective. The elective itself provides a broad overview of diagnostic radiology through an extensive series of lectures and rotations on various imaging subspecialties. During her first several years as elective director, Dr. Major attended all of the lectures in the various subspecialties, paying particular attention to what was being taught and what ultimately seemed to be of import to students who, for the most part, were interested in practicing specialties other than radiology. Through this experience she developed a very clear understanding of the kinds of information that all medical students need in order to more fully utilize diagnostic imaging effectively in the care of their patients. Her infectious enthusiasm and high energy were repeatedly recognized by our medical students and, since 1999, Dr. Major has been recognized for her teaching excellence by the graduating medical school class on four separate occasions. Fortunately she has, in this book, pulled together all the insights gathered during the past seven years to create a text through which she can share her observations with medical students outside the Duke University School of Medicine.

This textbook of educational gems, gathered from across the broad spectrum of diagnostic imaging, is written in the easy conversational tone which Dr. Major has used effectively to reach hundreds of students during the past seven years. In addition to the exquisite anatomic renderings, the text incorporates two features which are very helpful in ultimately mastering the material presented. The first of these is a summary of "Key Points" which highlights the critical teaching points in each chapter. These key points are accompanied by a series of "Tables" which again simplifies the information presented in the chapter and presents it in an easily understood highlighted format. These key points and tables, taken together, provided an easy to remember summary of each chapter which will help the interested student ensure that he or she has garnered the relevant information from each section. Finally, each chapter is color coded, so that it may be readily identified without having to leaf through the entire book to find the chapter of current interest.

This text represents a student-focused compendium of key points in diagnostic imaging. It is compiled by one of the country's most effective medical student teachers and written in a way that allows the reader to believe that he or she is conversing with Dr. Major herself. The innovations of key points, summary tables, and color coded chapters adds to the ease of use of this text and contributes significantly to its overall effectiveness. We are gratified that Dr. Major has undertaken this enormous effort as it will make available to all medical students the breadth and depth of knowledge which was heretofore available only to a select few.

Carl E. Ravin
Professor and Chairman
Department of Radiology
Duke University

Radiology has always been an important part of patient care. Numerous terrific textbooks have been written to guide the student through radiographic analysis in hopes of teaching the student about radiology as it relates to patient care. As the specialty of radiology has grown, so have the size of textbooks for the students! Fortunately for the student, not all of this information is necessary to learn. Unfortunately, how does the student know what is superfluous? The reality is only a small percentage of students in training will choose radiology as a specialty where the inclusion of extra information is useful and interesting. Regardless of your specialty choice (and radiology is a good one) most students will need to have some level of understanding of radiology to adequately perform patient care.

I have been teaching radiology to medical students for a number of years at Duke University Medical Center. During this time I have had the opportunity to see *how* students learn and *what* is necessary for the student to understand during the training process. My goals in writing this book for you were to include what was important to know as a student (and not everything I know as a radiologist), and present it in a format that is user friendly. Before every entry in this book, I asked "is this information absolutely necessary for the student to understand?" If the answer was *yes*, you will find it included. If the answer was *no*, it was left out, with reference to it in the suggested reading list.

My approach to everything in life is quite "practical" (with the most obvious exception being shoe purchases). Thus, the name of the book suits the design, intent and content well, and reflects the author's (my) approach to life. It is written with humor and is my preferred style of teaching.

The focus of this book is to expose the student to radiology as a specialty necessary for patient care, as well as to evaluate commonly encountered pathologic disorders and those abnormalities that may need to be addressed in a timely manner. All commonly used imaging modalities in radiology are covered. Emphasis is placed on the modalities that would be encountered in an on-call or clinic situation. To that end, for instance, there is no

discussion regarding interpretation of magnetic resonance imaging studies. You are more apt to have to evaluate a head CT in an emergency situation than an MRI of the brain. However, I have discussed when these types of studies would be appropriate to order.

The book is organized by the body system (for the most part), and within each system is a discussion of imaging modalities and how each modality is used (or not) in that particular system. I chose to organize this readable text by *organ system* rather than *imaging modality* because it makes sense for patient care, and many training institutions' radiology departments are organized by body part rather than imaging modality. As an example "Chapter 3, Abdominal Imaging" includes a discussion of barium studies and computed tomography for evaluation of the gastrointestinal tract as well as imaging of the genitourinary system.

Each chapter is color-coded for easy reference and contains **Key Points** and **Tables** that are also colorfully highlighted. The purpose of the **Key Points** is to provide lists of "findings" on an x-ray as well as discuss search patterns. These are take home points that are useful for evaluation of a radiology exam. The purpose of the **Tables** is to provide lists and indications of types of exams, as well as provide differential diagnoses when appropriate. Used together, the **Key Points** and **Tables** are a nice summary of the chapters.

Many figures are included in this text. Because of the size of the book, all possible examples of disease could not be included. But key examples are provided with adequate explanation.

One thing that is germane to understanding and interpreting radiology is knowledge of anatomy and tissue composition. Wonderful anatomy texts are available, and you likely have used many of these during your anatomy instruction. A complete review of anatomy cannot be put into a *Practical Approach*. But I thought it important that some normal anatomy be shown. To that end, each chapter has sketches of normal anatomy for your review in order to provide a reasonable understanding of anatomy that you will encounter on an x-ray image. I have tried to be consistent with the approach to anatomy and the use of the illustrations coupled with normal x-rays to improve your understanding of the anatomy on the x-ray. This knowledge of what is normal will allow you to be more comfortable understanding the pathology present in many of the examples in this book.

At the end of each chapter I have provided a suggested reading list, as I alluded to above. These additional textbooks will provide much more detail regarding the topics that are addressed in each chapter, as well as topics not discussed. The reading list is also useful for those who find radiology to be a terrific way to provide patient care and would like to read more about it.

In the end, I hope that you will find this *Practical Approach to Radiology* to be as much fun to read as it was to write.

I welcome any comments that you may have.

Nancy M. Major

Basic Concepts of Imaging Methods

A book that provides a practical overview for a student learning to interpret images shouldn't have too much of it dedicated to how the images are acquired. Nevertheless, it is important to understand how images are generated. In turn, you will understand the differences in imaging techniques and what studies might be necessary in caring for your patients.

The goal of this chapter is to review the basics of the primary diagnostic imaging methods and the principles used in interpreting them, with emphasis on the *language* for description of the methods. There will be very little discussion of physics. I will emphasize only what is necessary for film interpretation. Wonderful textbooks have been written (Wonderful physics textbooks—is that possible?) on how to make different types of x-ray images. My goal is to get you to know which studies should be performed to diagnose a patient's illness, how to recognize pathology, and what to do once the pathology has been identified. Therefore, no time for physics.

Conventional X-rays

Advancements in computer technology have revolutionized body imaging. As a result of the digital revolution, images can be obtained quickly and downloaded onto a computer screen within seconds. X-rays are photons that are formed within an x-ray tube (a type of cathode-ray tube). The x-rays are directed (collimated) by lead-lined shutters to an area requiring imaging. These x-rays pass through the human body and are attenuated by interaction with various tissues in the body. There are five basic *radiographic densities*: *air, fat, soft tissue/fluid, bone,* and *metal* (**Key Point 1–1**) (**Table 1–1**). Because air attenuates very little of the x-ray beam, the beam blackens the film. Bone and metal (bullets, barium, and so on) attenuate a large proportion of the x-ray beam, allowing very little of the beam to blacken the film. Thus bone and metal

Key	Point 1–1

Conventional X-ray Densities

Air

Fat

Fluid/soft tissue

Bone

Metal

Table 1–1 Language Used in Describing Radiographic Studies	
Type of Study	**Term Used**
Plain films	Density
Fluoroscopy	Density
Computed tomography (CT)	Attenuation
Ultrasonography	Echogenicity
Magnetic resonance imaging (MRI)	Signal Intensity
Nuclear medicine	Activity

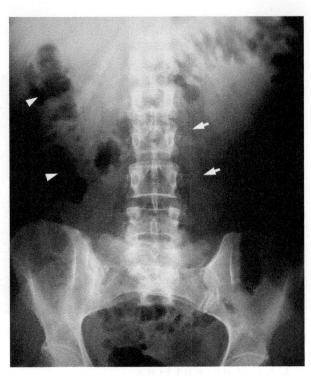

Figure 1–2 Normal x-ray of kidneys, ureters, and bladder (KUB). Conventional x-ray demonstrating the types of densities normally encountered on a KUB. Air (*black density*) is noted in the ascending colon (*arrowheads*). The spine and pelvis are visualized as white, and the psoas shadows are a soft tissue density (*arrows*).

appear white on an x-ray image (radiograph) (Figure 1–1).

Soft tissue and fluid are mentioned together because soft tissue structures are primarily water, and therefore their densities appear similar on an x-ray film. A joint effusion for example, has the same density as muscle. Soft tissue and fat attenuate intermediate amounts of the x-ray beam compared with air or metal. The result is a proportional degree of film darkening. Similarly, a thick structure (large patient, for instance) attenuates more radiation than a thin structure. These differences in attenuation result in differences in the level of exposure of the film.

Anatomic structures are seen on x-rays when tissues of different density outline them. In the abdomen, for example, fat density outlines the margin of the liver, spleen, and kidneys (which are soft tissue/fluid density), thus allowing these organs to be visualized. Bone and metal are of high density, and their detail can be visualized through overlying soft tissues (Figure 1–2).

We can use the principle of observation of different densities to diagnose disease states. For example, the silhouette sign (of Felson) in pulmonary radiology describes obliteration of a normal air–soft tissue interface, such as the cardiac silhouette with the adjacent right middle lobe. When fluid density (such as pus from pneumonia) fills the right middle lobe, the right heart border becomes obscured because it, too, is a soft tissue (fluid) density (Figure 1–3).

Fluoroscopy

Modifications to the x-ray technique allow a continuous stream of x-rays to be produced from

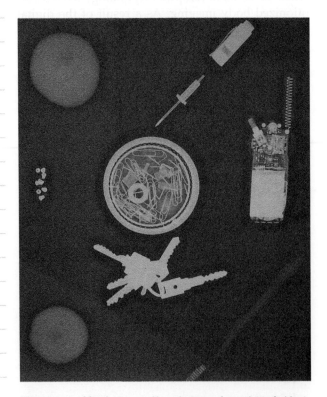

Figure 1–1 Metal on x-ray. X-ray images of a variety of objects demonstrating the property of metal imaging as very white on an x-ray. I suspect you can figure out what the different objects are in the image.

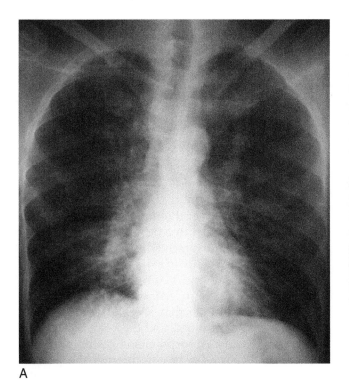

A

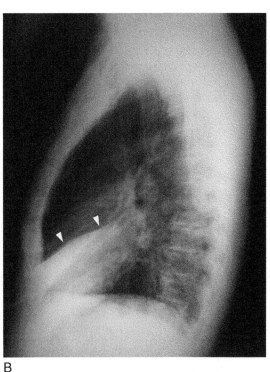

B

Figure 1–3   Silhouette sign. A, Frontal conventional chest x-ray shows a lack of definition of the right heart border compared with the left. This indicates a density (in this case pneumonia) of the right middle lobe. B, The lateral film shows the middle lobe superimposed over the heart, as evidenced by the increased density (more white) in this location (*arrowheads*).

the x-ray tube. Fluoroscopy allows real-time visualization of moving anatomic structures. A continuous x-ray beam passes through the patient, and the part of the beam that remains is captured: *physics happens*, and an image is projected on the television-like screen (Figure 1–4). The same terms used to describe a conventional x-ray are also used to describe a fluoroscopic image. Uses of fluoroscopy include evaluation of peristalsis, diaphragmatic motion, barium studies, catheter placement, and angiographic procedures.

Important concepts to keep in mind when observing or performing a fluoroscopy procedure are *distance* and *time*. The exposure to radiation using fluoroscopy decreases with the square of the distance from the radiation source (Key Point 1–2). Standing farther away from the fluoroscopy table (x-ray beam) decreases the exposure dramatically. Exposure to radiation increases with time. Ideally, the time required to perform a fluoroscopy procedure (fluoro time) should be only seconds. Obviously that is not always possible, so if you are observing a case that is taking a lot of fluoro time, standing as far from the table as possible is a good idea, and standing outside the room may be even better!

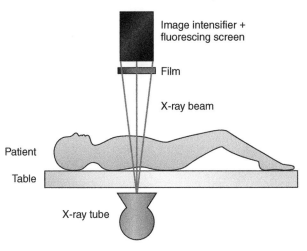

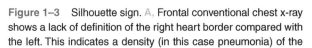

Figure 1–4   Diagram of the usual setup in the fluoroscopy suite. The x-rays come from below the table and penetrate the patient; the portion of the x-ray beam that gets through the patient is captured via film/image intensifier and screen. *Physics happens* and the image is then projected on a television-like screen.

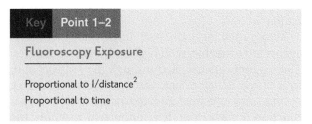

Key Point 1–2

Fluoroscopy Exposure

Proportional to $1/\text{distance}^2$
Proportional to time

Contrast Agents

It may be necessary to fill bowel loops or blood vessels with a substance that attenuates x-rays more than bowel loops or arteries do normally. Contrast materials take advantage of the density concept. Contrast agents are suspensions of barium or iodine (metals) that highly attenuate the x-ray beam and, therefore, can be used to outline anatomic structures.

A variety of contrast agents are used for radiology examinations. For example, contrast agents for computed tomography (CT) studies are not the same as for magnetic resonance imaging (MRI) examinations. Additionally, there are agents used to opacify bowel, and those are different for CT than for gastrointestinal (GI) studies using fluoroscopy.

Gastrointestinal Contrast Agents

Several types of nontoxic, high-density contrast agents are available for opacification of the bowel. The utility of each agent depends on what is being evaluated.

"Thick" and "thin" barium are used differently. Thin suspensions are used for single-contrast studies, which generally reveal function, whereas the thicker solution is used in conjunction with air (either ingested "fizzies" or insufflated air) and allows for mucosal evaluation (double-contrast or air/barium study). Finally, water-soluble iodinated agents are indicated if bowel perforation is suspected. Barium peritonitis is associated with high mortality. Low-osmolar agents may be safer if the patient is at risk for aspiration. Care must be taken when administering hypertonic water-soluble agents. Large volumes of such contrast agents in the GI tract may result in fluid shifts leading to hypovolemia, shock, and even death in infants and debilitated adult patients.

It is often necessary to inject contrast agents directly into arteries and veins. Iodine-based agents are chosen, because their high atomic mass allows for marked attenuation of the x-ray beam. Iodinated contrast agents are used for such procedures as CT, angiography, cystography, urography, and GI opacification. These agents are excreted via the urinary system and are safe and well tolerated by patients.

Two types of iodinated intravenous contrast agents are available, with high and low osmolalities. These agents are excreted through the kidneys and, to a much lesser extent, through the liver, biliary system, and intestinal tract (particularly when renal function is impaired). It is important to know the patient's renal function before ordering a CT that requires contrast administration. Agents with higher osmolality are associated with more adverse reactions than low-osmolality solutions. The cost differential can be as much as 15 times greater for low-osmolality agents.

Cross-sectional Imaging

Computed Tomography

CT was invented in the 1970s by Sir Godfrey Hounsfield (winner of the Nobel Prize for Medicine in 1979). Subsequently, there have been many generations (improvements) of CT scanners. A CT scanner obtains a series of axial images. A computer mathematically reconstructs a cross-sectional image of the body from measurements of x-ray transmission through thin slices of patient tissue. The patient lies on a bed, and the x-ray tube rotates around the body. Absorption and scatter attenuate the x-ray beam as it passes through the patient. Sensitive detectors on the opposite side of the patient measure x-ray transmission through the slice. These measurements are systematically repeated many times from different directions as the tube rotates around the patient (Figure 1–5). The gray scale used to determine tissue attenuation is measured in Hounsfield units (HU). Water is

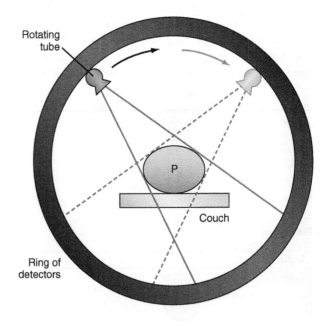

Figure 1–5   Diagram of the direction of x-ray beam in a CT unit. The patient (P) is on the couch, which is traveling through the gantry (opening) of the CT scanner. The x-rays travel around the patient by means of a rotating tube, and the ring of detectors measures the x-ray transmission through the slice. A computer reconstructs a cross-sectional image from the information.

CT Attenuation

Air	Black	–1024 HU
Bone/metal	White	+3000 to 4000 HU

Table I–2 CT Artifacts

Volume averaging
Beam hardening
Motion
Streak

assigned a value of 0 HU. Air images as black and therefore has an attenuation of –1024 HU. Very dense bone is very white on CT and therefore has an attenuation in the range of +3000 to 4000 HU (Key Point 1–3). Hounsfield units are not absolute values; they are relative units that vary from one CT system to another. Most CT systems allow slice thickness between 1 and 10 mm. The rapid scan acquisition along with the superior bone detail and the ability to demonstrate calcifications are some of the advantages of CT over other imaging modalities, including MRI. CT is acquired in the axial plane but can be reformatted or reconstructed to the sagittal or coronal plane or for three-dimensional (3-D) reconstruction (Figure 1–6).

Images are generally acquired in the axial plane and are viewed, by convention, as the observer looks from below upward toward the head. Therefore, the patient's right side is on the left side of the image. The upper portion of the image is anterior (unless otherwise indicated).

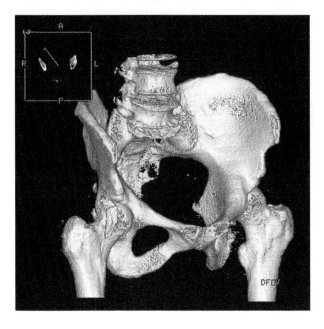

Figure 1–6 Three-dimensional reconstruction of the pelvis and acetabular fracture. Using the information obtained from the axial images, reconstruction can be performed for further evaluation. In addition to diagnostic information, reconstructions and reformations are often very useful for surgical planning.

The use of intravenous contrast can aid in the evaluation of lesions and distinguish pathology from the underlying parenchyma. The timing of the imaging after an intravenous bolus of contrast material facilitates this search. The earlier the images are obtained after injection, the greater the likelihood of arterial enhancement. As the time is delayed between injection and image acquisition, a venous phase and an equilibrium phase are also obtained. The administration of an oral contrast agent is necessary to opacify the bowel, in order to distinguish the bowel from lymph nodes, tumors, and hematomas.

It is necessary to understand a few artifacts, in order to not misinterpret films. These include *volume averaging, beam hardening, motion artifact, and streak artifacts. Volume averaging* is present in every CT image and must *always* be considered in interpreting an image. Assessment of the slices above and below the image being viewed is an excellent way to evaluate for volume averaging. Remember that taking a 3-D volume of tissue from a patient and creating a 2-D image requires averaging of the patient tissue in order to produce the image. *Beam hardening artifact* is seen as streaks of low density extending from structures of high x-ray attenuation. This often occurs around bone–soft tissue areas such as the petrous bone and shoulders. It results from greater attenuation of low-energy x-ray photons than high-energy photons as they pass through tissues. The mean energy of the x-ray beam is increased, resulting in less attenuation at the end of the beam than at its beginning. *Motion artifact* is demonstrated as streaks or a blurred or duplicated image that is a result of structures moving to different positions during image acquisition (for example, because of breathing or peristalsis). *Streak artifacts* emanate from high-density sharp-edged objects such as metallic hardware devices. Reconstruction or reformation of images affected by streak artifact is unsatisfactory (**Table 1–2**).

Ultrasonography

Ultrasonography is performed by using the "pulse-echo" technique, rather than electromagnetic radia-

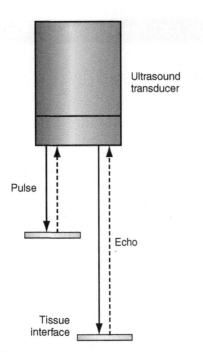

Ultrasound transducer

Pulse

Echo

Tissue interface

Figure 1–7 Diagram of pulse-echo technique utilized by ultrasound technology. The transducer sends out the pulse. The echoes travel through tissue and get reflected back to the transducer (which now functions as a receiver).

tion (Figure 1–7) (**Key Point 1–4**). The transducer converts electrical energy into a pulse of high-frequency sound energy, which is transmitted into patient tissues. Then the transducer changes jobs and becomes a receiver that detects echoes of sound energy reflected from body tissue. An average speed of sound in tissue is assumed to be 1540 m/sec. The depth of echo is determined by the time required for the round-trip pulse and returning echo. A powerful computer then interprets the sound waves, and a real-time image is produced. The transducers used for evaluation are high- and low-frequency transducers. A high-frequency transducer provides better spatial resolution and limited depth of penetration. High-frequency transducers are excellent for evaluation of superficial structures (thyroid, breast, testicles) and are in the range of 5 to 10 megahertz (MHz). Low-frequency transducers are in the range of 1 to 3.5 MHz and have lower resolution but better penetration of tissues. Low-

> **Key Point 1–4**
>
> Ultrasonography
> _____
>
> Pulse echo
> Not electromagnetic radiation

frequency transducers are most often used for abdominal, pelvic, and obstetric applications.

Ultrasound examinations are performed by applying the ultrasound transducer directly to the patient's skin, using a coupling agent (usually mineral oil or gel). The quality of the images produced is greatly influenced by the experience of the examiner. Ultrasound is a useful diagnostic tool when it is directed at solving a particular clinical problem, such as, is the mass cystic or solid? or are gallstones present?

Some problems that are encountered in ultrasound imaging occur when bone or gas-containing structures are near the area being evaluated. Bone almost completely absorbs the sound energy, making evaluation of tissues beyond the bone nearly impossible. Air almost completely reflects sound, leaving few echoes available to penetrate the tissues beyond this area. Evaluation of a mass near the lung or around bowel is difficult with ultrasound for this reason. Optimal visualization of many organs is performed through acoustic windows that allow adequate sound transmission, such as the distended bladder or amniotic fluid.

Doppler ultrasound takes advantage of the Doppler effect to evaluate moving objects such as blood flow. The Doppler effect is a shift in the frequency of returning echoes, as compared to the transmitted pulse, that is caused by reflection of the sound wave from a moving object. If blood flow is relatively away from the face of the transducer, the echo frequency is shifted lower. If blood flow is relatively toward the face of the transducer, the echo frequency is shifted higher. The amount of frequency shift is proportional to the relative velocity of the red blood cells. Therefore, Doppler ultrasound can detect not only the presence of blood flow but also its direction and velocity.

Color Doppler ultrasound combines gray scale and Doppler information in a single image. Stationary tissues are displayed in shades of gray, and blood flow and moving tissues with Doppler effect are displayed in color. Blood flow coming toward the transducer is usually displayed in shades of red. Blood flowing away from the transducer is displayed in shades of blue. Lighter shades of these colors imply higher flow velocities.

As with CT, there are artifacts that occur with ultrasound. The artifacts are not the same as those created with CT. These artifacts include *acoustic shadowing, acoustic enhancement, reverberation, mirror image,* and *ring down* artifacts. The more commonly encountered artifacts useful for interpretation of images will be discussed. *Acoustic shadowing* is a result of near-complete absorption or reflection of the ultrasound beam by bone, metallic objects, or air

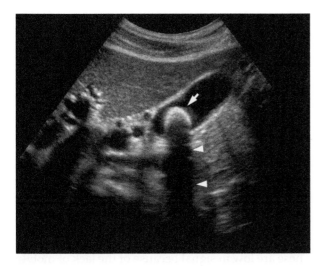

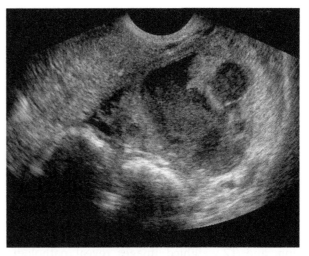

Figure 1–8   Acoustic shadowing. A large gallstone is demonstrated in the gallbladder. Note the increased echogenicity of the stone (*arrow*) and the acoustic shadowing (lack of echoes) beyond the stone (*arrowheads*). This artifact is useful for identification of different types of stones. (Courtesy of Barbara Hertzberg, MD.)

Figure 1–9   Lack of acoustic enhancement. This abscess located in the pelvis demonstrates some internal echoes (not black or *anechoic*). Instead it is filled with internal debris and lacks acoustic enhancement (white) on the opposite wall of the cyst. This is a finding that is seen in some cysts that are not simple fluid. (Courtesy of Barbara Hertzberg, MD.)

that obscures the deeper tissues. This artifact is very useful in identification of calculi (Figure 1–8). *Acoustic enhancement* causes the tissues deep to certain structures to be seen exceptionally well. This is true of fluid-filled structures. The other artifacts mentioned are useful to ultrasonographers for aid in identification of pathology but are not as commonly encountered by the novice who wishes to understand the basic concepts of fluid versus solid and identification of calcifications. Therefore, these additional artifacts are not discussed here (**Table 1–3**).

Solid tissues demonstrate *echogenicity* (speckles representing the tissue texture). Fat is highly echogenic (more white) than liver, kidney, or pancreas. Fluid-containing structures such as cysts, gallbladder, and distended bladder are *anechoic* (without internal echoes) and also demonstrate acoustic enhancement. Tissues with greater echogenicity are referred to as *hyperechoic*, and lesions of lower echogenicity compared with surrounding structures are termed *hypoechoic*. Potential confusion

can occur with cystic masses when they are filled with pus, blood, or mucin. These may cause some internal echoes within the cyst-like cavity. Acoustic enhancement may not be present (Figure 1–9).

Magnetic Resonance Imaging

The discussion of how to obtain a magnetic resonance (MR) image is beyond the scope of this book. Nevertheless, the student should be familiar with the types of images typically seen in medical imaging. The suggested reading list has references for a comprehensive review of the physics of MRI for those who are interested.

Radiowaves and magnetic fields are used to produce a tomographic image by measuring the signal produced from the strength, frequency, and time required for protons to return to their pre-excited state after excitation. A powerful computer analyzes these signals and creates an image.

The soft tissue contrast provided by MRI is substantially better than with any other imaging modality. Different tissues absorb and release radiowave energy at different, detectable, and characteristic rates. Terms that are part of the MRI vocabulary include *TR* and *TE*. The time allowed for protons to align with the main magnetic field is *TR*. The time allowed for absorbed radiowave energy to be released and detected is referred to as *TE*. Additional terms used in MRI are *T1*- and *T2*-weighted images. T1-weighted images are obtained by selecting a short TR (≤800 msec) and a

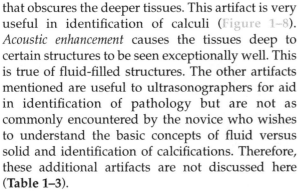

Table I–3   Ultrasonography Artifacts
Acoustic shadowing
Acoustic enhancement
Reverberation
Mirror image
Ring down

Table I–4 MRI Parameters		
Sequence	TR	TE
TI	Short	Short
Proton density	Long	Short
T2	Long	Long

short TE (≤20 msec). T2-weighted images are obtained with settings of a long TR (≥2000 msec) and a long TE (≥60 msec). Proton density-weighted images utilize a long TR (2000–3000 msec) and a short TE (20–30 msec) (**Table 1–4**). In general, T1-weighted images show good anatomic information, and T2-weighted images reveal pathologic information.

To perform an MRI examination, the patient lies on a table in a static, strong magnetic field. There are different field strengths of magnets. The strengths are measured in tesla (T) and are referred to as low-field (<0.3 T), mid-field (0.3–1.0 T), and high-field (>1.0 T) strength. The lower the magnetic field, the weaker the signal that is measured. Prolonged imaging time is often required, especially with low-field-strength magnets. The tomographic images can be obtained in any plane.

When interpreting MR examinations, *signal intensity* is the term used to describe the imaging sequences. To review, when discussing conventional x-rays and fluoroscopy, the term *density* is applied to the description of the image. When discussing CT, *attenuation* is used to describe the many shades of gray in the image, and the term *echogenicity* is used for ultrasound images. *High signal intensity* refers to something that is bright, such as fat on a T1-weighted image or fluid on a T2-weighted image (Figure 1–10). *Low signal intensity* (relative to the signal intensity of muscle) would be something like cortical bone, ligaments, or tendons. These are low in signal because of the lack of mobile protons in these structures. Most fluid is dark on a T1-weighted image (**Key Point 1–5**).

Important things to consider before sending a patient to an MR scanner are whether the patient has any electrically, magnetically, or mechanically activated implants. These include, but are not limited to, pacemakers, cochlear implants, and implanted pumps or stimulators. It is imperative to question a patient regarding these devices and then

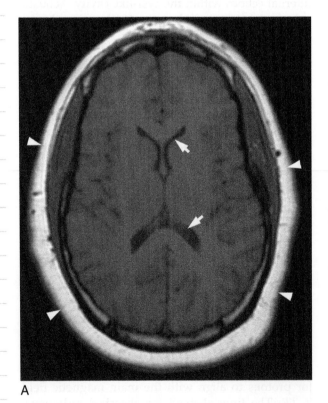

A

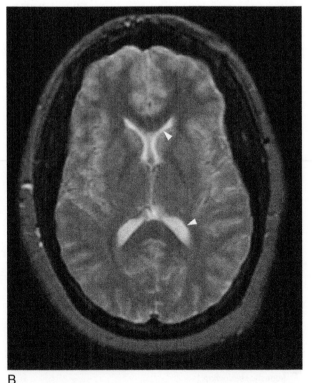

B

Figure 1–10 High signal intensity. A, Axial T1 weighted image through the brain demonstrates high signal representing the fat in the subcutaneous tissues (*arrowheads*). The CSF seen in the ventricles is low in signal (*arrows*). B, Axial T2 weighted image in the brain shows the high signal of the CSF (*arrowheads*). Note the cortical bone around the edge of the skull is black (low signal) because of the lack of mobile protons in cortical bone.

| Key | Point 1–5 |

MRI Signal Intensity

| High-signal intensity | Bright |
| Low-signal intensity | Dark |

to determine whether an implanted device, or hardware is MRI compatible. For instance, you must determine whether aneurysm clips are ferromagnetic or made of inert titanium. Bullets and shrapnel can induce electrical currents. This can lead to a burn in the patient as well as a projectile in the magnetic field. That is, they can dislodge. This, of course, is not a good thing. Metal workers and patients with a history of a penetrating eye injury should be screened with a conventional x-ray of the orbits to assess for metal. When in doubt, consult the radiologist or access the numerous websites available for safety issues.

As with the other imaging techniques, there are artifacts associated with this modality. These include *motion artifact, chemical shift misregistration artifact, truncation error,* and *aliasing.* The artifact that is most often identified by the clinician is *motion artifact* (**Table 1–5**). It is the one artifact that can most often be prevented ahead of time. Motion is often a result of claustrophobia or pain. It is imperative to make the patient as comfortable as possible. Claustrophobia is not a contraindication for MRI. There are medications available to allow the patient to be more comfortable during the examination as well as analgesics that will allow the patient to lie still. These can be prescribed ahead of time. It is extremely important that conspicuous notation of administration of this medication be made so the patient is appropriately monitored during the course of the study. Motion caused by cardiac rhythm and respirations can be minimized via MRI techniques called cardiac and respiratory gating. These techniques allow timing of image acquisition to match these physiologic motions. MRI can also be used to assess flow within vessels and to produce complex angiograms of the peripheral and cerebral circulation. Typically, MRI

contrast agents contain paramagnetic substances (gadolinium and manganese).

Contrast agents used for MRI studies are made of gadolinium solutions. These solutions are administered intravenously and are used similarly to iodinated intravenous agents in CT. The signal intensity increases as a result of T1 shortening, so T1-weighted imaging is performed after the administration of intravenous gadolinium solution. Imaging should be performed in a timely fashion after the administration of this contrast agent. Adverse reactions are uncommon. The paramagnetic solution is excreted through the kidneys.

Nuclear Imaging

Nuclear imaging is a very valuable tool for assessing physiologic function. The principle of nuclear radiology is straightforward. It is based on the detection of gamma rays and formation of an image demonstrating the distribution of a radioactive substance that has been previously administered to the patient. Gamma rays are produced from within the nucleus of an atom when an unstable nucleus decays. Knowledge of normal function is important in order to understand abnormal function.

Radioisotopes can be made from naturally occurring elements that are essential to normal biologic function (iodine-123) or an analog (technetium-99m pertechnetate). Properties necessary for a useful gamma ray emitter are listed in **Table 1–6**. More often, a radioisotope is combined with a physiologically "active" compound in vitro and administered intravenously or orally. After injection, and depending on how the radiopharmaceutical is absorbed, distributed, metabolized, and excreted by the body, images are obtained using a gamma camera (see Figure 8–1 in Chapter 8). Nuclear medicine studies give physiologic information, not anatomic information (**Key Point 1–6**). Tracer activity is described in terms of *uptake* of tracer. Areas that demonstrate increased radiotracer activity can be referred to as areas of *increased radiotracer activity,* although this is cumbersome, or as *hot* areas. The nuclear imaging chapter will go into more detail regarding the more commonly ordered nuclear studies.

Table 1–5 MRI Artifacts
Motion
Chemical shift misregistration
Truncation error
Aliasing

Table 1–6 Necessary Properties of Gamma Ray Emitters
Reasonable half life (6–24 hr)
Easily measured gamma ray
Energy deposition as low as possible in patient tissues

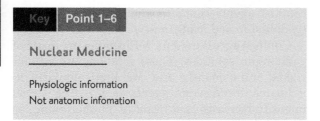

Key   Point 1–6

Nuclear Medicine

Physiologic information
Not anatomic infomation

Table I–7 Radiation Exposure		
Examination Background	Typical Effective Dose (mSv)	Equivalent Duration of Exposure
Chest radiograph	0.02	3 days
Abdomen	1.00	6 months
Intravenous urography	2.50	14 months
Head CT	2.30	1 year
Abdomen and pelvis CT	10.00	4.5 years

In conclusion, whenever a patient undergoes any of the aforementioned procedures, an expense is incurred. The more complex the imaging technique, the more expensive it is. Additionally, with the exception of MRI and ultrasonography, a radiation dose is given (**Table 1–7**). The dose should be as low as possible for a diagnostic image to be obtained. As a clinician, you must always keep in mind the risk/benefit ratio. Examinations should be performed based on sound clinical history and physical examination. Radiologists then interpret the images and aid in the care of patients. The following chapters should enable you to navigate through this process.

Suggested Reading List

Bushberg JT, Seibert JA, Leidholdt EM Jr, Boone JM: The Essential Physics of Medical Imaging, 2nd ed. Philadelphia, Lippincott Williams & Wilkins, 2001.

Huda W, Slone R: Review of Radiologic Physics, 2nd ed. Philadelphia, Lippincott, Williams & Wilkins, 2003.

MRIsafety.com: List of implants and devices tested for MRI safety. Available at http://www.MRIsafety.com. Accessed 05 March 2006.

Nickoloff EL, Ahmad N: Radiology Review: Radiologic Physics. Philadelphia, Elsevier, 2005.

Chest Imaging

Chapter outline

Methods of Imaging

Normal Anatomy

Mediastinum

Hilum

Pleura and Chest Wall

Diaphragm

Lungs

Cardiac Imaging

Emergencies

This chapter is more extensive than the others. This is by design. The majority of radiographs that you will view in training and during patient care are chest x-rays. Therefore, more examples of pathology are provided in this chapter. The outline here is quite ambitious for a basic imaging book. Refer to the suggested reading list at the end of the chapter for more information available to you for in-depth reading.

The goal for this chapter is to recognize normal anatomy in the various portions of the chest on conventional films, as well as some pathology. Examples of anatomy and pathology will be provided. You should also learn when to order a computed tomography (CT) study for further evaluation.

Methods of Imaging

Conventional radiographs are generally done in the form of posteroanterior (PA) and lateral projections. Generally conventional films ("x-rays") are the first study obtained in patients with suspected disease of the chest. The physics involved in this modality is not discussed here; for that additional information, you can refer to the suggested reading list at the end of the chapter.

Similar to examining a patient, you cannot formulate a differential diagnosis until after you have assessed the patient. First, don't just order an x-ray because that's "what my resident would do." An x-ray should be ordered if there is suspicion of disease and if the patient's treatment will be altered or determined by the result of the examination. This philosophy holds true for *all* radiographs. Order a study for your patient if you think it will aid in the patient's care. There is great temptation to order a study simply to "do something" for the patient, when in fact the study will add nothing to the information you already have. Think carefully before you order a study and ask yourself whether it will help you to help the patient. If the answer is "no," then you know not to order the study. Whenever you are in doubt, ask a radiologist. He or she will be happy to instruct you on what might be the best course of action for your patient.

Now, how do you know if the chest x-ray is satisfactory for interpretation? Start by assessing the four basic features: *penetration, rotation, inspiration,* and *motion* (**Key Point 2–1**). Adequate *penetration* is accomplished when there is faint visualization

11

Assessment of Posteroanterior Chest Radiograph for Adequacy

Penetration
Faint visualization of intervertebral disk spaces
Visualization of vessels superimposed over cardiac silhouette

Rotation
Spinous processes centered between clavicular heads

Inspiration
Apex of right hemidiaphragm projecting below right 10th posterior rib

Motion
Well-marginated borders of vessels, cardiac margin, and diaphragm

Table 2–1   Types of Radiographic Examinations for Evaluating Thoracic Disease

Posteroanterior (PA) and lateral chest x-ray
Portable chest x-ray
Decubitus chest x-ray
Computed tomography (CT)
Magnetic resonance imaging (MRI)
Positron emission tomography (PET)
Ventilation/perfusion (V/Q) scan

of the intervertebral disc spaces in the thoracic spine. Also, you should be able to identify vessels superimposed over the cardiac silhouette. *Rotation* can be quickly assessed by noting the relationships of the clavicular heads to the midline of the vertebral bodies (the spinous process). The two distances should be the same. Too much space on one side relative to the other suggests that the patient was rotated. Rotation affects the appearance of the structures in the chest film (Figure 2–1). Adequate *inspiration* is also quickly determined (depending

upon how long it takes you to count to 10!). The apex of the right hemidiaphragm should project below the right 10th posterior rib. *Motion* is determined by evaluating the borders of the structures in the film, such as the vessels in the lung parenchyma, the cardiac margin, and the diaphragm. If these structures are well-marginated, then the patient was able to halt respiration during the exposure.

In addition to the PA and lateral radiograph for evaluation, portable chest and decubitus films can be useful for evaluation of a patient with chest pathology (**Table 2–1**). Many of the chest x-rays that you will see during your career may in fact be portable chest x-rays. These are obtained from anterior to posterior and therefore are referred to as AP films. Generally, portable AP chest films are obtained for patients who are critically ill or who cannot be transported to the radiology department

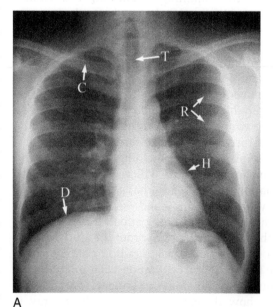

A

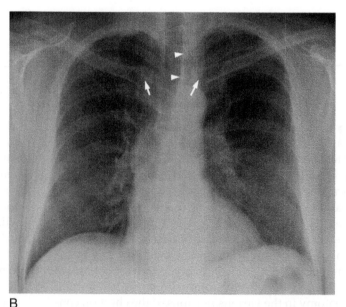

B

Figure 2–1   Normal frontal chest x-ray and rotation. A. Normal non-rotated appearance of a chest film. **T**–trachea, **C**–clavicle, **D**–diaphragm, **H**–heart, **R**–ribs. B. Rotation film shows the trachea no longer superimposed over the spinous processes (*arrowheads*), and the asymmetric space between the sternoclavicular joints (*arrows*).

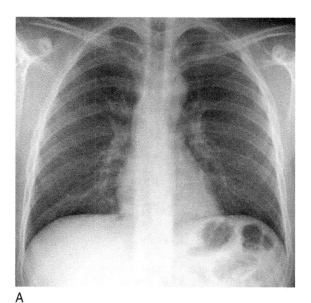

A

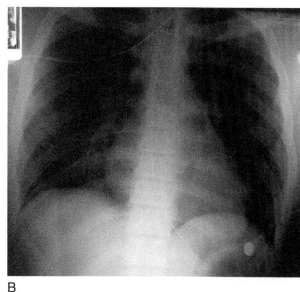

B

Figure 2–2   Normal and portable chest x-rays. A. Normal posteroanterior projection. B. Portable chest x-ray. Portable film shows enlargement of the cardiac silhouette and lower lung volumes.

(Figure 2–2). This is important to remember. It sometimes may be "quicker" to obtain a portable x-ray on your patient, and the temptation to get the examination done in an expeditious manner may exist. However, a portable examination does not include a lateral projection, and therefore you will not be able to precisely localize a pathologic density within the chest. Often a portable chest examination is used to determine interval changes in cardiopulmonary status or to assess line or tube placement. Pitfalls in the portable technique include the magnification of the cardiac silhouette, increase in motion artifacts due to the prolonged exposure, and decreased depth of inspiration, since many patients are supine during this exposure. This technique is not useful for identifying pleural effusions or a small pneumothorax. This is because fluid will remain dependent (posterior in a supine patient), making the assessment for fluid difficult with a portable technique. Pleural air in a pneumothorax rises to a nondependent area and becomes anterior in location. These pleural processes are more easily overlooked in a supine film. Another way that gravity plays a role is in the appearance of the blood vessels. The vessels at the base of the lungs are larger than those in the upper lobes on an upright chest x-ray. In the supine x-ray, the caliber of the vessels is nearly equal between upper and lower lung.

Decubitus films are extremely useful for determining whether a patient has a mobile pleural effusion. The patient is placed on the side with the suspected effusion. The x-ray beam is parallel to the table, and if the fluid is mobile it will move along the pleural space in the chest wall. As little as 50 mL of fluid can be demonstrated by this technique. This is a very useful technique for a patient who cannot tolerate an upright film. For instance, if a patient has an effusion and the lung parenchyma in that region cannot be assessed because of the effusion, then a decubitus film could be performed to assess that suspicious portion of the lung (Figure 2–3).

CT is being increasingly utilized as an imaging method for evaluation of the lung. Various techniques exist for evaluation of the lung parenchyma, including high-resolution CT (HRCT), for evaluation of parenchymal lung disease and bronchiectasis, and conventional CT, for evaluation of an abnormality identified on conventional x-ray, staging of lung cancer, assessment for pulmonary metastases, and differentiation of parenchymal- versus pleural-based processes (**Table 2–2**). Another common use of CT in the chest is to evaluate for a pulmonary embolus. In this case, the scan is timed to be performed when the intravenous bolus of contrast is in the pulmonary arterial system. The bright contrast in the vessels is indicative of blood in the vessels. An embolus resembles a "filling defect" or soft tissue density in the blood vessel (Figure 2–4).

The role of MRI continues to evolve. It is the imaging modality of choice for evaluation of congenital and acquired vascular disorders. Additionally, MRI is superior to CT in the diagnosis of chest wall or mediastinal invasion because of the high contrast between tumor and chest wall fat and musculature on MRI (Figure 2–5). MRI is a useful examination for staging of lung cancer in patients who are

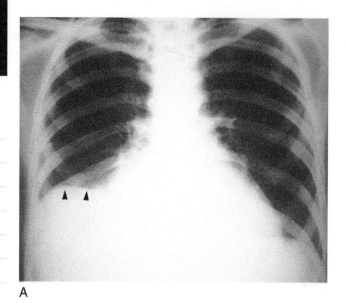

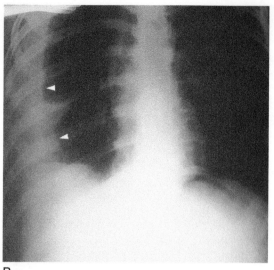

A

B

Figure 2–3   Subpulmonic effusion. A, Frontal projection shows apparent elevation of the right hemidiaphragm (*arrowheads*). B, Lateral decubitus film (right side down) shows layering in a mobile pleural effusion (*arrowheads*).

Table 2–2   Indications for Thoracic CT

Evaluation of parenchymal lung disease

Evaluation of bronchiectasis

Evaluation of chest x-ray abnormality

Staging of lung cancer

Assessment for pulmonary metastases

Assessment of parenchymal vs. pleural-based processes

Evaluation for pulmonary embolus

Evaluation for aortic dissection

Determination of biopsy approach

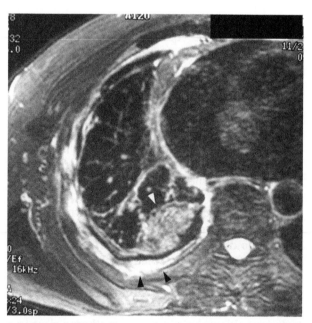

Figure 2–5   Mesothelioma. MRI axial T2-weighted image with fat suppression shows a mass in the lung (*white arrowhead*) with pleural involvement and extension to the chest wall (*black arrowheads*).

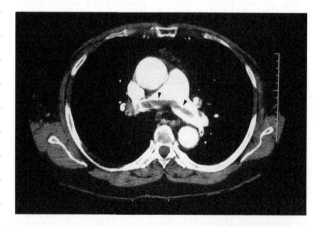

Figure 2–4   CT. Saddle embolus. Axial image through pulmonary arteries shows a low-attenuation (filling defect) thrombus straddling the pulmonary arteries (*arrowheads*).

unable to receive intravenous iodinated contrast for CT examination. MRI also nicely assesses posterior mediastinal masses (**Table 2–3**).

Finally, positron emission tomography (PET) and ventilation/perfusion (V/Q) scans are techniques utilizing nuclear medicine for the evaluation of lung cancer and pulmonary embolus, respectively.

Table 2–3 Indications for Thoracic MRI

Evaluation of congenital cardiac anomalies

Evaluation of vascular disorders (thoracic aortic aneurysm or dissection)

Diagnosis of tumor invasion into chest wall or mediastinum

Staging of lung cancer in patients with contraindication to iodinated contrast

Assessment of posterior mediastinal masses

Normal Anatomy

Bones

Numerous well written and much more complete texts about thoracic imaging are available. The discussion of anatomy in this chapter will cover the pertinent aspects that you will need to be familiar with as a beginner in x-ray interpretation.

In evaluation of the chest x-ray, the bones make up the framework that contains the lungs, pleura, and mediastinum. Chest x-rays are not the optimal way to evaluate bone structures. Nevertheless, the bones are an important part of the evaluation. Occasionally, the bones can give a clue as to the true pathology in the chest. For instance, a lytic lesion in the rib may accompany upper lobe interstitial disease and help make the diagnosis of eosinophilic granuloma. Rib notching can be seen in association with coarctation of the aorta (Figure 2–6). Although portion of the scapula can be seen on a chest x-ray, the detail to which this structure can be assessed is not optimal. Similarly, although a properly penetrated chest x-ray will reveal the thoracic spine and the spinous process, don't be tempted to think you have adequately assessed these structures (particularly in the setting of trauma) without good-detail bone films. This reminder is not to say "ignore the bones" or you "must get bone films on all patients"; rather, assess the patient and the x-ray to determine whether your patient needs additional imaging.

Trachea/Bronchi

The *trachea* on conventional x-rays is a vertical lucency. It appears as a lucency because it is air-filled. The right lateral wall should be examined on all x-rays and is referred to as the *paratracheal stripe.* The stripe is composed of mediastinal fat, lymph nodes, and pleura. The combination of these structures leading to the soft tissue density should not measure greater than 4 mm in thickness. If it is thicker than 4 mm, you must consider an abnor-

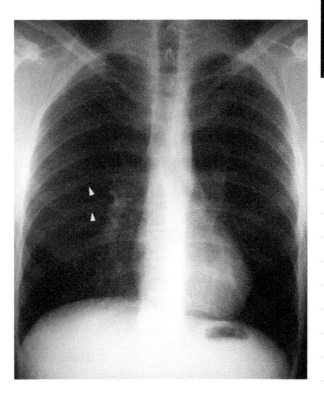

Figure 2–6   Coarctation of the aorta and rib-notching. Frontal chest x-ray demonstrates a small arch and abnormal contour to the ribs (*arrowheads*). This constellation of findings suggests a coarctation of the aorta.

mality in one of the comprising structures, such as lymphadenopathy. The left lateral wall usually is not visualized as a distinct structure. The posterior tracheal stripe measures about 3 mm and is composed of the posterior tracheal wall and adjacent fat. When air is present in the esophagus, the *tracheoesophageal stripe* can be seen (Figure 2–7). This represents the combination of the tracheal and esophageal walls and intervening fat. This stripe should measure less than 5 mm. If it is too thick, the cause is most often esophageal carcinoma.

The *bronchi* are also filled with air. The main bronchi arise from the trachea at the *carina* (crotch). The right main bronchus is shorter than the left. These are well visualized on the frontal film, and the bronchus intermedius is readily seen on the lateral film. There are three right-sided lobar bronchi (upper, middle, and lower) and two left-sided ones (upper and lower). There are 10 *segmental* bronchi on the right (3 right upper, 2 right middle, and 5 right lower), and 8 on the left (4 left upper and 4 left lower). These bronchi are air-filled and will appear as tubular or circular lucencies depending on whether they are seen in tangent or in cross-section. The lobar and segmental anatomy is shown in Figure 2–8.

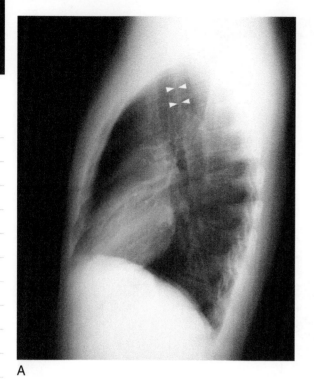

A

B

Figure 2–7 Tracheoesophageal stripe. A, Lateral film demonstrates the interface between the trachea and esophagus (*arrowheads*). Thickening of this stripe suggests disease in this location. B, Lateral coned down view of an abnormally thickened tracheoesophageal stripe (*arrowheads*) in a patient with squamous cell carcinoma of the esophagus.

Fissures

The lobes of the lung are enveloped in pleura. The interlobar *pulmonary fissures* are invaginations of the visceral pleura into the substance of the lung. These fissures completely or incompletely separate the lobes from one another. An incomplete lobe has important consequences for development or spread of consolidation and collateral air drift in patients with lobar obstruction.

Most patients have two interlobar fissures on the right and one on the left. The minor fissure separates the right upper from middle lobe and is incomplete in approximately 80% of individuals (Figures 2–9 through 2–11). There are a couple of accessory fissures, the inferior accessory fissure and the azygous fissure. The inferior accessory fissure is the most common accessory fissure, found in 10% to 20% of individuals. It separates the medial basal segment from the remaining basal segments. The azygous fissure is seen in 0.5% of individuals and represents an invagination of the right apical pleura by the azygous vein (systemic circulation) that has incompletely migrated to its normal position at the right tracheobronchial angle. The azygous fissure appears as a vertical curvilinear line, convex laterally, that extends from the lung apex to the

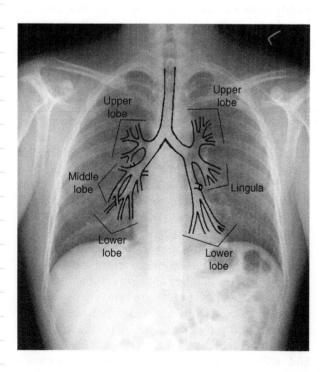

Figure 2–8 Schematic drawing superimposed over a normal frontal chest demonstrating the location of the segmental bronchi.

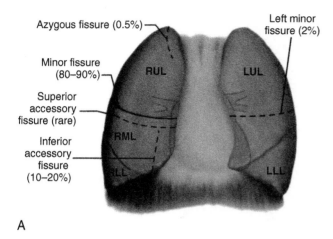

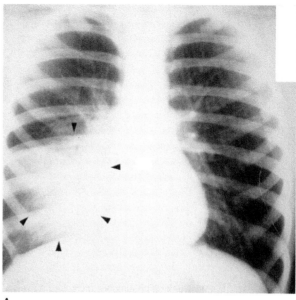

A

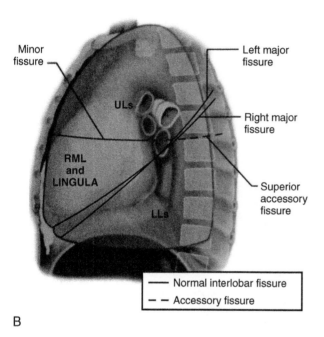

Figure 2–9   Schematic anatomic drawing of the fissures of the lungs as visualized in an anteroposterior A and lateral B direction.

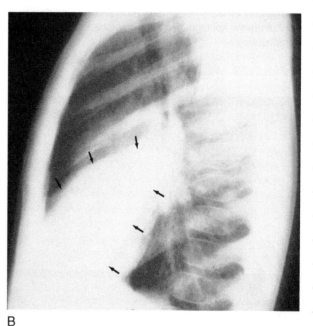

B

Figure 2–10   Right middle lobe pneumonia. Arrows point to the increased density of the right middle lobe pneumonia. Note loss of the right heart border on the frontal projection A, and the increased density (*arrows*) superimposed over the cardiac silhouette on the lateral projection B.

azygous vein (Figure 2–12). The fissure is important to prevent spread of apical lung disease and to exclude a pneumothorax from the apical portion of the pleural space.

Pulmonary Vessels

The *pulmonary arteries* image as a tubular soft tissue density within the hilum. The main pulmonary artery arises from the right ventricle anterior to the ascending aorta. It then bifurcates into right and left pulmonary arteries. The right and left pulmonary arteries are best visualized on the lateral chest film (Figure 2–13). The upper and lower divisions of the

pulmonary arteries are best seen on the frontal projection (Figure 2–14). The branches of the right and left pulmonary arteries accompany and divide along with the corresponding lobar, segmental and subsegmental bronchi. As the arteries divide, they diminish in caliber. You can see at the periphery of the lungs that the vessels are smaller compared with centrally.

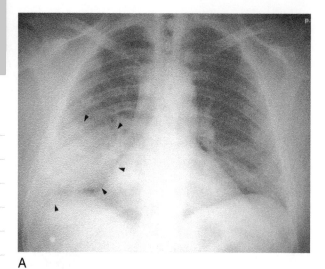

A

Figure 2–11   Right lower lobe pneumonia. Increased density is noted in the lower portion of the right hemithorax (*arrowheads*). Note the lateral aspect of the right hemidiaphragm is obscured because the density of the pneumonia is similar to the density of the right hemidiaphragm and the lower lobe is adjacent to the hemidiaphragm.

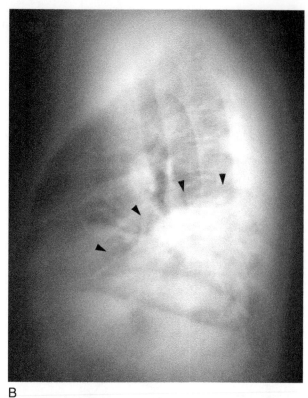

B

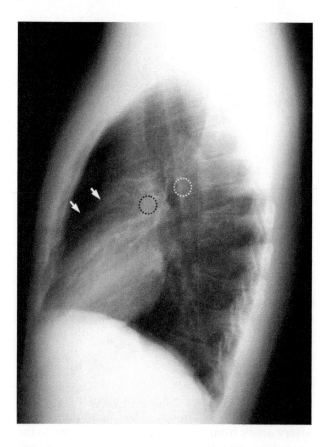

Figure 2–12   Azygous fissure. Frontal projection shows an accessory azygous fissure (*arrowheads*). Note the contour of the fissure is concave to the lung rather than the convex margin that would be seen with a pneumothorax.

Figure 2–13   Pulmonary arteries. Lateral film shows the pulmonary arteries. Dotted black circle indicates right pulmonary artery. Dotted white circle indicates left pulmonary artery. The *arrows* indicate the right main pulmonary artery.

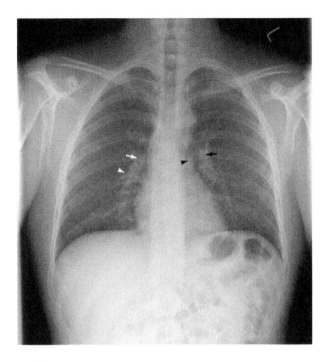

Figure 2–14   Pulmonary arteries. Frontal projection shows the main pulmonary artery (*black arrowhead*), left pulmonary artery (*black arrow*), right pulmonary artery (*white arrow*), and interlobar artery (*white arrowhead*).

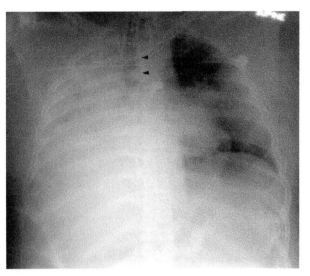

Figure 2–15   Right lung collapse. Frontal projection shows opacification of the right hemithorax with shift of the mediastinal structures to the right hemithorax (*arrowheads*). These findings indicate right lung collapse. Note the presence of a nasogastric tube.

The *pulmonary veins* arise within the interlobular septa from the alveolar and visceral pleural capillaries. These veins travel separate from the bronchoarterial system and ultimately drain into the left atrium. These vessels are also tubular and get larger as they approach the left atrium. The pulmonary veins are more horizontally oriented compared with the branching pulmonary arteries.

Interstitium

The tissue that holds the lung together is referred to as the *interstitium*. The interstitium provides support for the pulmonary vessels and the airways. It is a continuous structure arising from the region of the hilum and extending to the visceral pleura. The interstitium is part of the reason why the lung images as a soft tissue density in the setting of lobar or lung collapse (Figure 2–15). If the air is sucked out of the lung, the structures within the lung (bronchi, vessels, and interstitium) are what yields the soft tissue density (also perhaps some mucus within the bronchi). More about that later.

Analyzing the Chest Film

Now you should have a better idea of normal anatomy. Next let's focus on where these structures belong in the chest radiograph. I cannot emphasize to you enough that a consistent search pattern should be followed. For any x-ray that you are reviewing, if you proceed in a consistent fashion, and remember to look at *all* the structures, you will have done a thorough examination. Your search pattern doesn't need to be the same as your classmate's (or mine...although mine has worked pretty well throughout the years!), but it should be the *same* for you *every* time (Key Point 2–2).

One suggested method is to start by assessing the *bones*. Assess the shoulder joints, acromioclavicular joints, clavicles, ribs, and spine. You should be assessing for normal alignment of joints, evidence of degenerative disease, lytic or sclerotic lesions, and abnormal configuration of vertebral bodies.

Key   Point 2–2

Search Pattern for Examining Chest Radiographs

1. Bones
2. Soft tissues
3. Interfaces
4. Mediastinum (cardiac size, vertebral bodies)
5. Hilum
6. Pleura
7. Diaphragm
8. Cardiac silhouette

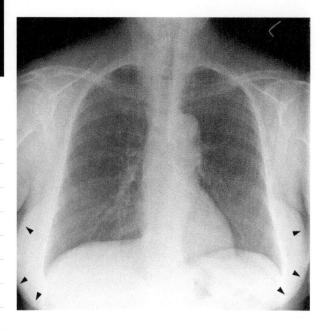

Figure 2–16   Breast shadows. Frontal projection shows breast shadows (*arrowheads*). Note the vague increased density in the costophrenic locations due to the superimposed soft tissues when compared with the density of the apices of the lung.

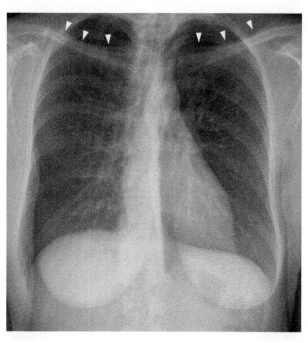

Figure 2–17   Companion shadow. Note the companion shadow adjacent to the clavicle (*arrowheads*). Loss of this shadow may suggest pathology in this location.

Assess the *soft tissues*. The soft tissues consist of skin, subcutaneous fat, and muscles. You can get an assessment of the state of the patient's health by assessing the soft tissues. Cachectic patients will obviously be very wasted and have thin subcutaneous tissue. When patients are extremely large, it can sometimes be very difficult to see small underlying structures such as the lung parenchyma (Figure 2–16). The soft tissues lateral to the chest wall should be symmetric in size and homogeneous in density. Breast tissue should be evaluated for symmetry. Asymmetry of breast tissue may suggest the presence of a mass or prior mastectomy. Fat density should be present in the supraclavicular fossa. Companion shadows of skin and subcutaneous tissue paralleling the clavicles helps to exclude a mass in this region (Figure 2–17). The pectoralis major is normally seen coursing to the axilla as it inserts on to the humerus. Absence of the pectoralis muscle can lead to a relative lucency of one hemithorax compared to the other. This should not be mistaken for disease in the contralateral hemithorax. Identifying that the pectoralis muscle is absent will lead to the correct diagnosis. Remember that the hardest thing to identify is what's not there! (Figure 2–18)

There are numerous locations where the mediastinum interfaces with the lung. Recognition of the normal *interfaces* will allow for identification of disease processes when present. There are quite a few interfaces. Refer to the figures for an understanding of these interfaces. The right-sided interfaces (**Table 2–4**) will be described first (Figure 2–19). The margin of the superior vena cava (SVC) is seen as a straight soft tissue density within the right upper lobe extending from the clavicle to the right atrium. This interface can be displaced by such processes as mediastinal mass or adenopathy, superior vena cava syndrome, or a tortuous aorta. The right paratracheal stripe is a combination of the wall of the trachea, adjacent lymph nodes, soft tissue, and the pleural surfaces. The normal thickness of the paratracheal stripe is less than 4 mm (Figure 2–20).

The interface between the azygous vein and the right upper lobe creates a round soft tissue density representing the azygous vein as it enters the posterior portion of the SVC. In a supine position, the vein may be enlarged, so interpretation of the size of this structure must take into account the position of the patient at the time of the exposure. The vein may be distended in patients with right-sided heart failure or obstruction of blood return to the right heart. Additional causes for "apparent" distention of this vein are masses in this location, such as adenopathy or neoplasm.

The right lung contacts the tissue immediately adjacent to the spine. This interface is referred to as the paraspinous interface. Masses in or adjacent to the spine will distort this interface (Figure 2–21).

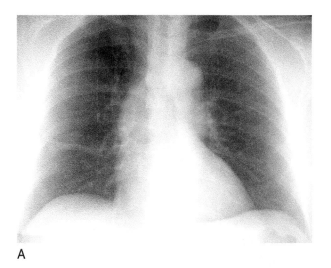

A

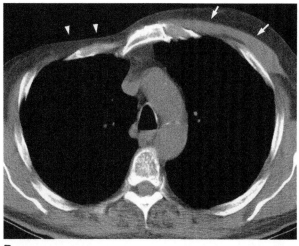

B

Figure 2–18 Poland's syndrome. A, Frontal chest x-ray demonstrates a relative difference in density. The right hemi-thorax appears more lucent when compared with the left. This is due to absence of the pectoralis muscle. B, Noncontrast CT image at the mid thoracic level shows absence of the pectoralis muscle (*arrowheads*) in comparison to the contralateral side (*arrows*). (courtesy of Michael Gotway, MD)

Another interface that allows for detection of disease is the azygoesophageal recess. This interface, as you probably figured out, extends from the arch of the azygous vein to the diaphragm along the course of the esophagus. Convexity at the superior third should suggest an abnormality in this location. Possible explanations for this convexity include a bronchogenic cyst, enlarged left atrium, or adenopathy. Inferior convexity should suggest lymph node enlargement or a hiatus hernia.

The right heart border interfaces with the medial segment of the middle lobe. Disease in this segment of the lung obscures the heart border, and in patients with right atrial enlargement, this interface becomes more prominent.

Proceeding to the left side, at the more superior portion of the left lung is an interface between the great vessels and the lung (Figure 2–22) (**Table 2–5**). This interface is much more apparent in older patients as these vessels become sclerotic and slightly more tortuous. They appear as a well-defined "tubular" soft tissue density that appears contiguous with the arch of the aorta. The trans-verse arch of the aorta creates a tubular, soft tissue density, convex in the left lung. The arch can also elongate and become more sclerotic with age, causing this interface to project in a more lateral

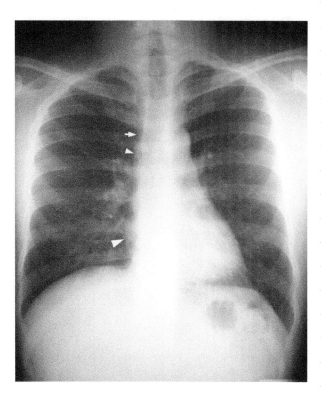

Figure 2–19 Normal chest x-ray with right-sided interfaces. Superior vena cava, straight margin (*arrow*). Azygous vein and right upper lobe (*small arrowhead*). Right heart border with right middle lobe (*large arrowhead*).

Table 2–4 Right-sided Mediastinal Interfaces
Superior vena cava
Right paratracheal stripe
Anterior arch of azygous vein
Right paraspinal interface
Azygoesophageal recess
Right heart border (right atrium)

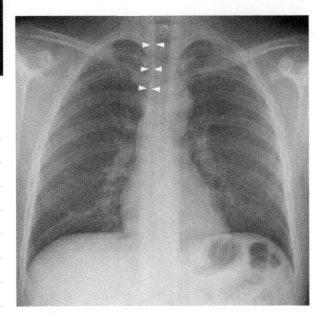

Figure 2–20 Normal frontal chest x-ray with normal paratracheal stripe. Normal thickness of the paratracheal stripe (*arrowheads*). Disease in this location will cause thickening of the soft tissues and widening of the paratracheal stripe.

location in this population. Similarly, aneurysmal dilatation or injuries to the arch will alter the appearance of this interface (Figure 2–23).

The aortopulmonary window (interface), located inferior to the arch of the aorta, represents the left

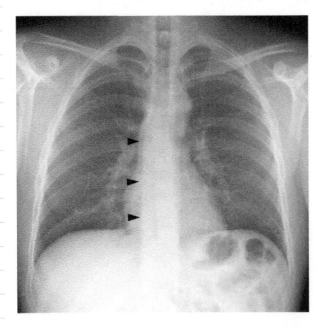

Figure 2–21 Normal frontal chest x-ray with normal paraspinous stripe. Normal thickness of the paraspinous stripe (*arrowheads*). Disease in this location will cause thickening of the soft tissues and widening of the paraspinous stripe.

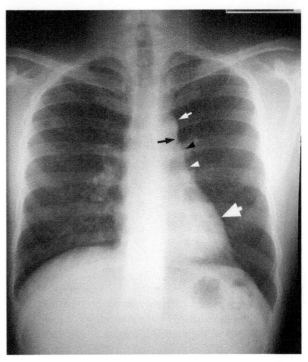

Figure 2–22 Normal frontal chest x-ray demonstrating left-sided interfaces. Aortic arch interfaces with the left upper lobe (*small white arrow*), the interface between the aortic arch and the main pulmonary artery is normal lung (aortopulmonary window, *black arrow*), the main left pulmonary artery interfaces with the lung (*small black arrowhead*), the left atrial appendage is noted and is seen to enlarge with mitral valve stenosis and left atrial enlargement (*small white arrowhead*), the left heart border interfaces with the lung (*large white arrow*).

upper lobe and its interface with the mediastinum. The normal appearance of this interface is concave to the lung. If it is convex in appearance, a mass or adenopathy should be considered as possible explanations for the appearance.

The left paraspinal interface represents the reflection of the left lung and paraspinal soft tissues. This interface is seen in the majority of patients. All tissues in this location can have abnormalities associated with them. A few differential possibilities for left paraspinal interface abnormalities include neurogenic tumors, hematoma, and medial pleural fluid.

Table 2–5 Left-sided Mediastinal Interfaces

Aortic arch
Main pulmonary artery
Aortopulmonary window
Left paraspinal interface
Left atrial appendage
Cardiac apex (left ventricle)

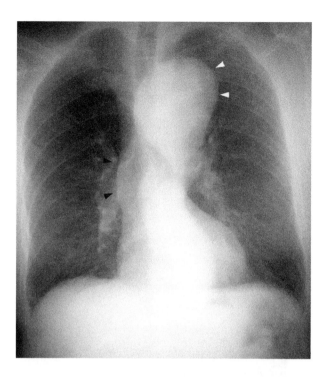

Figure 2–23   Thoracic aortic aneurysm. Distortion of left-sided interfaces is evident in this patient with a thoracic aortic aneurysm (*white arrowheads*). Ascending aorta is also prominent (*black arrowheads*).

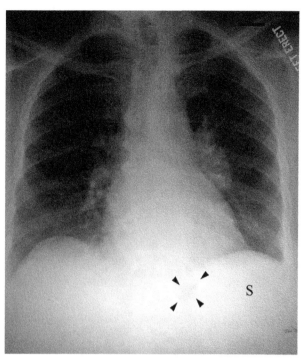

Figure 2–24   Splenomegaly. Frontal chest x-ray shows displacement of the gastric bubble to the midline (*arrowheads*) by an enlarged spleen "S" (soft tissue density in the left upper quadrant).

The left atrial appendage forms a concave interface below the main pulmonary artery. Straightening of this interface is usually due to left atrial enlargement from any cause.

Additional normal findings as part of your search pattern include visualization of the *diaphragm* and the upper portion of the *abdomen*. The right hemidiaphragm usually projects slightly higher than the left. The right hemidiaphragm appears contiguous with the liver because they both are of a soft tissue density, and they contact each other. The diaphragm will assume the configuration of the upper portion of the liver. The left hemidiaphragm is contiguous with the stomach.

Upper abdominal organs and abnormalities can often be identified on chest x-ray. This is why the search pattern includes evaluation below the diaphragms. Liver enlargement is in the differential diagnosis for apparent elevation of the right hemidiaphragm. Splenomegaly can be seen as a soft tissue density causing mass effect on the stomach and splenic flexure (Figure 2–24). Air and calcification within the liver are recognized as different densities against the background of the soft tissue density of the liver. For instance, calcifications may be seen in the gallbladder. Air can be seen in the biliary tree of the liver because it is of a different density than the liver.

As a reminder, the frontal radiograph shouldn't be used in isolation to determine anatomy and pathology. It is not possible to precisely localize an abnormality on an x-ray with just one view or projection. The lateral chest film should be evaluated in conjunction with the frontal film. Knowledge of the anatomy on the lateral film can help determine the location of the pathology (Figure 2–25). Familiarity with how the lateral x-ray is taken and knowledge of the densities seen on an x-ray allows determination of the right and left diaphragms. The left side of the chest is generally positioned against the x-ray cassette. The x-ray beam diverges, so objects further away from the cassette will appear bigger. Thus, the right hemidiaphragm will appear bigger than the left by extending in an anteroposterior direction beyond the margins of the left. Another clue to distinguish right and left is the heart will preclude the entire left lung from abutting the diaphragm. That is, the diaphragm and the heart will appear to be of a similar density and will blend together at the point where the heart abuts the diaphragm. If one of the diaphragms can be followed in its entirety, it is going to be the right. Finally, if you can identify the major fissures, the left major fissure will be more vertically oriented. Follow the fissure to the diaphragm. Since the fissures are not always so readily

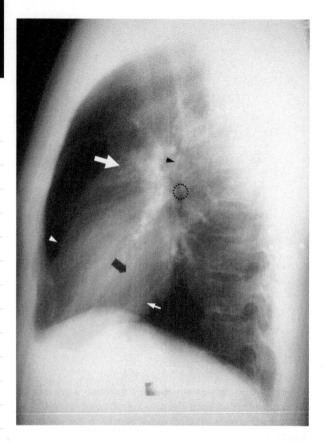

Figure 2–25   Normal lateral film anatomy. Ascending aorta (*white arrow*), anterior margin of right ventricle (*white arrowhead*), major fissure (*large black arrow*), inferior vena cava (*small white arrow*), carina (*circle*), posterior tracheal wall (*black arrowhead*).

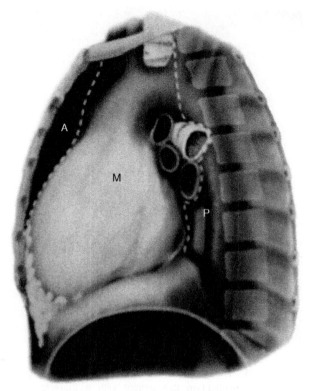

Figure 2–26   Compartments of mediastinum. Anatomic sketch demonstrating one of the common divisions into the anterior (A), middle (M) and posterior (P) mediastinum.

identified, this is not as helpful as the first two methods.

One of the great temptations in reviewing x-rays is that once you happen across an abnormality, you fail to search further. You must remember to be complete in your search pattern. It is said that up to 10% of all examinations have a second abnormality. For instance, you may identify an opacity in the lung resembling a pneumonia but fail to recognize the mass that leads to the postobstructive pneumonia or the lytic bone lesion that might be present in conjunction with the parenchymal process. This is referred to as "satisfaction of search."

Mediastinum

The mediastinum is arbitrarily divided into *anterior, middle,* and *posterior* portions and the *thoracic inlet,* based on creating a tidy differential diagnosis (Figure 2–26). As you read a variety of textbooks discussing the mediastinum, you may encounter variations in the structures included in the different compartments. The discussion here is the most

commonly used description of the mediastinum. When an abnormality is encountered on a chest x-ray, a determination is made (using frontal and lateral projections) of the location of the mass (lung, pleural space, mediastinum). There are no fascial boundaries between the mediastinal compartments. The lack of boundaries allows masses that arise in one compartment to communicate to another compartment. Often, once a mediastinal mass is noted, a CT examination is necessary to delineate the size and extent of the process, and often the tissue type can be determined. If a biopsy is necessary, the CT can readily identify the best location for the biopsy.

The thoracic inlet is the region of the upper thorax that is bounded by the first rib; it is the arbitrary divide between the neck and the thorax. The tissues within this region include mesenchymal tissue (fat and vessels) as well as thyroid tissue and lymph nodes.

Masses in this location include abnormalities in any of the tissue types mentioned. Thyroid masses, lymph node enlargement, and lymphangiomas are the most commonly encountered thoracic inlet masses.

The *anterior* (also referred to as the *prevascular*) mediastinum includes the structures that lie posterior to the sternum and anterior to the pericardium. Structures in this space include the thymus (usually not seen in normal adults), lymph nodes (these are located in all mediastinal compartments), and thyroid, as well as mesenchymal tissue (**Table 2–6**). Abnormalities in the anterior mediastinum include disorders associated with the tissues in this location (Figures 2–27, 2–28, and 2–29). Lymphoma is the most common primary mediastinal neoplasm in adults.

The *middle* (also referred to as the *vascular*) mediastinum is composed of the pericardium, great vessels, heart, trachea and bronchi, descending aorta, thoracic duct, esophagus, and lymph nodes. The hila can be considered extensions of the middle mediastinum. Many structures are present in the

Table 2–6   Differential Diagnosis of Anterior Mediastinal Mass

Sternum
    Osteomyelitis
    Metastasis
    Plasmacytoma/multiple myeloma
    Eosinophilic granuloma (children)
    Primary tumor
Thymus
    Hyperplasia
    Cyst
    Thymoma
    Thymolipoma
    Carcinoma
    Lymphoma
Germ cell tumor (incomplete migration during development)
Thyroid mass (passing through thoracic inlet)
Lymph nodal mass
Vascular or lymphatic mass

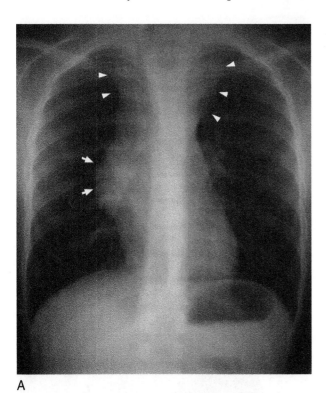

A

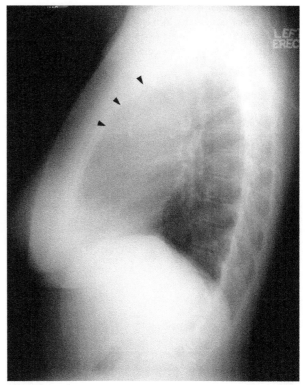

B

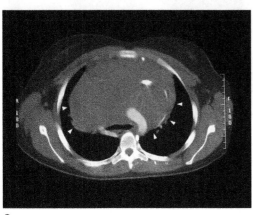

C

Figure 2–27   Hodgkins lymphoma. Frontal A and lateral B film showing lymphadenopathy involving the anterior portion of the mediastinum (*arrowheads*). Note also the adenopathy involving the right hilar region (*small arrows*). Axial CT scan (with contrast in the arterial phase) at the level of the carina C shows the extent of the adenopathy (*arrowheads*).

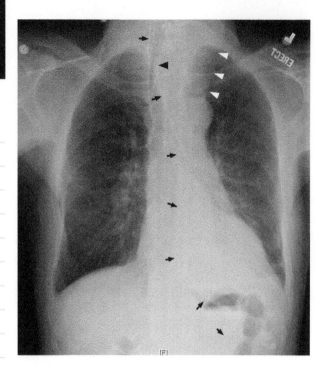

Figure 2–28 Mediastinal mass causing tracheal deviation. Frontal chest x-ray shows a mass in a mediastinal compartment (*white arrowheads*) that has resulted in mass effect on the trachea (*black arrowhead*). A nasogastric tube is also present and is deviated due to the presence of the mass (*black arrows*). The mass is affecting middle mediastinal structures (trachea and esophagus).

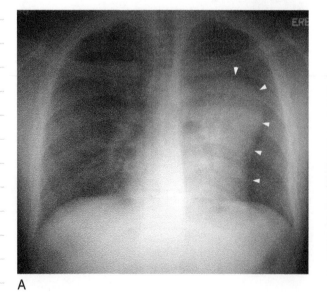

A

Figure 2–29 Teratoma. This large mediastinal mass is readily identified on the frontal A and lateral B chest x-rays (*arrowheads*). Note that on the lateral film the retrosternal airspace is opacified by the anterior mediastinal mass. The axial noncontrast CT at the level of the arch of the aorta C

middle mediastinum, and therefore many possibilities exist for a differential diagnosis of a middle mediastinal mass (**Table 2–7**). CT examination is extremely useful for evaluation of masses in this compartment (Figure 2–30). CT can evaluate the

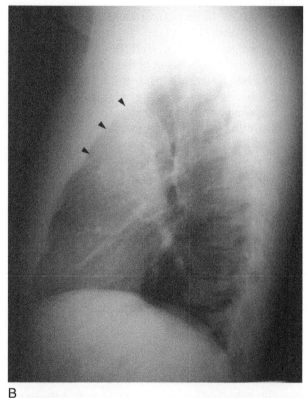

B

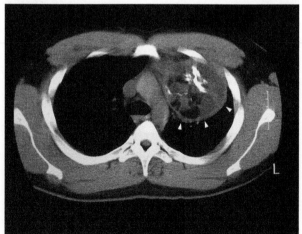

C

demonstrates a large mass (*arrowheads*) with a variety of attenuation characteristics. The low attenuation represents fat tissue, while the very high attenuation is a focus of calcification characteristic of a teratoma.

Table 2–7 Differential Diagnosis of Middle Mediastinal Mass

Bronchogenic tumor
Esophagus
   Hiatal hernia
   Dilated esophagus
   Esophageal diverticulum
   Esophageal tumor
   Esophageal duplication cyst
Pericardium
   Cyst
   Lipoma
Lymph nodal mass
Masses arising from heart
   Aneurysm
Vascular mass
   Great vessel aneurysm
   Great vessel rupture
   Aortic dissection

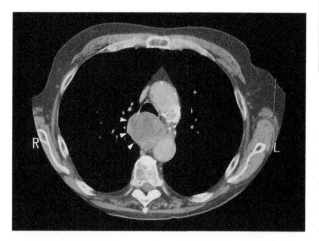

Figure 2–30 Middle mediastinal mass. CT with intravenous contrast shows a mass in the middle mediastinum adjacent to the descending aorta (*arrowheads*). CT is excellent for evaluating the extent of the involvement by mediastinal masses.

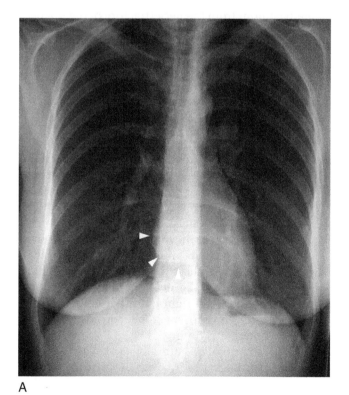

A

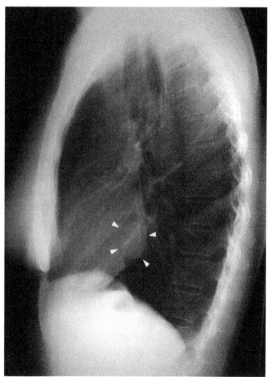

B

Figure 2–31 Bronchogenic cyst. Frontal A and lateral B film shows a well-defined soft-tissue mass in the middle mediastinum. The location near a main bronchus and the well-defined nature of the lesion should suggest a bronchogenic cyst. The soft tissue density is due to the fluid nature of this lesion (fluid and soft tissue same density on plain x-ray). A CT examination would show the low attenuation of fluid compared with a higher attenuation for soft tissue.

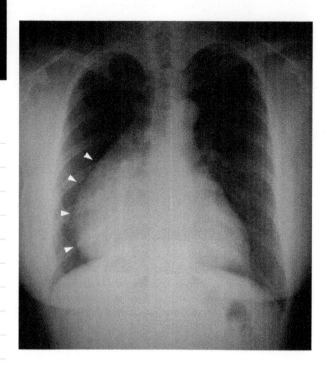

Figure 2–32 Pericardial cyst. Large mass that is contiguous with the right heart border (no normal right heart border identified). The frontal x-ray is not diagnostic of a cyst. A CT examination would characterize the density of the lesion as fluid, diagnostic of a pericardial cyst.

extent as well as the density of the masses. Examples of commonly occurring middle mediastinal masses are shown in Figures 2–31 through 2–35.

An important mediastinal mass to recognize is the injured aorta after high-speed deceleration injury or penetrating trauma. Keep in mind that penetrating trauma can include attempts at central line placement. Widening of the mediastinum is seen on plain radiographs. The normal contours as described previously are obscured (Figure 2–36). CT will demonstrate the abnormal soft tissue density within the mediastinum and can show the extent of the hemorrhagic collection. Acute clot is high in attenuation and is readily appreciated on CT.

The *posterior* mediastinum consists of the spine and neurogenic structures (spinal cord, nerve roots) as they exit the vertebral bodies. Lymph nodes are present again in the posterior mediastinum. Cross-sectional imaging studies (CT and MRI) are extremely useful in determining the origin of the mass and tissue types. Some of these masses have a characteristic appearance on MRI (**Table 2–8**). Some examples of posterior mediastinal masses are

seen in Figures 2–37 through 2–39 (Figures 2–37 through 2–39).

As a reminder, the advantage of performing CT in the setting of a mediastinal mass is that, not only does it demonstrate the extent of the pathology, but, because of the greater range of gray scale, different tissue types are readily appreciated. With your new knowledge of these tissue types, you can work through an appropriate differential diagnosis as listed in Table 2–8. For instance, perhaps you have never seen a case of mediastinal lipomatosis. Once you recognize the fat density, you can exclude aneurysm and acute hemorrhage from the differential diagnosis (Figure 2–40). In summary, for evaluation of a mediastinal mass, you must have a frontal and lateral projection, and in many cases a CT will be diagnostic.

Another pathologic process involving the mediastinum is a pneumomediastinum. Causes include positive-pressure ventilation, blunt chest trauma, and Valsalva maneuvers during strenuous exertion such as childbirth, weightlifting, or inhalational drug use. Air dissects centrally to the hilum and mediastinum (Figure 2–41). If the air dissects peripherally, it can rupture through the visceral pleura, leading to a pneumothorax. Pneumomediastinum can also result from air dissecting inferiorly into the mediastinum from the neck (fracture of the trachea) and superiorly into the mediastinum from the retroperitoneal space along the aortic hiatus or peritoneal cavity.

Hilum

Another portion of the x-ray that is evaluated is the *hilum*. Knowledge of the normal appearance allows for identification of disease processes. The hilum, simply stated, represents the junction of the lung with the mediastinum. The structures comprising the hila are demonstrated in Figures 2–13, 2–14. The right and left pulmonary arteries comprise the predominant portion of the hilar density on the frontal chest x-ray. The left hilum projects higher than the right on most chest x-rays. If the right hilum projects higher than the left, volume loss in the right upper lobe (elevated right hilum) or left lower lobe (lowered left hilum) must be considered as an explanation of this finding.

Hilar abnormalities are first recognized on conventional radiographs. As with mediastinal masses, cross-sectional imaging with CT or MRI further delineates the tissue type and extent of the pathology. Using your knowledge of the various densities, you can narrow the differential diagnosis after assessing the appearance on CT and conventional x-ray films (**Tables 2–9 and 2–10**).

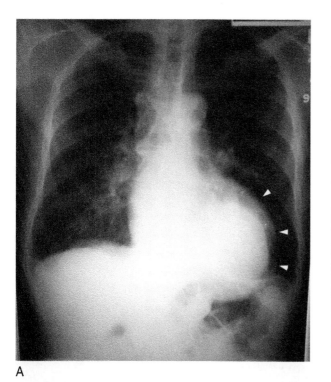

A

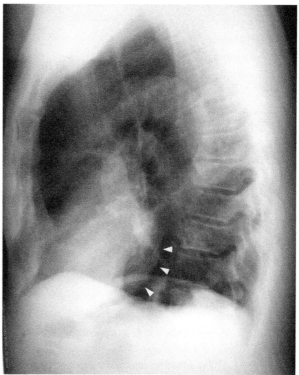

B

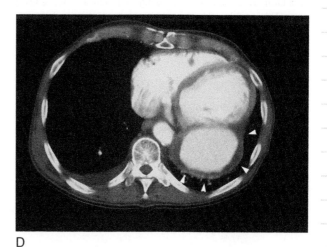

D

C

Figure 2–33   Left ventricular pseudoaneurysm. A, A density projects over the location of the left ventricle on the frontal film. Two left heart borders are noted (*arrowheads*). B, The lateral film is a comparison from several years before. Note the position of the left ventricle (*arrowheads*). C, The lateral film performed at the same time as A shows enlargement of the left ventricle (*arrowheads*) with an abnormal contour to the left ventricle. D, CT with contrast in arterial phase shows a pseudoaneurysm arising from the left ventricular wall (*arrowheads*). This is a result of a myocardial infarction that occurred several years previous to this examination. The double density on the frontal film is a result of the x-ray beam penetrating the left ventricle and the pseudoaneurysm. The abnormal left ventricular enlargement and contour seen on the lateral film is a result of the pseudoaneurysm attached to the left ventricular wall.

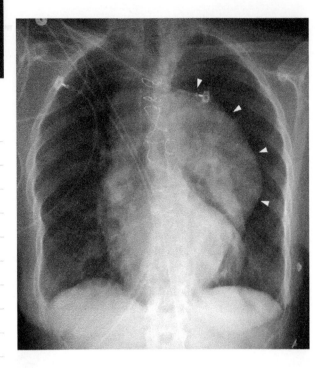

Figure 2–34 Thoracic aortic aneurysm. Frontal chest x-ray shows a soft tissue mass (*arrowheads*) contiguous with the arch of the aorta (don't see the arch as a separate and distinct structure). This mass also is contiguous with the descending aorta. This would qualify as a middle mediastinal mass, but a CT would determine the extent of the mass as well as the attenuation of the mass.

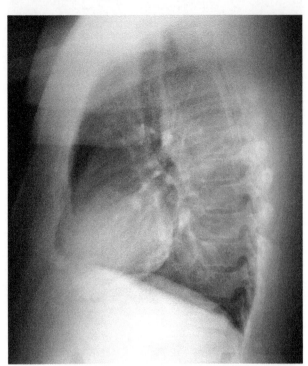

B

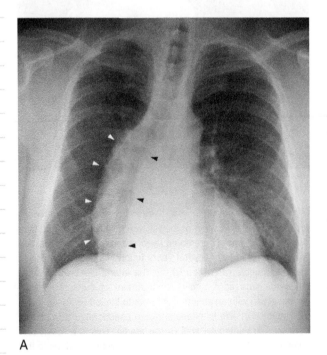

A

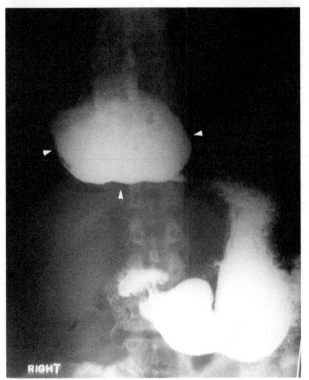

C

Figure 2–35 Achalasia. A, Frontal chest x-ray demonstrating the edge of the distended esophagus (*white arrowheads*) and normal right heart border (*black arrowheads*). B, Lateral x-ray shows increased density superimposed over the cardiac silhouette. C, The barium swallow shows barium collected in the distal esophagus resulting in the distention of the esophagus. The esophageal distention is the cause of the increased density over the cardiac silhouette.

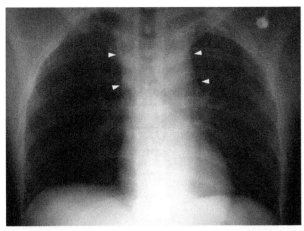

A

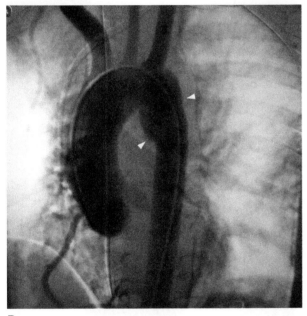

B

Figure 2–36   Mediastinal hematoma. A, Portable frontal chest x-ray shows a soft tissue density around the region of the arch of the aorta (*arrowheads*). This patient was in a motor vehicle collision. In the setting of acute trauma with this appearance in the mediastinum, an aortic injury must be considered, and the patient must have a CT examination for evaluation of injury to the aorta and the presence of a mediastinal hematoma. An angiogram will be useful to show the aortic injury, but the mediastinal hematoma or other associated injuries will not be assessed. B, Image from an angiogram in this patient showing the injury to the aorta (*arrowheads*).

This book is not designed to review all possible causes of unilateral or bilateral hilar enlargement. You can refer to the tables for a more complete differential diagnosis for the finding of unilateral or bilateral hilar enlargement. The more commonly encountered abnormalities will be described.

Table 2–8   Differential Diagnosis of Posterior Mediastinal Mass
Neural tumor
Ganglioneuroma
Ganglioneuroblastoma
Neuroblastoma
Paraganglioma
Dural ectasia
Schwannoma
Neurofibroma
Vertebral mass
Osteomyelitis with phlegmon
Metastasis, myeloma
Eosinophilic granuloma
Primary tumor
Extramedullary hematopoiesis
Disk-derived mass
Discitis with abscess
Lymph nodal mass
Vascular or lymphatic mass
Germ cell tumor

Unilateral Hilar Enlargement

One of the most common causes of unilateral hilar enlargement is malignancy, usually squamous cell carcinoma. This may reflect direct extension into the nodes or the centrally located mass. Metastatic lymph node involvement from small cell carcinoma can also cause unilateral hilar enlargement. This tumor spreads via the lymphatics and hematogenously, explaining involvement of the hilum in patients on presentation. In all patients with lung cancer, CT should be performed to evaluate nodal enlargement, determine extent of disease for staging, and assist in treatment planning.

Primary pulmonary tuberculosis is also associated with unilateral hilar enlargement. Parenchymal disease is seen in association with hilar nodal involvement in primary pulmonary tuberculosis.

Pulmonary artery enlargement can lead to a prominent hilum. Consider pulmonary artery aneurysm or poststenotic dilation as possible causes for vascular enlargement. Refer to Table 2–9 for additional causes of unilateral hilar enlargement (Figure 2–42).

Bilateral Hilar Enlargement

Causes for bilateral hilar enlargement include lymph node enlargement and pulmonary artery enlargement. Bilateral hilar enlargement from metastatic

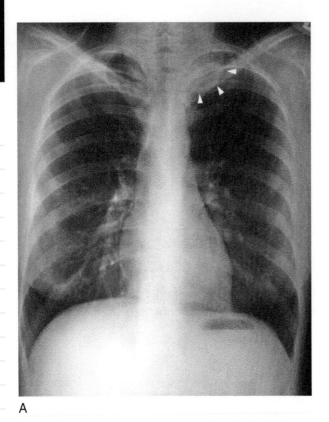

A

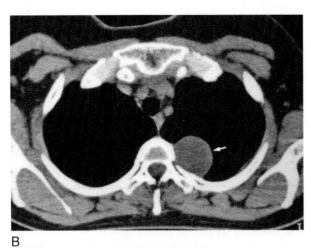

B

Figure 2–37 Schwannoma. A, Frontal chest x-ray demonstrates soft tissue density superimposed over the medial left clavicle (*arrowheads*). The lesion cannot be localized based on the frontal projection. B, Noncontrast CT at the level of the great vessels demonstrates a well defined soft tissue density in the posterior mediastinum (*arrow*). (Courtesy of Edward Patz, MD.)

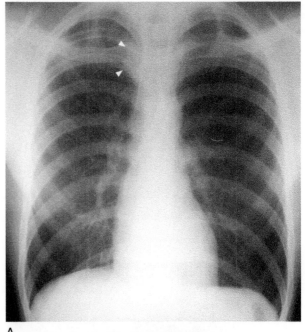

A

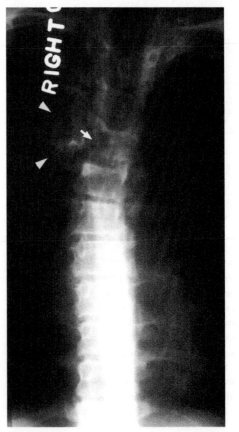

B

Figure 2–38 Osteochondroma thoracic spine. A, Frontal chest x-ray demonstrates increased density in the region of the right sternoclavicular joint (*arrowheads*). B, Thoracic spine image (technique for obtaining this image is different from a chest x-ray). Note the increased bone density in the upper thoracic spine (*arrowheads*). The osteochondroma has lead to the scalloped contour of the adjacent thoracic vertebral body (*arrow*).

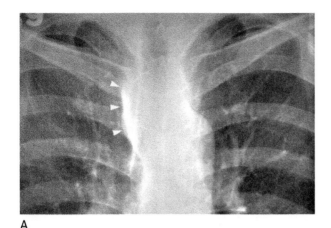

A

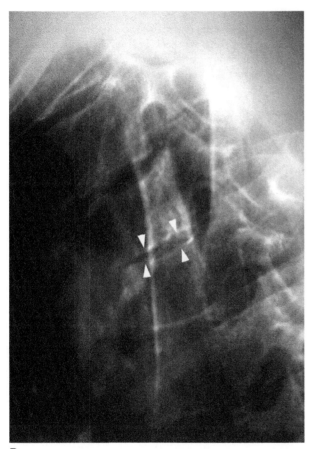

B

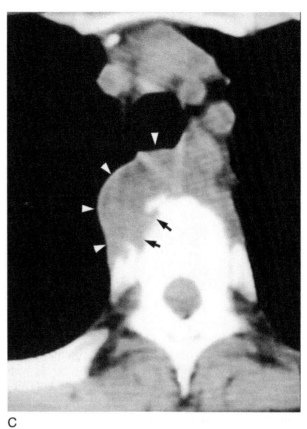

C

Figure 2–39   Osteomyelitis. A, Frontal coned down view of an upright chest x-ray demonstrates abnormal right paraspinal soft tissue density (*arrowheads*). B, Coned down lateral view of the thoracic spine demonstrates abnormal narrowing of the disk space (*arrowheads*) and irregularity of the endplates, compatible with diskitis/possible osteomyelitis. C, CT at the level of the great vessels demonstrating a paraspinous soft tissue density (*white arrowheads*) with slight erosion of the vertebral body (*black arrows*). (Courtesy of Edward Patz, MD.)

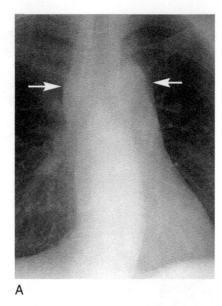

A

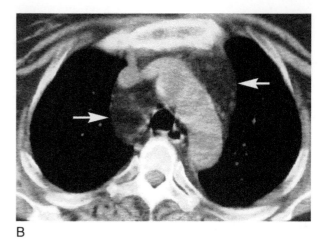

B

Figure 2–40 Mediastinal lipomatosis. A, Frontal coned down view of an upright chest x-ray shows widening of the mediastinum (*arrows*). B, CT with contrast at the level of the aortic arch demonstrates density consistent with fat (*arrows*), diagnostic of mediastinal lipomatosis. (Courtesy of Edward Patz, MD.)

disease is uncommon. Hodgkin's lymphoma is more likely to cause bilateral hilar enlargement than non-Hodgkin's lymphoma. Bilateral hilar lymph node as well as paratracheal lymph node enlargement can be seen in most patients with sarcoidosis. Causes of pulmonary artery enlargement include pulmonary artery hypertension, high-output states such as anemia, and chronic pulmonary diseases. Refer to Table 2–10 for additional causes of bilateral hilar enlargement (Figures 2–43 and 2–44).

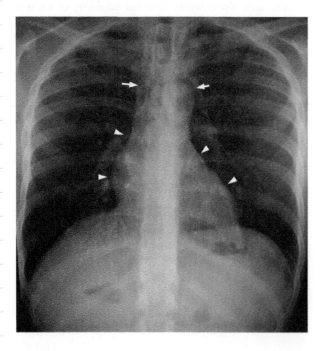

Figure 2–41 Pneumomediastinum. Frontal chest x-ray demonstrating very well defined cardiac and mediastinal structures (*arrowheads*). Note the air density around the aortic arch (*arrows*).

Table 2–9	Differential Diagnosis of Unilateral Hilar Enlargement

Lymph node enlargement
    Bronchogenic carcinoma
    Lymph node metastases
    Tuberculosis
    Histoplasmosis
    Coccidioidomycosis
Pulmonary artery enlargement
    Pulmonary artery aneurysm
    Poststenotic pulmonary dilation
    Pulmonary embolus (central or chronic)
Cyst
    Bronchogenic cyst

Table 2–10	Differential Diagnosis of Bilateral Hilar Enlargement

Lymph node enlargement
    Hodgkin's lymphoma
    Sarcoidosis
    Silicosis
    Angioimmunoblastic lymphadenopathy
    Malignancy
Pulmonary artery enlargement
    Pulmonary artery hypertension
    Left-to-right intracardiac shunt
    High-output states (anemia, thyrotoxicosis)
    Cystic fibrosis
    Chronic pulmonary disease

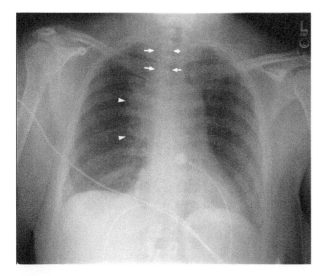

Figure 2–42   Lung cancer with hilar adenopathy. Frontal chest x-ray demonstrating a soft tissue density contiguous with the right hilum (*arrowheads*). In addition there is thickening of the right paratracheal soft tissues (*small arrows*).

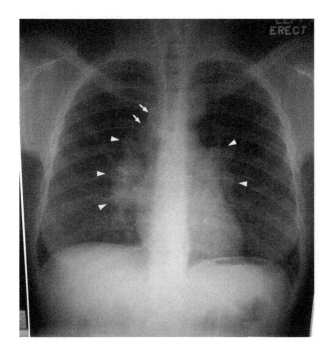

Figure 2–43   Sarcoidosis with bilateral hilar enlargement. Frontal chest x-ray demonstrating increase in soft tissue density around the hilar bilaterally (*arrowheads*). Additionally, a soft tissue density is also noted in the location of the azygous vein (*small arrows*).

Pleura and Chest Wall

The *pleura* is inspected on x-ray for abnormalities as well. Two layers make up the pleura: the visceral pleura and the parietal pleura. These are serosal membranes that envelop the lung. The visceral

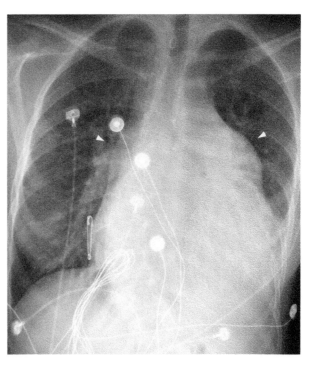

Figure 2–44   Primary pulmonary hypertension. Frontal chest x-ray showing large soft tissue density in the region of the origins of the pulmonary arteries (*arrowheads*). Pulmonary artery enlargement is present in patients with primary pulmonary hypertension.

pleura is adherent to the lung, and the parietal pleura is contiguous with the chest wall and the diaphragm. The pleural space is a potential space between the visceral and parietal pleurae. The normal amount of fluid in this space is about 5 mL.

The appearance of a pleural effusion on x-ray depends on the patient's position for the x-ray. A pleural meniscus results when the fluid collects in the lateral costophrenic sulcus, leading to a concave margin (Figure 2–45). A lateral decubitus film is useful for evaluation of a suspected pleural effusion. A large pleural effusion can cause passive atelectasis of an entire lung, leading to the appearance of opacification of a hemithorax. A helpful sign to distinguish a large effusion from a collapsed lung, which can also cause opacification of a hemithorax, is to evaluate the mediastinal structures. If you think about it, one of the aforementioned processes demonstrates mass effect and the other is caused by volume loss. So the mediastinum will shift away from the mass effect (large effusion) and toward the volume loss (complete collapse) (Figure 2–46). If both are present, it can be difficult to distinguish fluid from collapse. In this setting, CT can be used to determine effusion or atelectasis, because the differences in density are

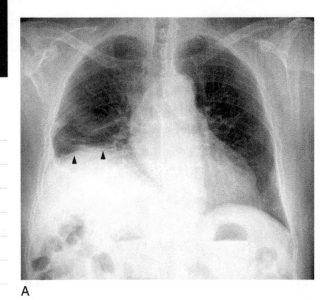

A

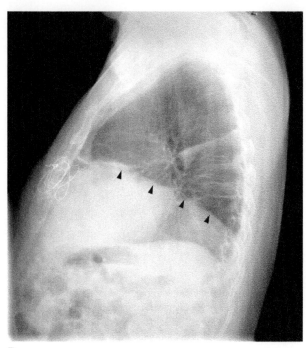

B

Figure 2–45 Right pleural effusion. A, Frontal chest film showing apparent elevation of the right hemidiaphragm (*arrowheads*). The pleural fluid (soft tissue density) is the same density as the diaphragm, and therefore, the diaphragm is not seen as a discrete structure. B, Lateral film shows the sizeable pleural fluid collection (*arrowheads*).

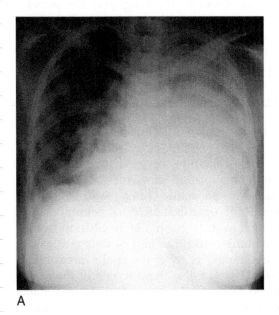

A

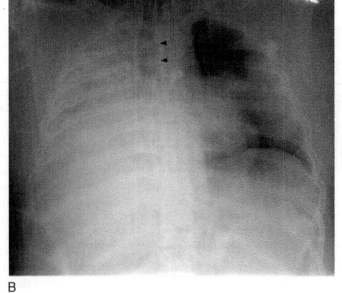

B

Figure 2–46 Opacification of a hemithorax. A, Frontal chest x-ray demonstrating a massive pleural effusion. The mediastinal structures are shifted away from the side of the effusion. B, Frontal chest x-ray of lung collapse. This lung is completely atelectatic or airless. It is of soft tissue density because the interstitial structures that are left behind are soft tissue structures. Note that the mediastinal structures are shifted toward the side of collapse in this setting (*arrowheads*). This patient also has an endotracheal tube and nasogastric tube.

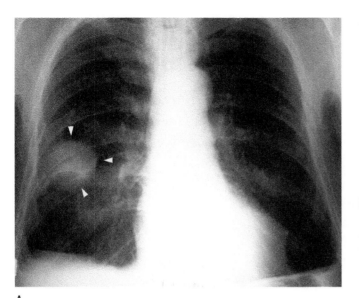

A

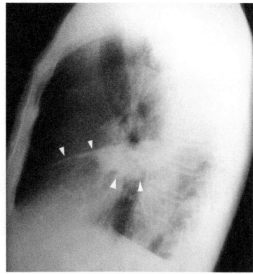

B

Figure 2–47   Pseudotumor of the lung. A, Frontal projection of a patient with loculated fluid in the major fissure (*arrowheads*). This causes a soft tissue mass-like appearance on the frontal chest film. B, The lateral film shows thickening of the major fissure from the fluid (*arrowheads*) and the presence of this loculation (*arrows*).

apparent. Ultrasound may also be useful to evaluate the presence and size of an effusion in these confusing cases. Ultrasonography can also be used as guidance for thoracentesis (draining of pleural fluid).

Fluid can also extend into the fissures. An elliptical opacity is then noted on the chest x-ray (soft tissue/fluid density) in the location of the fissures. This situation is most often seen in patients who have fluid overload. The loculated collections of fluid have been termed "pseudotumor" (Figure 2–47).

A subpulmonic effusion is seen when fluid accumulates between the lower lobe and the diaphragm. This appearance can sometimes be difficult to identify on an upright chest film. It appears as "apparent elevation of the hemidiaphragm." Clues on the frontal chest x-ray that might indicate a subpulmonic effusion include new elevation of the hemidiaphragm compared with a previous chest x-ray, a more laterally located dome of the diaphragm, appearance of the minor fissure close to the "diaphragm," and separation of the gastric air bubble from the base of the lung by increased soft tissue/fluid density. A lateral decubitus view is useful to show the mobility of the fluid collection (Figures 2–48 and 2–49) (**Key Point 2–3**).

Detection of pleural fluid in the supine patient can be difficult because the fluid accumulates in a dependent location (posterior). The x-rays have to penetrate fluid in addition to lung, so a relative "haziness" is present in one hemithorax compared

with the other. The diaphragm of the affected side may be obscured because the fluid density abuts the diaphragm (same density), making the diaphragm no longer visible. If the effusion is really large, it may be seen at the apex of the lung as fluid density. Fluid that collects medially may mimic mediastinal widening. This apparent widening is a reflection of the soft tissue/fluid density abutting the soft tissue density of the mediastinum (Figure 2–50). Causes of pleural effusions are listed in **Tables 2–11** and **2–12**.

Pneumothorax presents with abrupt onset of dyspnea and pleuritic chest pain as atmospheric air enters the pleural space (Figure 2–51). There are many causes of pneumothorax (**Table 2–13**), including penetrating injuries inflicted as a result of mean-spirited trauma (gun shot, knife wound) or as a result of meaningful intervention such as line placement. Blunt trauma to the chest can also result in a pneumothorax by acutely increasing intrathoracic pressure. Tracheobronchial laceration can result in a pneumothorax and a bronchopleural fistula. In fact, this is an injury to consider when chest tubes have been placed and the pneumothoraces persist with respiratory compromise (Figure 2–52).

The appearance of a pneumothorax is important to recognize, because its timely treatment can be life-saving for the patient. On an upright chest x-ray, a pneumothorax can be diagnosed when the pleural line is noted to be paralleling the chest wall, separating the partially collapsed lung from pleural air peripherally. Evaluation of the vasculature

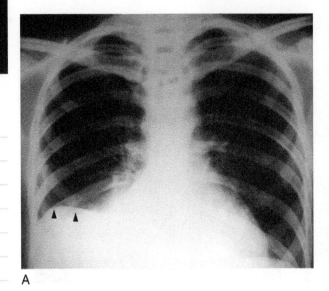

A

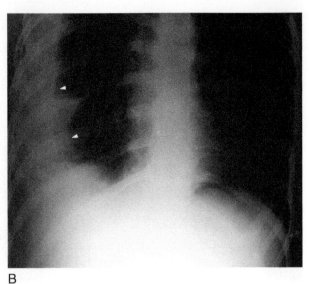

B

Figure 2–48 Right subpulmonic effusion. A, Upright, frontal chest x-ray demonstrates apparent elevation of the right hemidiaphragm (*arrowheads*). Note the slightly laterally located apex of the right hemidiaphragm (a not-so-easy identification). B, A lateral decubitus film shows the mobile nature of this collection of fluid (*arrowheads*).

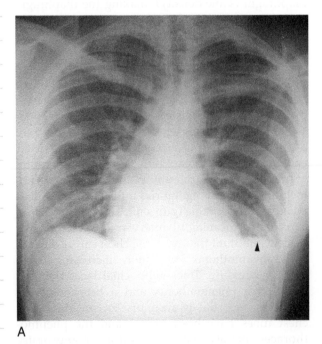

A

B

Figure 2–49 Left subpulmonic effusion. A, Upright, frontal chest x-ray demonstrating apparent elevation of the left hemidiaphragm (*arrowhead*). B, Left lateral decubitus film shows mobility of the subpleural effusion (*arrowheads*).

Clues to the Identification of Subpulmonic Pleural Effusion

New elevation of hemidiaphragm
Laterally located dome of the diaphragm
Minor fissure appears close to diaphragm
Increased soft tissue/fluid density between gastric bubble and lung

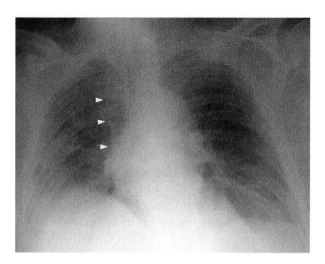

Figure 2–50   Medial collection of pleural fluid. Frontal chest x-ray in a recumbent patient demonstrating apparent mediastinal widening (*arrowheads*). This is a result of fluid extending along the structures of the mediastinum.

Table 2–11 Causes of Pleural Effusion

Increase in hydrostatic pressure
    Congestive heart failure
Decrease in osmotic pressure
    Cirrhosis
    Nephrotic syndrome
    Hypoalbuminemia
Increased capillary permeability
    Infection
    Neoplasm
    Autoimmune disease
Decrease in pleural pressure
    Atelectasis
Impaired lymphatic drainage
    Fibrosis
    Tumor
Transport of fluid from abdomen
    Ascites

Table 2–12 Transudative and Exudative Pleural Effusions

Transudative

Congestive heart failure
Cirrhosis
Nephrotic syndrome
Hypoalbuminemia

Exudative

Infection
    Lung infection
    Bloodborne infection
Autoimmune
    Immune complex disease
    Vasculitis
Neoplasm
    Lung neoplasm
    Pleural metastasis
    Mesothelioma
    Paraneoplastic
Other
    Lung infarct
    Trauma
Chylothorax

reveals that lung markings are not seen at the peripheral margins of the film. Films obtained in expiration will allow for easier identification of the pneumothorax (Figure 2–53). Loculated pneumothoraces (air in pleural space trapped between adhesions) and subpulmonic pneumothoraces (air collected between lung and diaphragm) can occur as well.

In the setting of a rib fracture, it is not as important to document the rib fracture as it is to identify the pneumothorax. Therefore, don't waste your time or the patient's time by ordering a rib series when concerned about a rib fracture. Instead, get a film that you can act on—a chest x-ray.

Because most portable chest x-rays are obtained in a supine position in the high-risk critically ill patient, you will have to have some practice in evaluation for pneumothorax in this view. Remember that the free air will rise to the top. In a supine patient, the nondependent portion of the pleural space is anterior and anteromedial. Small pneumothoraces may not produce a visible pleural line. Look for asymmetry in the density of the lung. The affected lung may be hyperlucent compared with the unaffected lung (just the opposite from pleural effusion). Additionally, it may appear that the mediastinal structures are very well defined

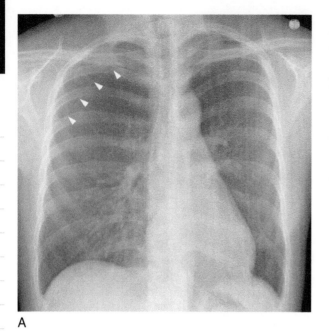

A

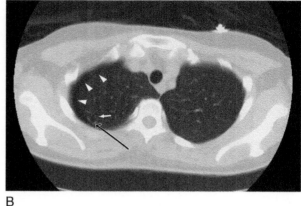

B

Figure 2–51   Right apical pneumothorax. A, Upright, frontal chest x-ray demonstrating a pneumothorax (*arrowheads*). Notice the absence of lung markings beyond the pleura in the apex of the right lung. B, CT filmed in lung windows showing the architecture of the lung parenchyma. The right-sided pneumothorax is noted (*arrowheads*). In addition, a small bleb is noted in the right lung (*arrow*).

because of sharply marginated edges due to the air-soft tissue interface. Finally, the "deep sulcus sign" describes air in the lateral costophrenic sulcus giving the appearance that the lateral sulcus is abnormally deep (Figure 2–54) (Key Point 2–4).

If after evaluation of the supine film you have concern for an anterior pneumothorax, further evaluation should be performed. These patients usually cannot be positioned upright—otherwise, you'd have done that in the first place. How else can you get the x-ray beam parallel to the air collection? A lateral decubitus film is a great answer! Put the affected side up (air floats to the top). Certainly you can always perform CT, but a conventional film may be obtained more quickly. The CT is helpful when other problems need to be addressed in addition to determining whether the patient has a pneumothorax.

Tension pneumothorax is a result of air entering but not exiting the pleural space. The pressure exceeds atmospheric pressure, resulting in complete lung collapse and impaired venous return to the heart (Figure 2–55). Clinically, these patients are compromised in their respiration and circulation. They will demonstrate tachypnea, tachycardia, hypotension, and cyanosis. Radiographically, you can think of a tension pneumothorax as the lung being under mass effect. The mediastinal structures are shifted away from the side of the pneumothorax. The lung will be collapsed and the diaphragm inverted. The diagnosis of a tension pneumothorax remains a clinical one, and because of the circulatory compromise, immediate action is required. Evacuation of the pleural space can be done with a needle, catheter, or chest tube in a timely manner.

Confusion may occur in evaluation for a pneumothorax (Key Point 2–5). Skin folds resulting from the compression of redundant skin may be mistaken for a pneumothorax. The x-ray appearance of the skin fold produces an *edge*, rather than the *line* that is seen with a pneumothorax (Figure 2–56). A clue that helps determine a skin fold is following the edge in its entirety. It will often extend beyond the chest wall. More confusing is determining whether a bulla (air-filled cavity) is present

Table 2–13   Causes of Pneumothorax
Penetrating trauma
Gun shot
Stabbing
Rib fracture
Central line placement
Improper feeding tube placement
Thoracentesis
Biopsy or surgery (lung, pleura, esophagus)
Increased intrathoracic pressure
Positive-pressure mechanical ventilation
Parenchymal disease
Infection
Neoplasm
Cystic lung disease (sarcoidosis, cystic fibrosis)
Obstructive pulmonary disease (emphysema, asthma)

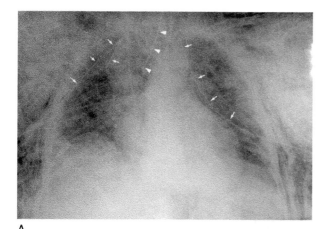

A

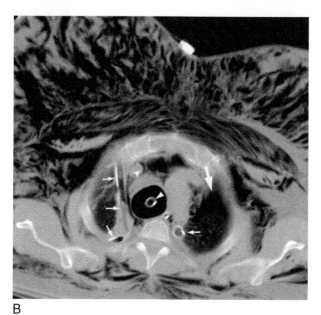

B

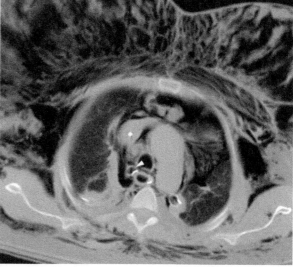

C

Figure 2–52 Tracheal laceration. A, Frontal, portable, supine chest x-ray demonstrates an endotracheal tube (*arrowheads*) and bilateral chest tubes (*small arrows*). Note the massive amount of subcutaneous air. Persistent pneumothoraces can be difficult to identify on supine imaging. The endotracheal tube has an aberrant course. B, CT at the level of the arch shows the massive soft tissue emphysema. Endotracheal tube (*arrowhead*) is noted in a markedly distended trachea. Chest tubes are present (*small arrows*). Note the presence of a left sided pneumothorax (*large arrow*). C, CT image slightly more distal shows the endotracheal tube no longer within the trachea (*arrowhead*). (Courtesy of Michael Gotway, MD.)

versus a pneumothorax. The bulla can also demonstrate hyperlucency, but often the bulla will have margins that are concave to the chest wall, whereas a pneumothorax has margins that are convex to the chest wall. In difficult cases, CT is useful because it will show the surrounding lung parenchyma in better detail.

Processes causing pleural-based diseases are listed in **Table 2–14**. CT is an excellent modality for evaluation of pleural-based processes. It can readily demonstrate the extent of the disease process as well as the density of the process, helping to narrow the differential diagnosis. Chest wall lesions are best evaluated with CT. Refer to **Table 2–15** for a list of some of the processes affecting the chest wall.

Diaphragm

The *diaphragm* is generally visualized as a discrete structure only when it is surrounded by air. The diaphragm appears as round densities on either side of the spine on x-rays. It is a musculotendinous structure that separates the thoracic and abdominal cavity. The diaphragm is apposed to the liver on the right and to the spleen and stomach on the left. At the periphery of the diaphragm is the pleural surface. The nodularity seen in some diaphragms is caused by contraction of slips of the muscle. This appearance increases with increasing age of the patient. The diaphragm has insertions on the xiphoid process, ribs, upper lumbar vertebral bodies, and transverse processes. Through the diaphragm travel the aorta, the thoracic duct, and the azygous and hemiazygous veins (aortic hiatus). The esophageal hiatus is the opening for the esophagus as well as the vagus nerves.

A few different types of hernias through the diaphragm are worth noting. The *hiatus hernia* is most common and represents herniation of the stomach through the esophageal hiatus (Figure 2–57). This

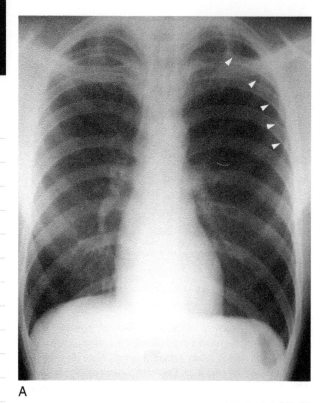

A

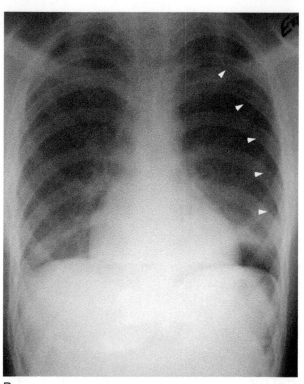

B

Figure 2–53 Pneumothorax. A, Upright, frontal chest x-ray demonstrating a pneumothorax (*arrowheads*). This film was obtained during inspiration. B, Upright, frontal chest x-ray obtained with expiration. Notice the apparent enlargement of the pneumothrax as it becomes more conspicuous (*arrowheads*).

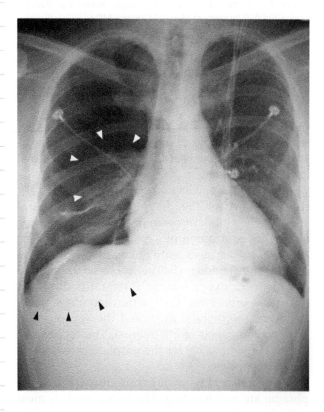

Figure 2–54 Large pneumothorax with deep sulcus sign. Upright, frontal chest x-ray demonstrating a large right-sided pneumothorax with air density visible along the right costophrenic sulcus (*black arrowheads*). Note the collapsed lung (*white arrowheads*).

Key   Point 2–4

Features of Pneumothorax on Supine Chest Radiograph

Hyperlucent lung
Sharply marginated mediastinal border
Hyperlucent costophrenic sulcus

Key   Point 2–5

Pitfalls in Diagnosing a Pneumothorax

Skin folds
Clothing/starched bed sheets
Bullae
Scapula
Chest wall abnormalities
Tubing artifacts

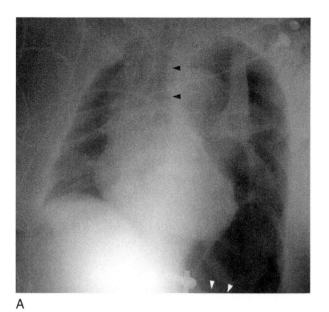

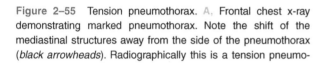

A

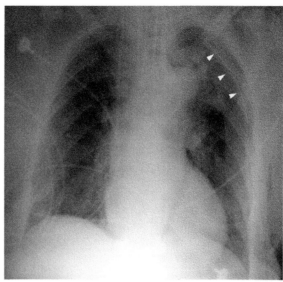

B

Figure 2–55   Tension pneumothorax. A, Frontal chest x-ray demonstrating marked pneumothorax. Note the shift of the mediastinal structures away from the side of the pneumothorax (*black arrowheads*). Radiographically this is a tension pneumo-thorax, but the diagnosis is a clinical one. A deep sulcus is suggested (*white arrowheads*). B, Note resolution of pneumo-thorax after placement of chest tube (*white arrowheads*).

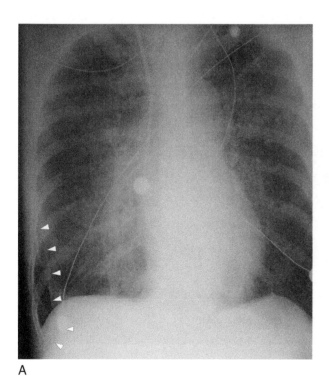

A

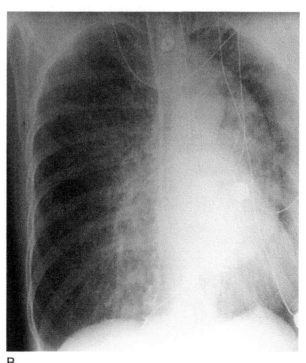

B

Figure 2–56   Skin fold mimicking pneumothorax. A, Patient with interstitial lung disease and a concern for a loculated lower right basilar pneumothorax (*arrowheads*). This is a skin fold. Note that lung markings are present lateral to the edge. B, Repeat image shows the skin fold disappears with repositioning the patient. Skin folds are most often encountered with portable films as the skin gets rolled on the x-ray cassette.

Table 2–14   Focal Pleural Disease
Opacities that mimic focal pleural thickening
Apical cap
Companion shadows of first and second ribs
Subpleural deposits of fat
Thickening
Pneumonia
Pulmonary infarct
Trauma
Asbestos exposure
Calcification
Hemothorax
Empyema
Asbestos exposure
Pleural/extrapleural mass
Fibroma
Lipoma
Neurofibroma
Metastasis
Mesothelioma
Loculated pleural effusion
Empyema
Hematoma

Table 2–15   Chest Wall Lesions
Tumors
Neurofibroma
Lipoma
Hemangioma
Desmoid
Fibrosarcoma
Liposarcoma
Metastases
Melanoma
Bronchogenic carcinoma
Infection
Abscess
Tuberculosis
Trauma
Hematoma

type of hernia is identified by noting a mass in the region immediately superior to the left hemidiaphragm on a frontal radiograph and projecting behind the heart on the lateral x-ray. Occasionally, you might be lucky enough to see an air-fluid level within the mass. A *foramen of Bochdalek hernia* is the result of a defect in the posterior portion of the diaphragm (Figure 2–58). Large Bochdalek hernias can present in the neonatal period with respiratory distress and a hypoplastic lung. These hernias can be diagnosed during a prenatal ultrasound screening examination. In adults, these hernias are predominantly located on the left side. A CT examination can identify the herniated mass. A *foramen of Morgagni hernia* is right-sided and usually incidentally discovered as a mass in the cardiophrenic angle (Figure 2–59).

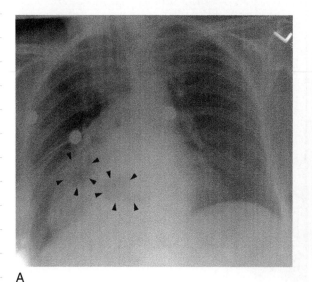

A

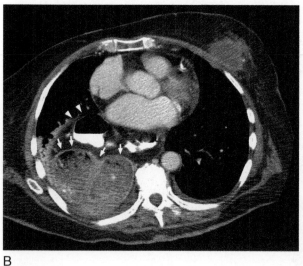

B

Figure 2–57   Hiatus hernia. A, Frontal, upright, slightly rotated (look at the sternoclavicular joints) chest x-ray demonstrates an abnormal contour to the right side of the cardiac silhouette. Air is noted within the density adjacent to the right heart border (*arrowheads*). B, CT scan after intravenous and oral contrast demonstrates oral contrast in the anterior aspect of this mass (*arrowheads*). The remainder of the stomach and contents are noted slightly posterior to the portion with oral contrast (*small arrows*).

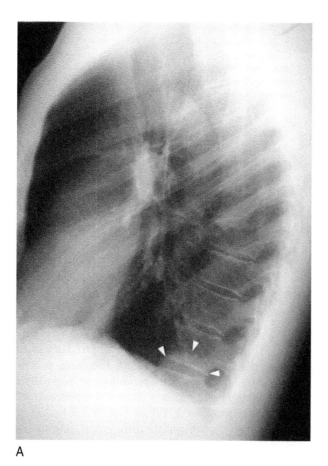

A

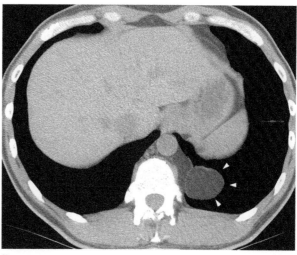

B

Figure 2–58   Bochdalek hernia. A, Upright lateral chest x-ray shows a density in the region of the posterior lung or mediastinum (*arrowheads*). B, Axial noncontrast CT shows the fat density of the hernia (*arrowheads*). Note the similar density to the paraspinous fat. A Bochdelak hernia is recognized from its posterior herniation in the diaphragm. This is the most common congenital hernia (Courtesy of Michael Gotway, MD).

Traumatic hernias can occur after blunt and penetrating trauma and are most often left-sided. If the left hemidiaphragm is indistinct or elevated or gas loops are noted in the left hemithorax (bowel), along with the appropriate clinical history, diaphragmatic

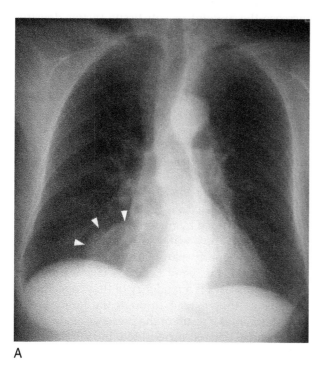

A

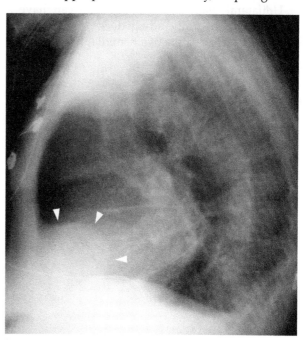

B

Figure 2–59   Morgagni hernia. A, Frontal chest x-ray shows a well defined soft tissue density at the right cardiophrenic angle (*arrowheads*). B, Lateral view demonstrates the anterior location of the Morgagni hernia (*arrowheads*).

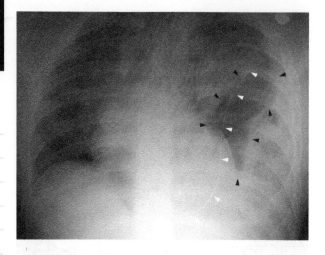

Figure 2–60   Traumatic diaphragmatic hernia. Portable frontal chest x-ray obtained after motor vehicle crash. Patient suffered blunt chest trauma. A loculated air density is noted in the left hemithorax (*black arrowheads*). No left hemidiaphragm is visualized. A nasogastric tube is coursing along the esophagus and into the left hemithorax within the air collection (*white arrowheads*). The stomach has herniated through the diaphragm into the left hemithorax.

rupture should be considered (Figure 2–60). Many times this diagnosis is overlooked in the acute setting due to associated injuries. CT can diagnose the associated injuries as well as identifying the herniated structures.

Unilateral diaphragmatic elevation can have a number of causes, including those leading to the appearance of elevation of a hemidiaphragm. These are listed in **Table 2–16**.

Table 2–16   Causes of Unilateral Diaphragmatic Elevation
Eventration
Diminished lung volume
Hypoplastic
Lobar/lung atelectasis
Pulmonary resection
Paralysis/injury to phrenic nerve
Upper abdominal mass
Hepatomegaly
Splenomegaly
Gastric/colonic distention
Ascites
Diaphragmatic hernia
Subpulmonic pleural effusion

Lungs

Now that all the other structures in the chest have been evaluated, the lung parenchyma can be discussed. The focus of this chapter is not to discuss all possible diseases that can affect the lung parenchyma. For that, you can refer to the suggested reading list. However, a systematic approach to evaluation is presented. Tables have been included for reference for appropriate differential diagnoses.

Start by determining whether the parenchymal process causes an increase or a decrease in lung density. Remember that the normal density is a result of the amount of air-filled bronchi, bronchioles, and soft tissue density. Processes that increase the amount of soft tissue (water density) will increase the density of the parenchyma. Processes that destroy the blood vessels and parenchyma will lead to a relative increase in lucency (decreased density).

Abnormal pulmonary opacities may be divided into air-space disease, atelectasis, interstitial disease, nodular or mass-like processes, and branching opacities. Recognizing these patterns of opacity will allow for an appropriate differential diagnosis (**Key Point 2–6**).

Air-space opacity develops when the air that is normally present within the terminal air spaces of the lung is replaced by material of soft tissue (fluid) density (blood, pus, water, or tumor cells). Initially, the process is poorly marginated due to an irregular interface with the x-ray beam. A characteristic of air-space diseases is a tendency of these opacities to coalesce as they extend through the lung. An air bronchogram is a result of the presence of air within the bronchi that is surrounded by intra-alveolar cellular material (blood, pus, water, or tumor cells). These tubular lucencies are now conspicuous due to the surrounding soft tissue density (Figure 2–61). A "bat's wing" or "butterfly" appearance is a finding

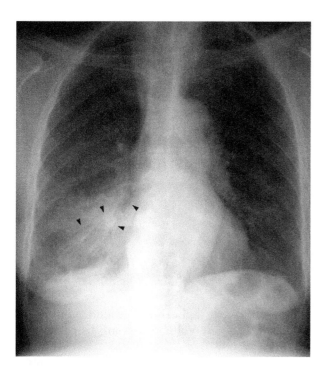

Figure 2–61   Air bronchograms. Upright, frontal chest x-ray demonstrated linear lucencies (*arrowheads*) in a focus of air-space disease. In this case the intra-alveolar cellular material is tumor cells. The patient has bronchoalveolar carcinoma. Those with a keen eye might also recognize the adenopathy present along the mediastinal contour.

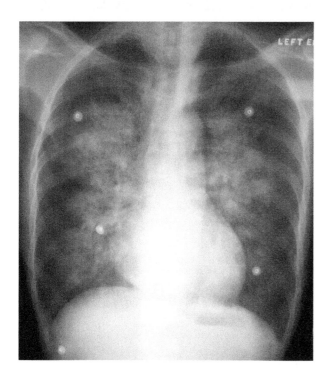

Figure 2–62   Pulmonary edema (bat's wing). Upright portable chest x-ray demonstrating increased opacity characteristic of air-space disease.

seen only with air-space disease, typically with pulmonary edema or hemorrhage (Figure 2–62). Finally, on serial chest x-rays, air-space disease will show rapid change in appearance over short intervals. (As a reminder, atelectasis and progressing

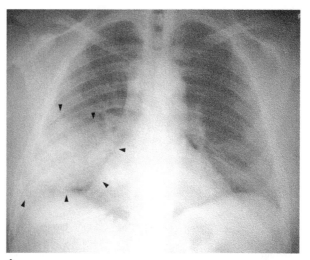

A

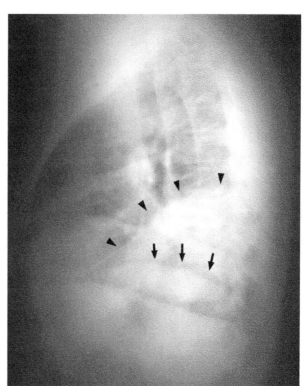

B

Figure 2–63   Right lower lobe consolidation. A, Frontal projection demonstrating opacification in the right lower lung (*arrowheads*). Note loss of the lateral aspect of the right hemidiaphragm. B, Lateral film identifies the location of this density to be in the right lower lobe (*arrowheads*). Note the right hemidiaphragm is not visualized. Horizontal linear lucencies represent folds of skin (*arrows*) in this somewhat obese individual.

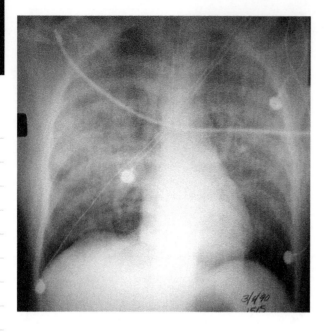

Figure 2–64   Pulmonary hemorrhage. Upright frontal chest x-ray demonstrating the typical bat's-wing distribution due to pulmonary hemorrhage. Note the presence of an endotracheal tube and nasogastric tube.

interstitial pulmonary edema can change quickly, too) (Figures 2–63 through 2–65) (Key Point 2–7) (Table 2–17).

Atelectasis is a condition in which there is loss of lung volume. Different types of atelectasis are listed in **Table 2–18**. Atelectasis can affect an entire lobe (lobar), a segment of a lobe (segmental), or a subsegment of a lobe (subsegmental or plate-like), or it

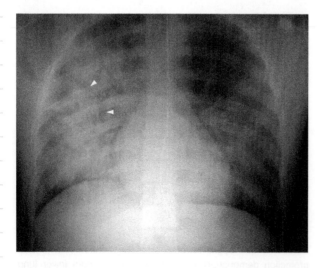

Figure 2–65   Near drowning. Frontal chest x-ray demonstrating asymmetry of the air-space disease. Air bronchograms are noted (*arrowheads*). The right lung is more involved with this process than the left lung.

may be round in appearance (round atelectasis). Signs that suggest volume loss are listed in **Key Point 2–8** (Figure 2–66).

Interstitial disease is diagnosed when the interstitial compartments of the lung thicken. This can be caused by blood, pus, edema (water), or tumor cells (**Table 2–19**). The interstitial opacities can occur in different types of patterns. These are

Table 2–17   Differential Diagnosis of Air-space Disease

Infection
  Bacterial
  Tuberculosis
  Mycoplasma
  Viral
  Fungal
Vascular
  Pulmonary contusion (trauma)
  Pulmonary embolism
  Pulmonary edema
  Hemorrhage
  Goodpasture's syndrome
  Wegener's granulomatosis
  Hemosiderosis
Chronic infiltrating lung disease
  Bronchiolitis obliterans-organizing pneumonia
  Pulmonary alveolar proteinosis
  Eosinophilic pneumonia
Neoplasm
  Bronchoalveolar cell carcinoma
  Lymphoma
Inhalation
  Aspiration
  Lipoid pneumonia

Table 2-18 Types of Pulmonary Atelectasis

Type	Example
Obstructive	Bronchogenic carcinoma
Passive	Pleura effusion
Compressive	Bulla
Cicatricial	Postprimary tuberculosis
Adhesive	Respiratory distress syndrome of the newborn

Table 2-19 Differential Diagnosis of Interstitial Lung Disease

Idiopathic pulmonary fibrosis
Pulmonary edema
Collagen vascular disease (rheumatoid lung)
Lymphangitic carcinomatosis
Sarcoidosis
Asbestosis
Silicosis
Coal worker's pneumoconiosis
Miliary tuberculosis

Key Point 2-8

Signs of Atelectasis

Displacement of interlobar fissure
Increased density of atelectatic lung
Ipsilateral mediastinal shift
Hilar elevation (upper-lobe atelectasis)
Hilar depression (lower-lobe atelectasis)
Compensatory hyperinflation of adjacent lobe
Crowding of vessels
Shifting granuloma
Small hemithorax
Elevated hemidiaphragm

Thickening of the peripheral interstitium of the lung produces linear opacities that are obliquely oriented, are 2 to 6 cm long, and less than 1 mm in thickness, and course through the substance of the lung toward the hila (Kerley's A lines). These correspond to lymphatic communications between the perivenous and bronchoarterial circulation. Shorter (1–2 cm), thin lines coursing perpendicular to the pleural surface are Kerley's B lines and represent thickened peripheral subpleural interlobular septa (Figure 2–67).

You may consider further evaluation of a patient with interstitial lung disease with high-resolution

reticular, reticulonodular, nodular, and linear as defined on conventional x-rays. The predominant pattern of interstitial opacity depends on the nature of the underlying disease and the portion of the interstitium affected.

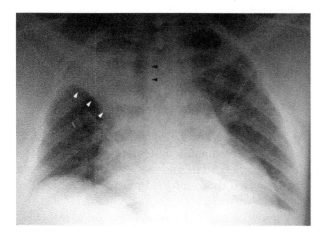

Figure 2–66 Right upper lobe collapse. Frontal chest x-ray demonstrates opacification of the right upper portion of the lung. The minor fissure is elevated (*white arrowheads*) and the trachea is shifted to the right hemithorax (*black arrowheads*). These are associated findings of volume loss.

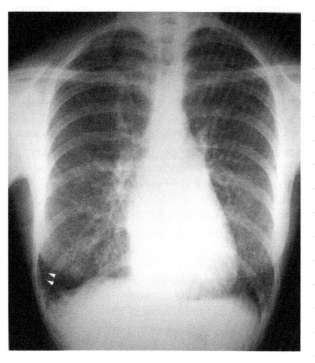

Figure 2–67 Interstitial pulmonary edema. Frontal chest x-ray demonstrates thickening and prominence of the interstitium. Kerley's B lines (*arrowheads*) are noted along the chest wall. The presence of Kerley's B lines confirms interstitial lung disease.

CT (HRCT). The pattern of interstitial disease abnormalities as seen with HRCT can offer a more specific differential diagnosis, depending on which portion of the interstitium is affected. To describe the patterns of appearance on HRCT is beyond the scope of this book, but recognize that HRCT is available to you and your patient for further evaluation of this disease process. In addition to characterizing parenchymal abnormalities, HRCT may be used for biopsy planning and for managing and following patients with interstitial lung disease.

Emphysema

Emphysema is a pathologic diagnosis that is defined as an abnormal, permanent enlargement of the air spaces distal to the terminal bronchiole, accompanied by destruction of alveolar walls and without obvious fibrosis. Three different types of emphysema exist. *Centrilobular emphysema* is the most common form and has a tendency to affect the upper lobes. *Panlobar emphysema* has a tendency to affect the lower lobes. *Paraseptal emphysema* is seen in the immediate subpleural regions of the upper lobes. It may coalesce to form apical bullae. Rupture of these bullae into the pleural space can lead to spontaneous pneumothorax.

Frontal and lateral chest radiographs are the initial radiographic examinations performed in patients with suspected emphysema. Hyperinflation is the most important plain radiographic finding and reflects the loss of elastic recoil.

The abnormal increase in lung volume is best detected by noting inferior displacement and flattening of the normally convex superior hemidiaphragms, obtuse angles at the costophrenic angles and an increase in the AP diameter of the chest (Figure 2–68). The effects of emphysema and chronic hypoxemia on the right heart may be appreciated on an x-ray as enlargement of the central pulmonary arteries and right ventricle, particularly when there is accompanying pulmonary artery hypertension.

Bullae are thin-walled cystic spaces exceeding 1 cm in diameter that are found within the lung parenchyma. Bullae represent contiguous areas of emphysematous lung (Figure 2–69). Diseases in which bullae may be identified on a chest radiograph are included in **Table 2–20**.

Solitary Pulmonary Nodule

This section would be a reasonable place to discuss identification and evaluation of the solitary pulmonary nodule (SPN). The limited number of pages available in this book precludes discussion

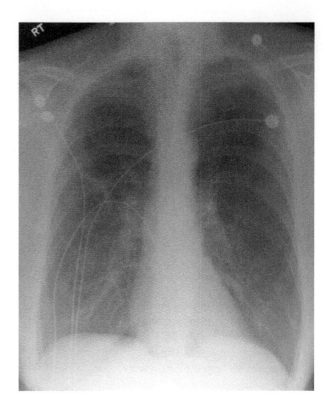

Figure 2–68   Emphysema. Frontal chest x-ray in a patient with a 77-pack-year history of smoking. Note the pathologic increase in lung volumes. In this example the elongated cardiac silhouette is consistent with the increased lung volumes.

of the SPN. However, it is an important concept to understand, and it is necessary to know how to perform a workup for a patient with SPN. An algorithm has been provided for the evaluation of SPN. It is worth noting that identification of an SPN is not always straightforward, even for the chest radiologist (Figure 2–70).

Cardiac Imaging

The *heart* is a middle mediastinal structure. Because cardiac-related diseases can present on x-ray, I felt it was worthwhile to have a separate section on cardiac disease and imaging. A basic approach to the radiographic evaluation of cardiac diseases is presented. The included reference list has books that are well written and easy to understand and include much more information regarding cardiac diseases.

A stepwise approach will allow you to not overlook any abnormalities (Key Point 2–9). A systematic and logical approach, done consistently, will help you identify the abnormalities and offer a diagnosis. Remember that you have already looked at the noncardiovascular structures (soft tissues and bones). If rib-notching is identified, for example,

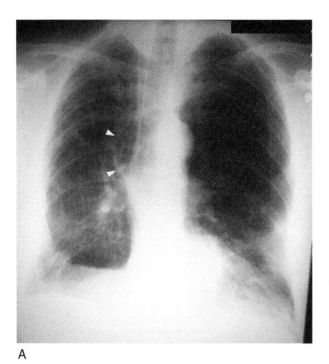

A

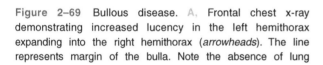

B

Figure 2–69 Bullous disease. A. Frontal chest x-ray demonstrating increased lucency in the left hemithorax expanding into the right hemithorax (*arrowheads*). The line represents margin of the bulla. Note the absence of lung markings within the bulla. B. Lateral radiograph demonstrates inversion of the diaphragms (*black arrowheads*) and increase in the retrosternal airspace (*white arrowheads*), findings consistent with emphysema and bullous disease.

you are likely to be thinking appropriately that your patient may have coarctation of the aorta.

Evaluation of the size of the cardiac silhouette will help further in identifying the possible cause of the patient's cardiac abnormality. The average normal cardiothoracic ratio in adults as visualized on an upright chest radiograph is 0.45. Quite frankly, are you going to take out a ruler and a calculator to do this? If you are tempted, you are pursuing the wrong field. Let's call it 0.5 or half and make it easier to evaluate. A ratio greater than 0.5 indicates cardiomegaly. Remember that this is a PA chest film that we are talking about.

Assess the aorta for anomalies. Associated congenital heart disease can be present with a right-sided aortic arch.

Table 2–20 Diseases with Bullae as a Manifestation

Lower lobe interstitial fibrosis
Sarcoidosis
Pulmonary histiocytosis X
Ankylosing spondylitis

What did the pulmonary vascularity look like? Under usual circumstances, in the upright position, there is more blood flow to the lower lung vessels than to the upper (gravity!). Recognizing normal distribution of flow becomes an important observation (**Table 2–21**). Cephalic blood flow (increased to the apices) is seen in pulmonary venous hypertension as a result of mitral stenosis, left ventricular failure, or mitral insufficiency (**Table 2–22**). A centralized pulmonary blood flow pattern is indicative of pulmonary arterial hypertension (**Table 2–23**).

Rather than have you memorize which chamber enlargement occurs with which valvular disorder, understanding blood flow function and physiology is paramount to understanding chamber enlargement. Therefore, it is worthwhile to work through this process if your patient has cardiac issues. The first inclination of an abnormality is often on the chest film (perhaps accompanied by physical examination findings). MRI has become more widely employed for cardiac anomalies and evaluation of cardiac pathology. A working differential of cardiac abnormalities can be made from the plain x-ray, however.

The circulating blood volume determines the cardiac size. In a situation where there is volume overload, such as renal failure or an arteriovenous

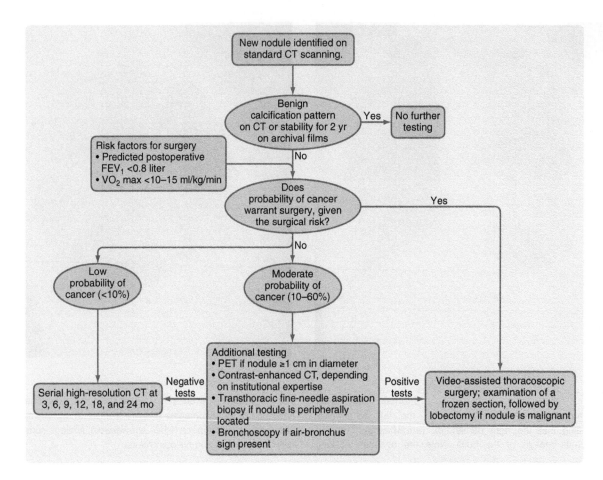

Figure 2–70   Algorithm for workup of a patient with a solitary pulmonary nodule. Entire textbooks and entire chapters have been devoted to SPN. The algorithm is presented for your reference.

FEV_1, forced expiratory volume in 1 second; PET, positron emission tomography; VO_2 max, maximum oxygen consumption.

malformation, volume overload is demonstrated by generalized enlargement of the heart and vessels in the systemic and pulmonary circulations. Specific chamber enlargement occurs as a result of regional volume overload, such as valvular insufficiency or left-to-right shunts. Let's try a few exercises: Mitral valve insufficiency will cause what chamber (or chambers) to enlarge? If you said left ventricle and left atrium you are correct! How about aortic insufficiency? Good guess… left ventricle and aorta (above the valve).

What about the effects of pressure overload (not volume overload)? This is encountered when there is a distal obstruction. Take, for example, stenosis of the aortic valve. The blood is being pumped through the valve from the left ventricle. If the valve is stenotic, then the left ventricle has to work hard at pumping the volume of blood through that tight

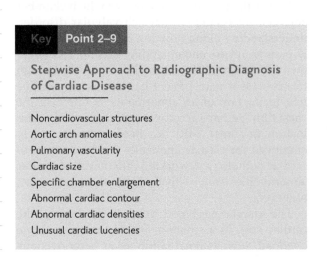

Key   Point 2–9

Stepwise Approach to Radiographic Diagnosis of Cardiac Disease

Noncardiovascular structures
Aortic arch anomalies
Pulmonary vascularity
Cardiac size
Specific chamber enlargement
Abnormal cardiac contour
Abnormal cardiac densities
Unusual cardiac lucencies

Table 2–21   **Normal Pulmonary Blood Flow**
Gradual and smooth branching pattern
Caudalization at rest
Right descending pulmonary artery diameter 10–15 mm in males, 9–14 mm in females
Artery-to-bronchus ratio of 1.0–1.2

Table 2-22 Abnormal Distribution of Pulmonary Blood Flow

Cephalization

Pulmonary venous hypertension
    Mitral stenosis
    Left ventricular failure
    Mitral insufficiency

Centralization

Pulmonary arterial hypertension
    Idiopathic pulmonary hypertension
    Eisenmenger's syndrome
    Thromboembolic disease
    Pulmonary hypertension secondary to lung disease

Lateralization

Unilateral increase in pulmonary vascular resistance or jet effect

Collateralization

Diffuse decrease in pulmonary vascular resistance provokes systemic collateral flow

Combination

Combined vascular abnormalities involving volume and distribution

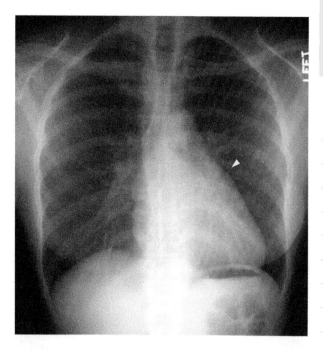

Figure 2–71   Left atrial enlargement in mitral stenosis. Note the abnormal convexity of the left heart border due to the left atrial enlargement (*arrowhead*). The double density sign is not present nor is there splaying of the carina in this example.

valve. Therefore, the ventricle hypertrophies (thickens); it does not dilate. The overall size of the left ventricle doesn't enlarge that much. If you identified cardiac enlargement, then volume overload would be present as a result of congestive heart failure from the weakened chamber.

Earlier, when discussing evaluation of the chest on radiographs, I referred to this portion of the chapter for evaluation of the cardiac silhouette for specific chamber enlargement. Again, no specific diseases will be discussed, but with your new knowledge about pressure overload versus volume overload, you will be able to draw logical conclusions.

Right atrial enlargement is identified on a PA chest x-ray by noting that the right heart border is more than 5.5 cm from the midline of the chest.

Right ventricular enlargement on a PA chest x-ray displaces the left-sided chambers leftward and superiorly, forming a more convex left upper cardiac border. On the lateral view, a taller and more convex anterior cardiac border is noted and displaces the left ventricle posteriorly.

Left atrial enlargement displaces the esophagus to the right and the descending aorta to the left on the PA view. It can also form a lateral bulge on the left cardiac border (Figure 2–71). A double density may be seen to the right side of midline. The lateral view shows displacement of the left lower-lobe bronchus and esophagus (best appreciated when there is contrast in the esophagus).

Left ventricular enlargement results in displacement of the chamber inferiorly and downward on a PA view. The gastric air bubble is displaced inferiorly, and the lateral film shows, in addition, enlargement of the cardiac contour posteriorly.

Pericardial effusion is considered when there is enlargement of the pericardial stripe. The normal pericardium is thin, measuring less than 2 mm. The reason it can be identified (seen only on the lateral film) is that the density of the pericardium is soft

Table 2-23 Causes of Pulmonary Arterial Hypertension

Idiopathic pulmonary hypertension
Eisenmenger's syndrome
Pulmonary thromboembolic disease
Pulmonary hypertension secondary to lung disease
Pulmonary venous hypertension (mitral stenosis)
Vasculitis (rheumatoid arthritis, polyarteritis nodosa)

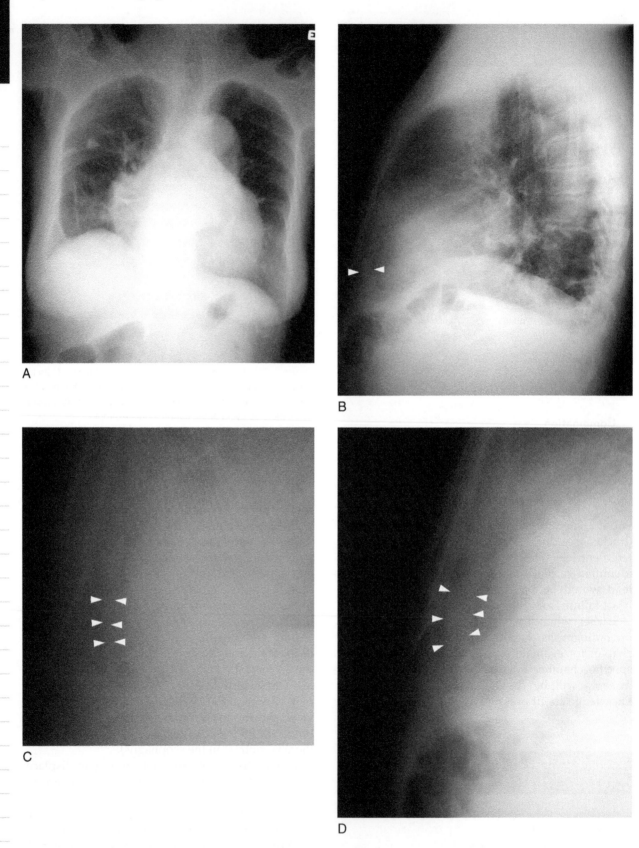

Figure 2–72 Pericardial effusion. A, Frontal chest x-ray demonstrating global and globular enlargement of the heart. No particular chamber enlargement is appreciated. B, Lateral film demonstrates fluid density between the fat pads around the pericardium (*arrowheads*). The normal thickness of the pericardium is a couple of millimeters. C, Close up of the normal pericardium. Abnormal thickness of the pericardium can be appreciated when there is fat density surrounding both sides of the pericardium. D, Coned down abnormally thick pericardium due to an effusion (*arrowheads*).

Table 2–24 **Commonly Encountered Lines, Tubes, and Devices on Chest Radiographs**		
Line or Tube	Origin	Destination
Endotracheal tube	Oropharynx or tracheostomy	Trachea superior to carina
Nasogastric tube (orogastric tube)	Nose	Stomach
Feeding tube	Nose	Descending to third portion of duodenum
Chest tube	Chest wall	Pleural space
Internal jugular central line	Internal jugular vein	Superior vena cava
Subclavian central line	Subclavian vein	Superior vena cava
Pulmonary artery catheter (Swan-Ganz catheter)	Internal jugular vein or subclavian vein	Pulmonary artery
Peripherally inserted central catheter (PIC[C]) line	Forearm vein	Brachiocephalic vein or superior vena cava
Pacemaker or internal defibrillator	Subcutaneous chest	Leads in right ventricle

tissue, and it is surrounded by the mediastinal fat stripe and the subepicardial fat stripe. Thickness measuring greater than 10 mm suggests an effusion (Figure 2–72). Measurements between 3 and 5 mm raise concern for an effusion or thickening or both. Suspected effusions can be further evaluated with ultrasonography or echocardiography.

Emergencies

There are many disease processes or interventions that can ultimately lead to a life-threatening emergency. In this section, a few of the more commonly encountered abnormalities that require immediate intervention will be presented.

Lines and Tubes

Lines and tubes are discussed here because, after placement of a line, a chest x-ray must be obtained to assess for adequate placement. Evaluation for lines and tubes is a critical portion of the chest evaluation. In this abbreviated portion of the chapter, many examples of different types of lines and tubes will be presented for you to evaluate. It is imperative that you be in the habit of tracing all lines and tubes from the origin of the tube to the final destination. That is only part of the search. You must also know where the line is actually supposed to be and compare that with the findings on the x-ray. Finally, you must remember to evaluate for a pneumothorax—keeping in mind that many of the patients will be supine, with the x-ray done portably. (Do you remember where free air collects in this situation?)

Commonly encountered lines are included in **Table 2–24** (Figures 2–73 through 2–76). It is imperative, to reiterate, that lines should be traced along the course as they project on the film. Avoid the temptation of looking at the beginning and the end. You will then overlook potential catastrophes, as in the example in Figure 2–77.

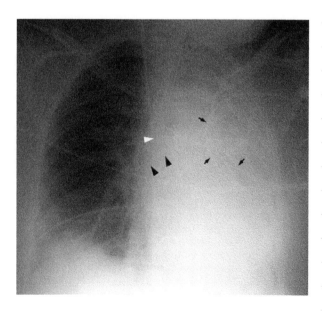

Figure 2–73 Abnormal endotracheal tube placement. Portable frontal chest x-ray demonstrating an endotracheal tube with tip in right mainstem bronchus (*white arrowhead*). This resulted in collapse of the left lung (opacified). A pulmonary artery catheter is also present with the tip in the normal location of right pulmonary artery (*black arrowheads*). The coiled lines are on the patient's skin and represent part of the leads for his EKG pads (*small arrows*).

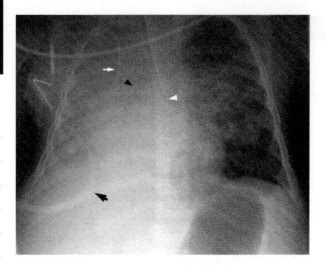

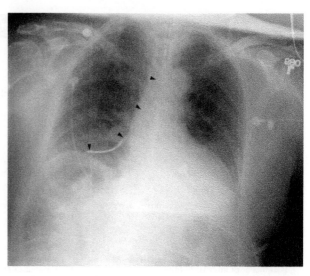

Figure 2–74   Endotracheal tube in left mainstem bronchus. Portable chest x-ray in a newborn infant. The tip of the endotracheal tube is in the left mainstem bronchus (*white arrowhead*). The right mainstem bronchus is readily visualized as it is surrounded by collapsed lung (soft tissue density) and the bronchus is air-filled (*black arrowhead*). A central venous catheter is in the middle of the right hemithorax. This is a result of the mediastinal structures shifting to the area with volume loss. The tip of the catheter is in the superior vena cava which is shifted due to the volume loss (*small white arrow*). The large-bore tube is external to the patient (*large black arrow*). Note the gaseous distension of the stomach. Likely an orogastric tube was placed shortly after this exam.

Figure 2–75   Misplaced feeding tube. Frontal chest x-ray shows the course of this tube following the trachea and right mainstem bronchus (*arrowheads*). The caliber and appearance of the tube with the presence of the radioopaque tip indicates a feeding tube. The ideal location of this tube is in the duodenum....not the right lung! The radioopaque tip is not particularly flexible and its caliber is larger than the peripheral bronchi. Concern should exist for the development of a pneumothorax.

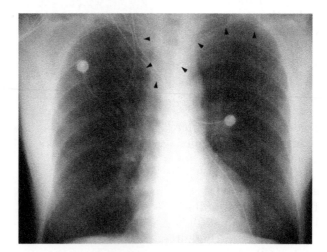

Figure 2–76   Misplaced central venous catheter. Frontal chest x-ray shows a line coursing along the expected location of the left subclavian vein. However, when the catheter approaches the superior vena cava, it turns away from the heart (*arrowheads*). This catheter is in the innominate (brachiocephalic) vein. Leads are noted on the chest.

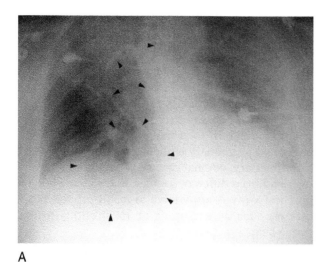

A

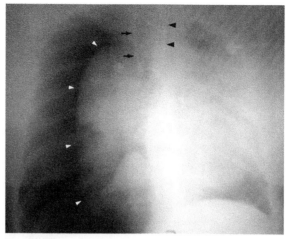

B

Figure 2–77   Misplaced feeding tube. A, Frontal chest x-ray shows a feeding tube coursing along the trachea and right mainstem bronchus, coiled in the right pleural space, resembling a figure of eight (*arrowheads*). B, Frontal chest radiograph demonstrating a tension pneumothorax after removal of the feeding tube. The right hemidiaphragm is dramatically inverted (not seen). *Arrowheads* point to the collapsed right lung. A central venous catheter (*black arrows*) and endotracheal tube (*black arrowheads*) have been placed.

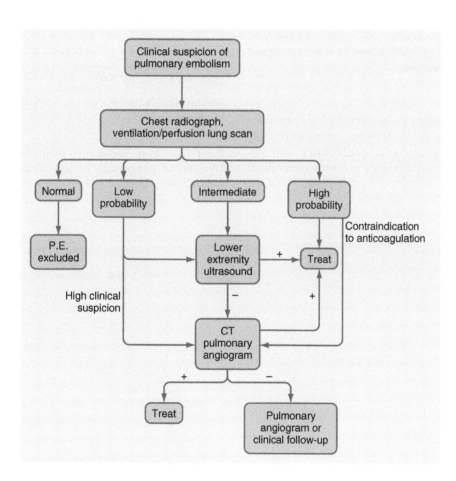

Figure 2–78   Pulmonary embolus (P.E.) protocol guidelines. Algorithm describing evaluation for suspected pulmonary embolus.

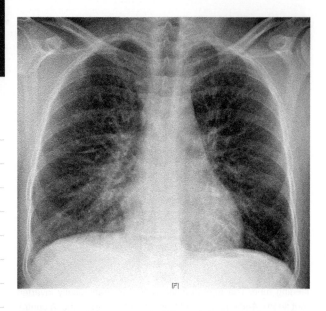

Figure 2–79   Emergent action! Frontal chest x-ray in a patient with shortness of breath demonstrates abnormal interstitium. The clinical picture in this example suggested interstitial pulmonary edema. Without clinical history, the findings could be chronic. All studies should be matched with the clinical scenario. Don't treat an x-ray. Treat the patient. Don't order an x-ray unless it changes your management. If you order an x-ray, check on the film! Be in the habit of looking at all your own films (with the radiologist if possible) and learn something!

Additional emergency situations include pneumothorax, particularly a tension pneumothorax; pulmonary embolus; and pulmonary edema. Recognition of such pathology requires immediate attention.

Pneumothorax and tension pneumothorax require immediate action and placement of a chest tube or, in the setting of patient compromise, placement of a device such as an angiocatheter or Heimlich valve followed by a chest tube.

A pulmonary embolus can be harder to identify on an x-ray. The x-ray may appear normal. Refer to the flow diagram for evaluation of a patient with suspected pulmonary embolism (Figure 2–78).

Pulmonary edema can be a result of volume overload from different sources. Recognizing edema on chest x-ray is imperative to instill proper medications, such as a diuretic or medications to improve heart function (Figure 2–79).

Suggested Reading List

Fraser RS, Colman NC, Muller NL, Pare PD: Synopsis of Diseases of the Chest, 3rd ed. Philadelphia, WB Saunders, 2005.

Hansell DM, Armstrong P, Lynch DA, McAdams HP: Imaging of Diseases of the Chest, 4th ed. Philadelphia, Mosby, 2005.

Webb WR, Higgins CB: Thoracic Imaging: Pulmonary and Cardiovascular Radiology. Philadelphia, Lippincott Williams & Wilkins, 2005.

Murray JF, Nadel JA, Mason: Textbook of Respiratory Medicine, 3rd ed., Volumes 1 and 2. Philadelphia, WB Saunders, 2000.

Reed JC: Chest Radiology: Plain Film Patterns and Differential Diagnosis, 5th ed. Philadelphia, Mosby, 2003.

Abdominal Imaging

Chapter outline

T his chapter is somewhat lengthy because of what I've chosen to include. This chapter covers structures below the diaphragm and above the pubics rami. Therefore, you will find information about the gastrointestinal (GI) tract as well as an introduction to genitourinary radiology. Improvements in technology, particularly imaging with computed tomography (CT), has revolutionized evaluation of intra-abdominal pathology.

Imaging Modalities

Plain films are utilized for evaluation of abdominal pathology. These plain film techniques include the *"KUB," upright, lateral decubitus,* and *cross-table lateral views.* The supine view of the abdomen is referred to as a kidneys, ureter, and bladder (KUB) film, because these structures are included on this view (Figure 3–1). The upright or erect view is used to assess free air and air/fluid levels (Figure 3–2). This view also allows evaluation of the lung bases. A lateral decubitus view is performed when the patient cannot stand upright and there is a need to assess for free air or air/fluid levels. Similarly, a cross-table lateral view will demonstrate air/fluid levels as well as free air and is most often used in infants (Figure 3–3) (**Table 3–1**).

Many of the studies utilized to evaluate the GI and genitourinary systems use a combination of fluoroscopy and plain films with the addition of a contrast agent. A *barium swallow* provides anatomic evaluation of the entire esophagus, including the hypopharyngeal and laryngeal areas (Figure 3–4). The mucosal surface is evaluated with an air contrast study. Dense barium is used to coat the mucosal surface. A *modified barium swallow* can be performed to aid in the evaluation of aspiration. This is often used for stroke patients and is referred to as a *speech swallow* study. It provides physiologic evaluation of swallowing and evaluation for tracheal aspiration. This study is performed in conjunction with a speech pathologist and requires the patient to attempt to swallow barium-impregnated foods of various consistencies to help determine the patient's level of swallowing function. This study is often videotaped for further evaluation.

An *upper gastrointestinal (UGI) series* evaluates the esophagus below the level of the cricopharyngeus,

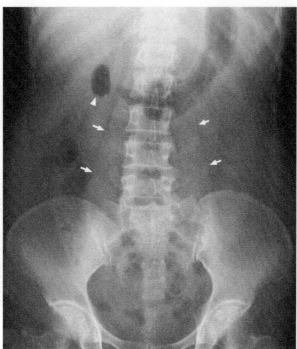

A

Figure 3–1   A, Normal kidneys, ureter, and bladder (KUB) film. Arrows point to psoas shadows. Arrowhead identifies air-filled small bowel in the region of the right upper quadrant. The stomach is also seen filled with air. Five non–rib-bearing lumbar vertebral bodies are present. B, Sketch demonstrating the normal frontal anatomy as would be seen on a KUB..

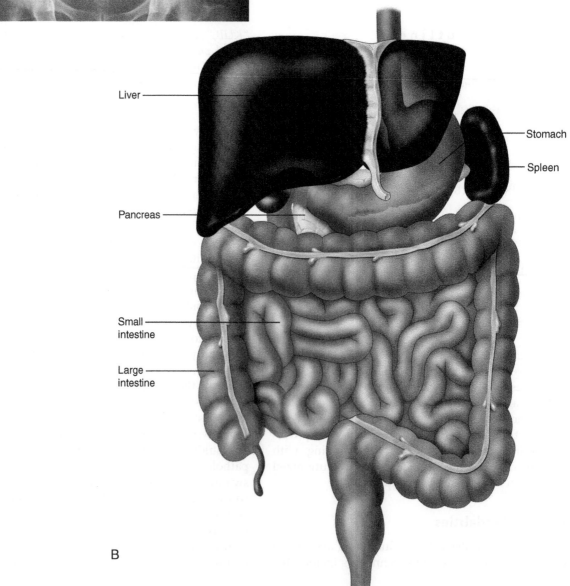

Liver

Stomach

Spleen

Pancreas

Small intestine

Large intestine

B

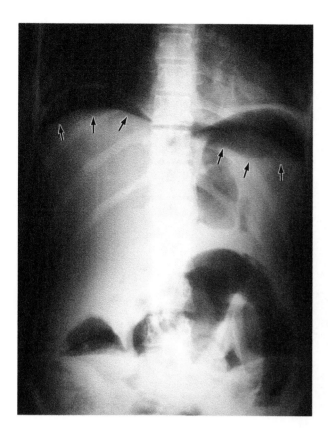

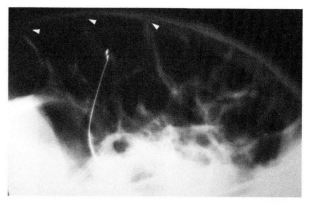

Figure 3–3   Free air. Cross-table lateral view in a pediatric patient demonstrates free air in the upper portion of the abdomen, as indicated by small white arrowheads.

Table 3–1   Plain Film Techniques for Abdominal Imaging
Supine
Upright
Cross-table lateral
Decubitus

Figure 3–2   Free air. Upright examination demonstrates free air in the upper portion of the abdomen, as indicated by arrows. The air is contained within the abdomen by the diaphragm. The thickness (or "thinness") of the diaphragm is easily identified because it is surrounded by air.

as well as the stomach and duodenum. This study is performed with either double contrast (dense barium with air mixture) or single contrast (thin barium only) (Figure 3–5).

A *small-bowel follow-through (SBFT)* is performed as a single-contrast study to evaluate the entire small bowel (duodenum, jejunum, and ileum). Another way to evaluate the small bowel is with enteroclysis. This double-contrast study to evaluate the entire small bowel requires insertion of a naso-duodenal tube, followed by instillation of a mixture of barium and methylcellulose (Figure 3–6).

A *barium enema* evaluates the rectum and the entire colon. Air contrast is administered per rectum along with dense barium to evaluate the mucosa. A single-contrast study is used for evaluation of function and obstruction (Figure 3–7). A well-performed barium enema has the perfect mixture of air and barium. A rectal tube is placed, and the rectum is insufflated with barium in retrograde fashion, followed by air. The preparation for this examination is more difficult for the patient than the actual study. The patient must evacuate the colon entirely before the study. When performing the study,

multiple views are obtained to identify the entire mucosal surface as well as levels of function of the GI tract. It is important that the patient be properly prepared for contrast studies of the GI tract. For an UGI study, it is ordinarily sufficient that the patient have taken nothing by mouth since the previous evening. Achieving a clean colon for barium enema is more difficult. Most preparations include a 2-day clear-liquid diet, a moderately powerful cathartic (patients can't be too far from a restroom), and an early-morning suppository on the morning of the study. It is imperative to have a clean colon. Retained feces can resemble polyps.

An advantage of the double-contrast barium enema compared with a single-contrast study is in the evaluation of mucosal detail. Double-contrast studies require the patient to be mobile. Single-contrast studies with thinner barium concentration are done for less mobile patients and for the evaluation of distal obstruction. If bowel perforation is suspected, a water-soluble contrast agent (iodinated contrast material) is recommended, because barium can cause peritonitis if a perforation is present. Similarly, ionic, iodinated contrast material can cause a chemical pneumonitis if it is aspirated. Therefore, if you are caring for a patient who is at risk for aspiration and may have a perforation,

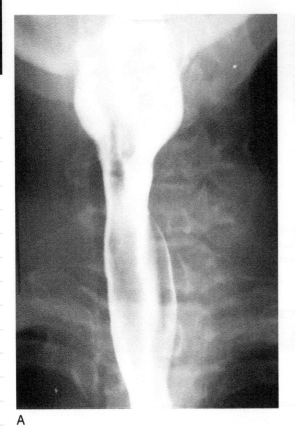

A

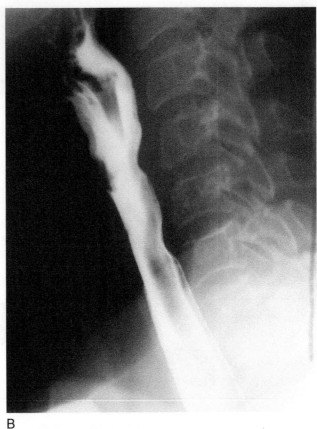

B

Figure 3–4   Normal barium swallow. A, Frontal examination demonstrating normal mucosa and appearance of the pharynx after air contrast barium swallow. B, Lateral film from air contrast barium swallow demonstrating normal appearance of the oropharynx. The cervical spine is also identified.

nonionic iodinated contrast is recommended. If perforation is suspected but not revealed on initial studies, a follow-up KUB a few minutes after the procedure may show a dense urogram. The urogram is a result of iodine in the contrast material being absorbed by the peritoneum, implying perforation of bowel.

Anatomic structures evaluated by CT in the abdomen and pelvis include the liver, biliary tree, vessels and lobes of the liver, gallbladder, spleen, kidneys, adrenal glands, pancreas, aorta, inferior vena cava, psoas muscles, bowel, bladder, bones, and anterior abdominal musculature (Figure 3–8).

Magnetic resonance imaging (MRI) can be used to evaluate liver ductal anatomy and to better characterize liver masses and pancreatic abnormalities. MRI technology continues to advance and allows studies to be performed without significant motion artifact from respiration, aortic pulsation, and bowel peristalsis.

Abdominal ultrasonography is a helpful study for evaluation of the liver, pancreas, gallbladder, kidneys, and reproductive organs. Ultrasound is a useful imaging tool to answer a "yes" or "no" question. For example, is obstruction present or not? Ultrasound is often used to assess for gallstones in the biliary tree and to evaluate obstruction of the bile ducts or ureteropelvic collecting systems. It is not a useful imaging modality to evaluate a patient with abdominal pain of unclear etiology, but it is excellent, for example, when the patient's history is concerning for gallstones.

Evaluation of the KUB

As with the evaluation of the chest x-ray, having an organized approach to reading abdominal films is important so as not to overlook pathology. An approach that I was taught in medical school stays with me even today (although that wasn't *that* long ago). "Bones, stones, gases, and masses" is a useful rhythmic reminder.

Included in the evaluation of the "bones" is mineralization, assessment for fracture or dislocation, arthropathy changes, and neoplastic changes.

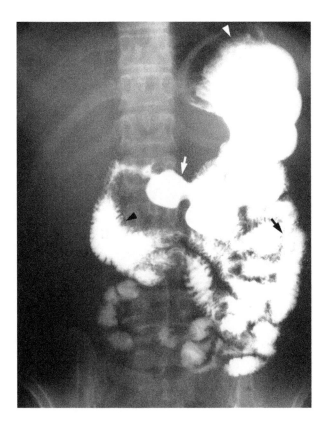

Figure 3–5   Upper gastrointestinal (GI) series. Air contrast barium upper GI series with small-bowel follow-through demonstrates barium within the stomach and duodenum. The fundus (*white arrowhead*), the antrum (*white arrow*), the descending portion of the duodenum (*black arrowhead*), and the feathery appearance of the jejunum (*black arrow*) are demonstrated in this image.

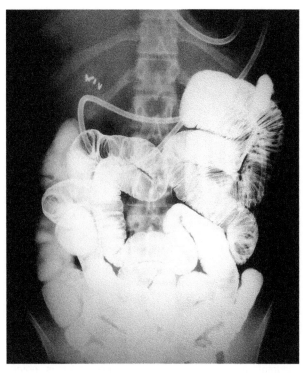

Figure 3–6   Enteroclysis. Image from enteroclysis demonstrates the contrast mixture and the feathery appearance of the jejunum in the upper portion of the abdomen, with the rather featureless ileum in the lower portion of the abdomen. A tube is present for administration of the methylcellulose mixture.

The term "stones" refers to those in the gallbladder as well as those in the genitourinary system, including the kidneys, ureter, and bladder. About 85% of stones in the genitourinary system are radiopaque. The search pattern includes evaluation of the renal shadows as well as along the expected course of the ureters into the bladder. Ureteral stones tend to obstruct at areas of narrowing, including the ureteropelvic junction (UPJ), the pelvic brim, and the ureterovesical junction (UVJ) (Figure 3–9). Further evaluation of suspected ureteral stones can be performed with ultrasonography, noncontrast abdomen/pelvis CT, or intravenous pyelogram (IVP), although the IVP is largely being replaced by the other two imaging modalities. CT to evaluate for stones is performed as a noncontrast study because contrast is high in attenuation, as is the stone. A stone could therefore be obscured in a study performed with the use of intravenous contrast material (Figure 3–10).

Gallstones are not as readily apparent as renal stones. Only about 25% of gallstones are radio-

paque. These stones will often be identified in the right upper quadrant, in the expected area of the gallbladder. Gallstones have a typical appearance on plain films, with a lucency in the center of the stone resembling a "Mercedes Benz" symbol (Figure 3–11). Recognition of this typical appearance will allow you to identify a gallstone in an unusual location. For instance, a gallstone that has left the gallbladder and wandered into the GI tract can lead to an ileus (Figure 3–12).

Other calcifications may be present, giving insight into the patient's pathology. Pancreatic calcifications suggest chronic pancreatitis (Figure 3–13). Arterial calcifications can provide indications into the severity of atherosclerosis or renal failure. In the pelvis, phleboliths (venous calcifications) are often noted and can be difficult to distinguish from ureteral stones. Clinical history is important.

After evaluating for stones, search for air ("gases") in abnormal locations. Free intraperitoneal air (pneumoperitoneum) is seen better on upright or decubitus views than on a supine film. An upright chest x-ray (when the diaphragms are included) is the best plain film technique for identifying free air. On the left lateral decubitus film (left side down), air will be noted lateral to the liver

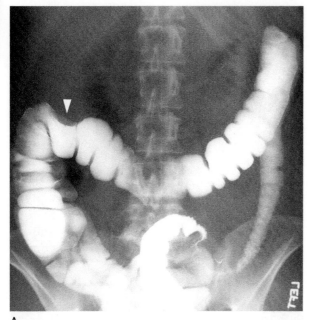

A

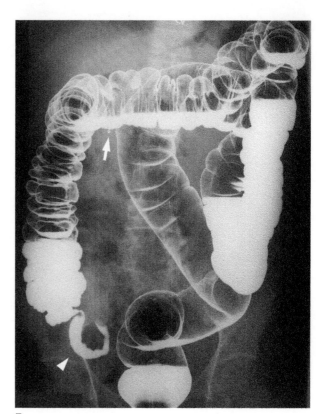

B

Figure 3–7   Barium enema. Single-contrast barium enema demonstrates large bowel. In the region of the right upper quadrant, an impression from the gallbladder is noted, demonstrating a slight mass effect on the hepatic flexure (*arrowhead*). A, The descending colon demonstrates peristalsis. B, Air contrast barium enema demonstrates air/fluid levels that indicate an upright film. Contrast is seen filling the appendix (*arrowhead*) in the right lower quadrant. A small diverticulum is noted at the inferior surface of the transverse colon (*arrow*).

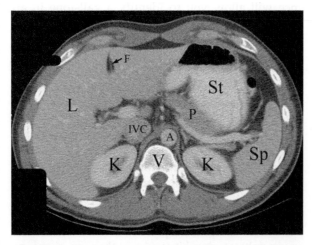

Figure 3–8   Normal CT. Axial image through the midportion of the abdomen after administration of intravenous contrast material. A, aorta; F, falciform ligament; IVC, inferior vena cava; K, kidney; L, liver; P, pancreas; Sp, spleen; St, stomach; V, vertebral body.

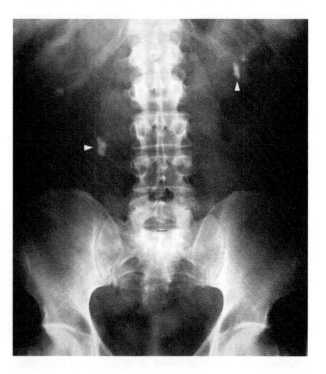

Figure 3–9   Staghorn calculus. Large calcifications superimposed over the kidneys (*arrowheads*) indicate staghorn calculus. These are large calcifications in the collecting system of the kidneys bilaterally.

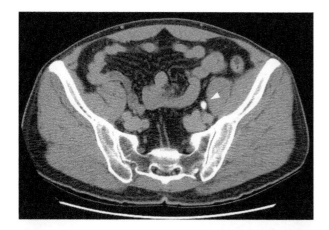

Figure 3–10 Ureteral stone. Axial CT through the region of the iliac crest without contrast enhancement. Calcification in the left lower quadrant demonstrates a stone within the distal left ureter (*arrowhead*).

(Figure 3–14). Supine signs of free air are not as sensitive but include the football sign, which is a large lucency in the middle of the abdomen (seen more often in children) (Figure 3–15); Rigler's sign, which is present when air is noted on both sides of

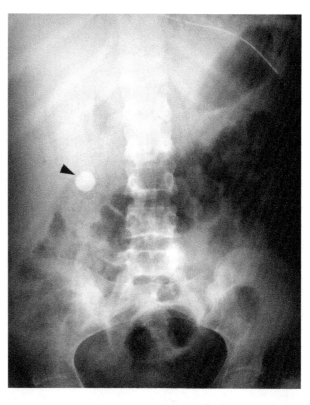

Figure 3–12 Gallstone ileus. Round calcific density in the right upper quadrant is evidence of a large gallstone (*arrowhead*). Bowel gas pattern suggests an ileus. Note is made of a nasogastric tube in the left upper quadrant with tip in stomach.

the abdominal wall (Figure 3–16); visualization of the falciform ligament; the continuous diaphragm sign; and a well-defined inferior hepatic edge (**Key Point 3–1**).

Pneumoperitoneum is most often associated with perforated bowel, usually from a duodenal or gastric ulcer. There are other causes of pneumoperitoneum (**Table 3–2**). Postoperative pneumoperitoneum should resolve in 3 to 4 days. Failure of resolution should suggest persistent leak of a bowel anastomosis or sepsis. CT can be useful in detecting free air in the peritoneal cavity (Figure 3–17). Adjusting the image to "lung windows" and assessing for air outside the bowel is helpful when a small amount of air is present.

Keep in mind that there are pitfalls in the evaluation of pneumoperitoneum; these are listed in **Key Point 3–2**.

Continuing the search through the "gases," assess the bowel gas pattern. Small bowel should measure less than 3 cm in diameter, large bowel less than 6 cm, and cecum less than 9 cm. Small bowel has valvulae conniventes (plicae) and is usually more centrally located than the large bowel, which has haustra and is usually more peripheral in location.

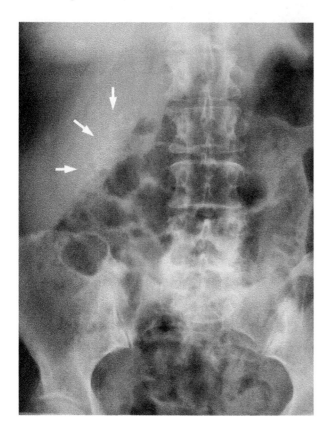

Figure 3–11 Gallstones. Coned-down view of a KUB examination in the right upper quadrant demonstrates calcification with a characteristic appearance of gallstones in the right upper quadrant (*arrows*).

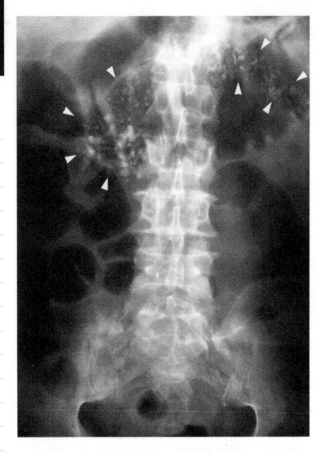

Figure 3–13 Pancreatic calcifications. Multiple calcifications are noted along the course of the pancreas and the upper portion of the abdomen (*arrowheads*). This is a finding that can be seen in patients with chronic pancreatitis, most often due to chronic alcoholism.

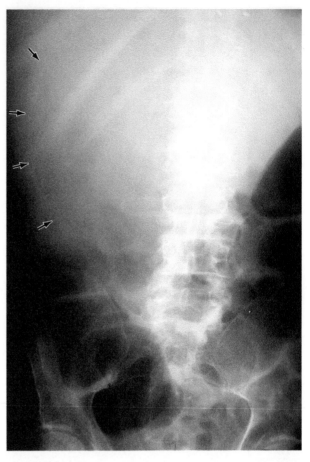

Figure 3–15 Free air. Supine x-ray demonstrates free air within the abdomen. Peritoneal outline is identified by small black arrows. This has been referred to as the "football sign." This is evident as generalized lucency over the midportion of the abdomen. Because air is nondependent, it will float to the anterior portion of the abdomen.

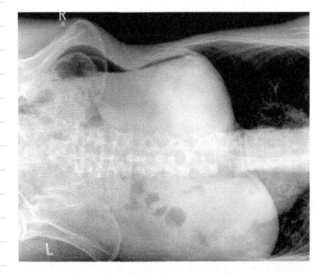

Figure 3–14 Pneumoperitoneum. Left lateral decubitus view demonstrates air in the peritoneum seen above the liver margin. This examination can be done if the patient cannot tolerate an upright x-ray.

Evaluation of "masses" should include mass effect on bowel loops, bowel loops being pushed away, or a paucity of bowel gas within the abdomen. Psoas shadows should be identified on all x-rays. Inability to visualize these shadows may suggest a retroperitoneal mass.

For a detailed description of abdominal anatomy and a more complete discussion of some of the diagnoses mentioned, refer to the suggested reading list at the end of the chapter. Analysis of the x-ray will indicate whether your patient has an abnormality, and an understanding of indications for the different types of examinations will help determine if an additional study is necessary to further characterize your patient's pathology. Compartmental anatomy of the abdomen will not be discussed, but I have provided illustrations that will help you to understand the communications between peritoneal and retroperitoneal compartments.

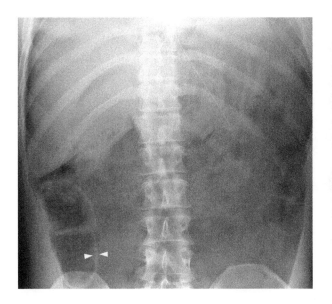

Figure 3–16 Free air. Rigler's sign. The bowel on initial inspection demonstrates a well-defined bowel wall (*arrowheads*). This is due to air on both sides of the bowel wall and is seen with free air in the abdomen, Rigler's sign. Also identified is a nasogastric tube with tip in the region of the stomach.

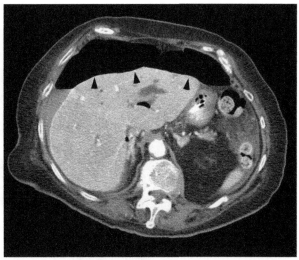

Figure 3–17   Free air. Axial CT image after the administration of intravenous contrast material (arterial phase) at the level of the midportion of the liver. Free air is identified in the anterior portion of the abdomen (*arrowheads*). Colon would not be expected to be present on this image. Evaluation of additional images would show this to be free air.

Key | Point 3–1

Plain Film Signs of Pneumoperitoneum

Upright
   Air beneath domes of diaphragms
Left lateral decubitus
   Air lateral to liver
Cross-table lateral
   Air outlining liver
Supine
   Midabdominal lucency (football sign)
   Air on both sides of abdominal wall (Rigler's sign)
   Visualization of falciform ligament
   Continuous diaphragm sign
   Well-defined inferior hepatic edge
   Localized right upper quadrant extraluminal gas

Key | Point 3–2

Pitfalls in Diagnosing Pneumoperitoneum

Irregular diaphragm contour
Basal lung plate-like atelectasis
Chilaiditi's syndrome (colonic interposition)
Subphrenic fat
Subphrenic abscess
Pneumatosis
Hepatic gas
Renal gas
Urinary bladder gas

Knowledge of these communications is necessary to understand the spread of disease in the abdomen (Figure 3–18).

Peritoneal Cavity

Peritoneal fluid has many origins (**Table 3–3**). Plain film findings associated with fluid in the peritoneal cavity are listed in **Key Point 3–3** (Figure 3–19). CT is often helpful in the evaluation of peritoneal fluid. The amount of peritoneal fluid is better appreciated on CT than on plain radiography, and the Hounsfield units (HU) may provide an indication as to the cause. Ascitic fluid with HU –10 to + 10 suggests serous fluid (water); exudative ascites will

Table 3–2 Causes of Pneumoperitoneum

Ruptured viscus
Trauma
Recent surgery
Infection
Pneumothorax
Peritoneal dialysis
Mechanical ventilation
Uterine instrumentation

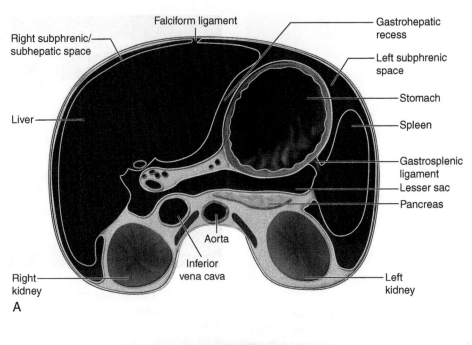

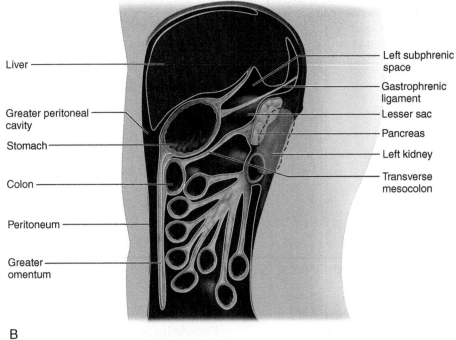

Figure 3–18   A, This sketch of the peritoneal cavity in cross-section notes important structures of the peritoneum and indicates how disease can spread through the peritoneum. B, Sagittal diagram demonstrating peritoneal reflections.

be greater than 15 HU, and acute bleeding will average more than 45 HU. Ultrasonography can evaluate ascitic fluid. A search in the dependent portion of the peritoneal cavity is mandatory. On ultrasound, serous ascites is sonolucent (few echoes). However, exudative or malignant ascites may demonstrate echoes reflecting debris within the fluid. Septations within the ascites suggest an inflammatory etiology.

Upper Gastrointestinal Tract

It is important to be able to identify the normal anatomy before you can identify pathology. A brief review of relevant anatomy follows. The esophagus is a muscular tube, formed by an outer longitudinal muscle layer and an inner circular muscle layer, that is lined by stratified squamous epithelium. Because the esophagus lacks a serosal layer, there is rapid

Table 3-3 Causes of Free Intraperitoneal Fluid

Ascites

Cirrhosis
Budd-Chiari syndrome
Right-sided heart failure
Constrictive pericarditis
Ovarian carcinoma
Peritoneal metastases
Hepatoma

Hemorrhage

Trauma
Ectopic pregnancy
Ruptured aneurysm

Infection

Appendicitis
Diverticulitis
Necrotizing enterocolitis
Peritonitis
Pelvic inflammatory disease

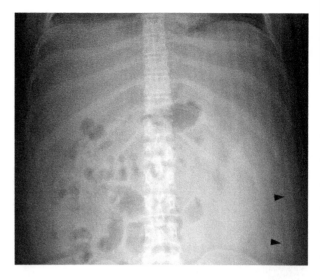

Figure 3–19 Ascites. Patient with autoimmune hepatitis and ascites. Note how bowel is collected in the midportion of the abdomen. Bulging flank stripe is noted on the left (*arrowheads*). These are findings that are seen on a KUB examination with ascites.

spread of tumor into adjacent tissues. The proximal third of the esophagus is striated muscle, and the remainder of the distal aspect is smooth muscle. There are six indentations in the esophagus as it courses from the pharynx into the abdomen. These are listed for you in **Table 3–4**. On cross-sectional imaging, the esophagus appears as an oval, soft tissue density surrounded by fat. It may have air in the lumen. The wall should not exceed 3 mm in thickness.

Normal peristalsis will clear the esophagus with each swallow. There are three types of peristaltic waves. *Primary* peristalsis moves the bolus along in the esophagus from top to bottom. *Secondary* peristalsis is initiated by distention of the esophagus. This wave starts in the midesophagus and spreads up and down the esophagus to clear any bolus left behind or reflux of contents. *Tertiary*

waves are nonproductive. Irregular contractions follow one another from the top to bottom of the esophagus at close intervals. These nonfunctional, nonperistaltic contractions lead to a corkscrew appearance.

Esophageal motility disorders are listed in **Table 3–5**. *Cricopharyngeal achalasia* occurs due to the failure of relaxation of the upper esophageal

Table 3-4 Indentations in Esophagus (Superior to Inferior)

1. Cricopharyngeus muscle—posteriorly at level of C6
2. Thoracic inlet
3. Aortic arch—level of T4–T5
4. Left mainstem bronchus
5. Descending aorta proximal to diaphragmatic hiatus
6. Esophagogastric junction

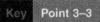

Key   Point 3–3

Plain Film Findings of Free Intraperitoneal Fluid

Fluid-density opacity in pelvis
Displacement of colon away from flank stripes
Indistinct liver, spleen, psoas margins
Separation of gas-filled small bowel loops
Bulging of flanks

Table 3-5 Esophageal Motility Disorders

Cricopharyngeal achalasia
Esophageal achalasia
Diffuse esophageal spasm
Neuromuscular disorders
Scleroderma
Postoperative states
Esophagitis
Gastroesophageal reflux (GER)

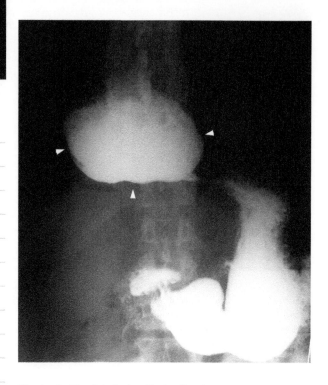

Figure 3–20 Achalasia. Single film from an upper gastro-intestinal series demonstrates marked distention of the distal esophagus (*arrowheads*). Narrowing of the esophagus is noted immediately distal to this dilation (tapered beak). This is a characteristic finding seen in achalasia.

sphincter. This can result in dysphagia and aspiration. On barium studies, a shelf-like indentation is present at the level of the fifth and sixth cervical vertebrae (C5–C6). *Esophageal achalasia* has a constellation of findings, including absence of peristalsis in the esophagus, increased resting pressure of the lower esophageal sphincter (LES), and failure of the LES to relax with swallowing. Pathologically, an absence of the myenteric plexus (Auerbach's plexus) is associated with this entity. The radiographic findings are logical given the characteristics of the disease. Uniform dilation of the esophagus is present with an air/fluid level, absence of peristalsis, a "tapered beak" deformity at the LES, and increased incidence of epiphrenic diverticula and esophageal carcinoma (Figure 3–20). Carcinoma generally involves a segment of the distal esophagus and may have an associated mass effect. *Diffuse esophageal spasm* is associated with multiple tertiary esophageal contractions, thickened wall, and chest pain. The most common cause is *neuromuscular disorders* such as cerebrovascular disease and stroke. *Scleroderma* is a systemic disease characterized by progressive atrophy of smooth muscle and progressive fibrosis. Absent peristalsis is seen in the distal portion of the esophagus, as well as delayed esophageal emptying, a stiff dilated eso-

Table 3–6 Esophageal Diverticula
Zenker's diverticulum
Midesophageal diverticulum
Epiphrenic diverticulum
Sacculations

phagus, and a gaping LES with free gastro-esophageal reflux. *Postoperative states* involving the mouth or pharynx can lead to impaired swallowing as well as altered morphology of the upper GI tract. *Esophagitis* is associated with tertiary contractions. *Gastroesophageal reflux* (GER) is a result of incompetence of the LES. The resting pressure of the LES is decreased and fails to increase with intra-abdominal pressure. Consequently, gastric contents are allowed to reflux into the esophagus. Because about 20% of normal individuals demonstrate reflux and patients with GER may not demonstrate reflux during exam, the best way to make the diagnosis is monitoring with a pH probe for 24 hours.

A *hiatus hernia* is a protrusion of any portion of the stomach into the thorax. The most common type is a sliding hiatal hernia, in which the gastro-esophageal (GE) junction is noted more than 1 cm above the esophageal hiatus. A paraesophageal hiatus hernia is not common and can be distinguished by noting a normal location of the GE junction with a portion of the stomach herniated above the diaphragm. The presence of a hiatal hernia needs to be accompanied by clinical symptoms for it to be a significant finding.

Additional abnormalities of the esophagus include abnormal contours and mucosal abnormalities. **Table 3–6** lists diverticula that can be seen in the esophagus. Food and liquid can get trapped in the posteriorly located *Zenker's diverticulum*. Symptoms include halitosis, dysphagia, and regurgitation of food.

Esophagitis has many causes, as listed in **Table 3–7**. Good-detail double-contrast studies can help diagnose esophagitis. Radiographic findings seen with esophagitis include thickened esophageal folds (>3 mm), limited esophageal distensibility, abnormal motility, and mucosal plaques, nodules, erosions, and ulcerations (Figure 3–21). Strictures can develop as a result of esophagitis.

Mass lesions and filling defects are well demonstrated with barium studies. Once they are identified, the extent of disease can be thoroughly evaluated with CT. Squamous cell carcinoma accounts for most cases of esophageal carcinoma. The remaining cases are adenocarcinoma arising in Barrett's esophagus (Figure 3–22).

Table 3–7 Causes of Esophagitis
Reflux
Infectious
Candida albicans
Herpes simplex
Cytomegalovirus
Human immunodeficiency virus (HIV)
Tuberculosis
Drug-induced
Aspirin
Tetracycline
Doxycycline
Quinidine
Potassium chloride
Indomethacin
Corrosive ingestion
Acidic agents
Alkaline agents (lye)
Crohn's disease
Radiation

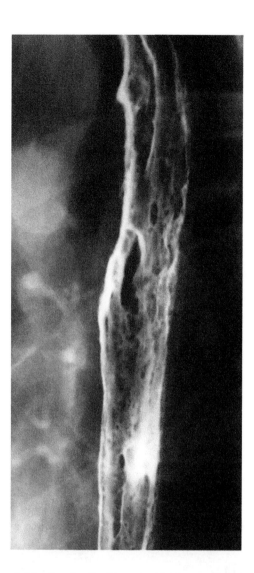

Figure 3–21 Esophagitis. Air contrast barium swallow demonstrates a shaggy appearance of the esophagus with irregularities along the mucosa. This is a finding of *Candida* esophagitis.

Esophageal perforation can result from endoscopic procedures or dilating instruments. Boerhaave's syndrome refers to rupture of the esophageal wall due to forceful vomiting. The tear is almost always the left posterior wall, near the left crus of the diaphragm. This can be associated with pneumomediastinum, pneumothorax, and/or pleural effusion. After contrast administration, contrast medium can be seen in the mediastinum or pleural space or both.

The distinction between Boerhaave's syndrome and a *Mallory-Weiss tear* is the extent of involvement of the esophagus. A Mallory-Weiss tear involves only the esophageal mucosa. Although this type of injury can be missed on an UGI series, it is usually seen with endoscopy. Mallory-Weiss tears should be considered in a patient who presents with copious hematemesis after forceful vomiting.

Evaluation of the stomach and duodenum can be done with a few different techniques (Figure 3–23). Air contrast, single-contrast, and CT examinations can be performed to evaluate the gastric and duodenal mucosa and walls. CT can also assess the extent of extraluminal disease. It is important to distend the stomach for accurate CT interpretation, because normal nodular thickening can mimic disease if not adequately distended. This is particularly true in the region of the GE junction. On CT, the normal gastric wall should measure less than 5 mm in thickness, and the normal duodenal wall is less than 3 mm thick.

An ulcer is defined as a full-thickness defect in the mucosa. About 95% of ulcers are benign. All gastric ulcers should be examined either endoscopically or followed to resolution radiographically (UGI series) (Figure 3–24). The findings on a double-contrast UGI series suggesting an ulcer include a barium-filled crater if the ulcer is on the dependent wall and a ring shadow due to barium coating the edge of the crater if it is on the nondependent wall. If the base of the ulcer is broader than the neck, a double ring shadow is seen, and if the ulcer is seen in tangent, a crescentic line may be seen (Figure 3–25). Some distinguishing characteristics of a benign ulcer are intact mucosa to the edge of the crater, smooth ulcer mound with tapering edges, overhanging mucosal edges, and depth of the ulcer greater than the width. As a

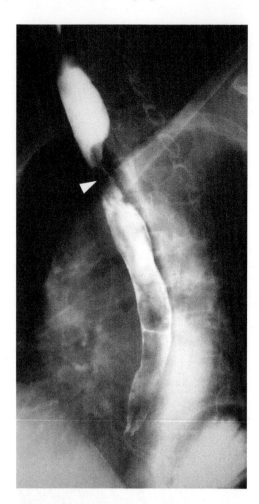

A

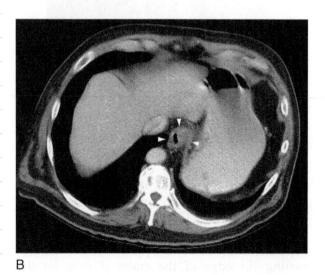

B

Figure 3–22   Esophageal carcinoma. A, Air contrast barium swallow demonstrates circumferential narrowing (*arrowhead*) of the proximal one-third of the esophagus. A string sign is noted, representing residual lumen. B, Axial CT after the administration of intravenous contrast material demonstrates thickening of the esophagus (*arrowheads*) due to esophageal carcinoma. Remember that the esophagus does not have a serosal layer, so disease spreads quickly.

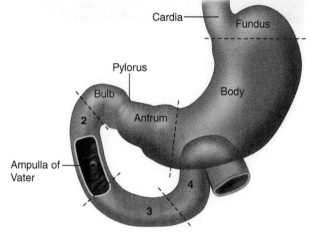

Figure 3–23   Sketch demonstrates the portions of the stomach and duodenum.

reminder, some benign-appearing ulcers can still be malignant; this is why it is imperative to follow the ulcer to resolution or to biopsy the ulcer. The differential diagnosis of benign ulcers is listed in **Table 3–8**.

Malignant ulcers have irregular tumor mass, eccentric location in the tumor mound, shallow

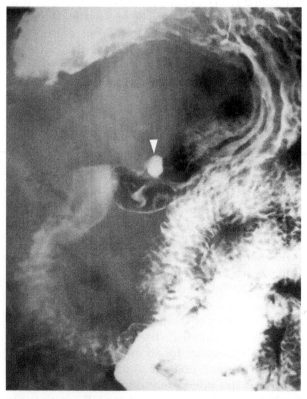

Figure 3–24   Benign gastric ulcer. Air contrast upper gastro-intestinal series demonstrates focal outpouching of barium (*arrowhead*), indicating a gastric ulcer.

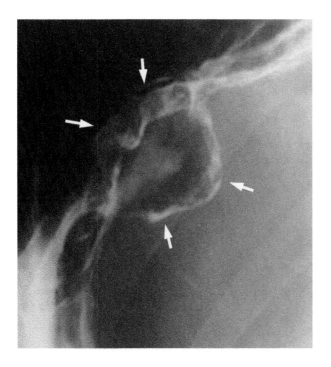

Figure 3–25 Benign gastric ulcer. Coned-down image of the stomach after air contrast upper gastrointestinal series shows ring shadow of gastric ulcer (*arrows*).

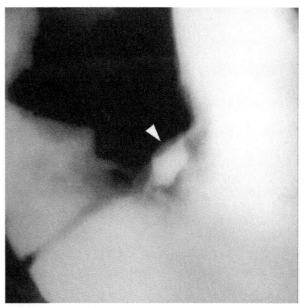

Figure 3–26 Malignant ulcer. Coned-down image of distal stomach after single-contrast upper gastrointestinal series demonstrates focal collection of contrast (*arrowhead*). Mucosal thickening around the ulcer is evident as relative lucency surrounding the barium collection. (Courtesy of William Thompson, MD.)

depth, width greater than depth, and irregular, shouldered edges (Key Point 3–4) (Figure 3–26). The differential diagnosis of a malignant ulcer includes gastric adenocarcinoma, lymphoma, leiomyoma, and leiomyosarcoma. CT is recommended for further evaluation of depth of involvement of the gastric wall and extent of disease.

Table 3–8   Differential Diagnosis of Benign Gastric Ulcers
Helicobacter pylori peptic disease
Gastritis
Hyperparathyroidism
Radiotherapy
Zollinger-Ellison syndrome

Key   Point 3–4

Features of Malignant Gastric Ulcers

Irregular tumor mass
Eccentric location in tumor mound
Shallow depth
Width greater than depth
Irregular edges
Shouldered edges

Ulcers that affect the duodenum occur more frequently than those affecting the stomach. These ulcers are associated with acid hypersecretion. The ulcers are typically seen in the bulb on the anterior wall. When large, a duodenal ulcer may resemble a diverticulum or a deformed bulb. Postbulbar ulcers are far less common. Complications of these ulcers include obstruction, bleeding, and perforation (remember to consider duodenal ulcer as a cause of pneumoperitoneum).

Filling defects and mass lesions can also affect the stomach and duodenum. Gastric carcinoma is the third most common GI malignancy after colon and pancreatic carcinoma. Filling defects can be seen in the gastric lumen (Figure 3–27). Infiltrative masses may produce thickened folds or cause the stomach to take on the shape of a water bottle, referred to as "linitis plastica." Malignancy is only one cause of linitis plastica. Other causes are listed in **Table 3–9**. Other filling defects seen on UGI or CT examinations include lymphoma, leiomyoma, and leiomyosarcoma (remember that these can be associated with ulcers), metastatic disease (usually from melanoma, breast, and lung malignancies), Kaposi's sarcoma, and polyps protruding into the lumen.

The appearance of a polyp on GI studies is entirely dependent on its location (dependent or

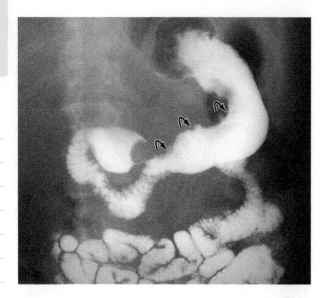

Figure 3–27 Gastric carcinoma. Marked thickening and irregularity of the folds along the lesser curvature of the stomach (*arrows*). This is a finding seen with gastric carcinoma.

nondependent). You might read in other literature that the polyp may appear as a *bowler hat* or a *Mexican hat*. Not being a hat aficionado, I find it easier to just think logically about where the barium would collect around a polyp if the base were viewed or if it were viewed end on. Most gastric polyps encountered are *hyperplastic polyps* that are less than 15 mm in diameter, are not neoplastic, and do not have malignant potential. *Adenomatous polyps* are true neoplasms with malignant potential. These are typically found in the antrum and are greater than 2 cm in diameter. *Hamartomatous polyps* occur in Peutz-Jeghers syndrome and have no

Table 3–9 Causes of Narrowed Stomach
Neoplastic
Gastric adenocarcinoma
Lymphoma
Metastases
Kaposi's sarcoma (AIDS)
Inflammatory
Helicobacter pylori gastritis
Corrosive ingestion
Radiotherapy
Cryptosporidium (AIDS)
Extrinsic compression
Pancreatitis
Pancreatic carcinoma

Table 3–10 Differential Diagnosis of Gastric and Duodenal Filling Defects and Mass Lesions
Neoplastic
Gastric adenocarcinoma
Duodenal adenocarcinoma
Duodenal adenoma
Metastases
Lymphoma
Leiomyoma
Leiomyosarcoma
Lipoma
Kaposi's sarcoma
Adenomatous polyps
Non-neoplastic
Lymphoid hyperplasia
Gastric mucosal prolapse
Brunner's gland hyperplasia
Ectopic pancreas
Extrinsic mass
Hamartomatous polyps
Hyperplastic polyps

malignant potential. Food and ingested foreign bodies image as filling defects as well. Extrinsic masses can produce a filling defect as the wall of the stomach or duodenum is displaced. CT is excellent for further characterization of the extrinsic mass. A list of additional filling defects and mass lesions is found in **Table 3–10**. When a mass is identified in the bulb, 90% of the time it will be benign. In the second and third portions of the duodenum, 50% of the time the lesion will be malignant, and in the fourth portion most tumors are malignant. It is not possible to determine the tissue type by imaging alone, and these lesions warrant a biopsy for accurate diagnosis.

Finally, the folds of the stomach and duodenum can become thickened from pathologic processes. Folds are generally considered to be thickened if they exceed 1 cm in the region of the fundus, 5 mm in the region of the antrum, or 3 mm in the region of the duodenum (including the second portion and remainder of the small bowel) (Figure 3–28). These processes are listed for you in **Table 3–11**. An additional important cause of thickened folds in the duodenum is intramural hemorrhage due to anticoagulation or trauma, particularly in the third segment, because it is fixed in the retroperitoneum. Blunt trauma renders this segment susceptible to compression against the spine. Pancreatitis and

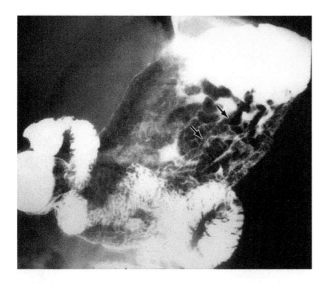

Figure 3–28 Focal gastritis and thickened folds. Image from an upper gastrointestinal air contrast study demonstrates thickening of the folds along the greater curvature (*arrows*). This is due to focal gastritis. (Courtesy of William Thompson, MD.)

cholecystitis can lead to paraduodenal inflammation, resulting in thickened folds, and parasitic overgrowth in the duodenum and jejunum (particularly giardiasis) is also a cause of thickened duodenal folds. Varices appear as smooth, lobulated filling defects that resemble thickened folds (Figure 3–29). CT can confirm varices as well as demonstrate the cause.

The duodenum can also have diverticula. These are usually incidental findings on a UGI series (Figure 3–30). These are most commonly seen along the inner aspect of the descending duodenum but may form in any portion of the duodenum. Mucosal folds will be seen to enter the neck of these frequently encountered diverticula. This helps to distinguish them from ulcers.

Table 3–11 Causes of Thickened Gastric and Duodenal Folds
Varices
Gastritis
Duodenitis
Neoplasm
Crohn's disease
Normal variant
Intramural hemorrhage
Pancreatitis
Cholecystitis
Giardiasis

Small Bowel

Unlike pathology involving the upper GI tract, which is often diagnosed by gastroenterologists and use of endoscopy, diagnostic radiology has the primary responsibility for evaluation of disease suspected of arising in the small bowel. Enteroclysis is the preferred method of examination of the small bowel. Unlike SBFT, this study provides uniform distention of the bowel, even distribution of barium, and superior anatomic detail. Clinical signs and symptoms that might suggest a small bowel etiology include colic, diarrhea, malabsorption, and occult bleeding.

The jejunum is considered to be roughly the proximal two-fifths of the small bowel. This portion of the small bowel has a feathery mucosal appearance, prominent valvulae conniventes, a wider lumen, and a thicker wall (Figure 3–31). The distal aspect of the small bowel is the ileum. This portion of the bowel on SBFT has less of a feathered mucosal pattern, thinner and less frequent folds, a narrower lumen, and thinner walls. There is no abrupt transition from jejunum to ileum. The small bowel is attached to the posterior abdominal wall by mesentery.

The small bowel is subject to erosions and ulcerations. The more commonly encountered entities include Crohn's disease, tuberculosis, Behçet's syndrome, and enterocolitis from *Yersinia enterocolitica* or *pseudotuberculosis.* Radiographic hallmarks of Crohn's disease are listed in **Key Point 3–5**. Fibrosis and progressive thickening of the bowel wall, especially at the terminal ileum, has been referred to as the "string sign" (Figure 3–32). Complications of Crohn's disease are best evaluated with CT. Behçet's syndrome is an uncommon, multisystem vasculitis. When Behçet's syndrome affects the terminal ileum, it mimics Crohn's disease. Similarly, tuberculosis is an uncommon entity that can mimic Crohn's disease. It should be remembered in the differential diagnosis of small bowel disease, even in the absence of an accompanying active pulmonary process. Bowel involvement by tuberculosis is best evaluated with CT. Identification of mesenteric adenopathy, peritoneal thickening, and high-density (exudative) ascites is diagnostic of tuberculosis.

Filling defects and mass lesions that can occur in the small bowel include those listed in **Table 3–12**. Only the more commonly encountered lesions will be discussed here. Carcinoid is the most common neoplasm of the small bowel. These lesions are considered low-grade malignancies that can recur locally or metastasize to lymph nodes, liver, or lung. Complications associated with carcinoid tumors

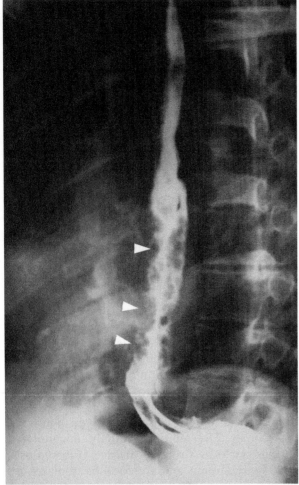

A

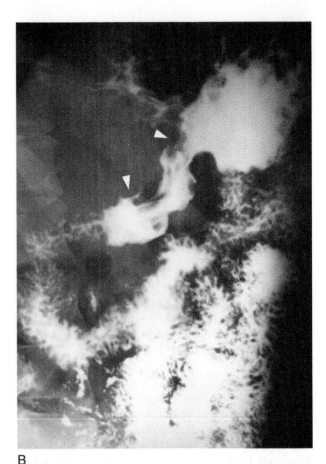

B

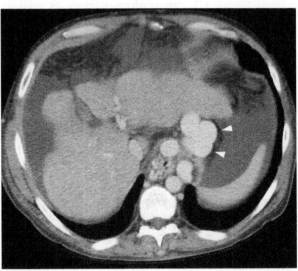

C

Figure 3–29 Esophageal varices. *A,* Air contrast upper gastrointestinal series demonstrates apparent filling defects which represent a mass impression from dilated veins along the distal aspect of the esophagus (*arrowheads*). *B,* Multiple indentations are noted along the stomach and first portion of duodenum (*arrowheads*). This is an effect of dilated veins with impression upon the stomach. *C,* Axial CT after the administration of intravenous contrast material at the level of the midportion of the liver. Multiple dilated veins (*arrowheads*) are noted and are consistent with varices. Note is also made of a nodular and small liver, as can be seen with cirrhosis. Additionally, ascites is present.

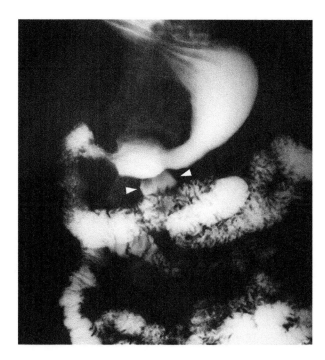

Figure 3–30   Duodenum diverticulum. Single image from air contrast upper GI series demonstrates outpouching from the third portion of the duodenum (*arrowheads*). This is an incidental finding and does not cause symptoms.

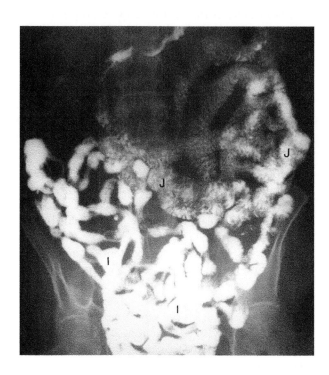

Figure 3–31   Single image from small-bowel follow-through demonstrates a feathery appearance of the jejunum (J) and the featureless ileum (I).

Radiographic Features of Crohn's Disease

Thickened, distorted folds
Contractures
Stenosis
Skip lesions
Involvement of the mesentery
Fistula and sinus tract formation

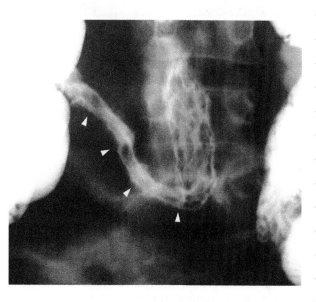

Figure 3–32   Crohn's disease. Coned-down image of barium study demonstrating a string sign (*arrowheads*) of the terminal ileum with irregularity of the mucosa, as seen in Crohn's disease.

Table 3–12   Differential Diagnosis of Filling Defects and Mass Lesions of the Small Bowel
Carcinoid
Adenocarcinoma
Lymphoma
Nodular lymphoid hyperplasia
Metastasis
Kaposi's sarcoma
Leiomyoma
Leiomyosarcoma
Adenoma
Lipoma
Hemangioma
Polyposis syndromes
Ascariasis

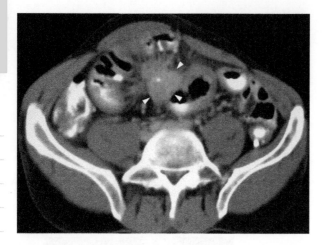

Figure 3–33 Carcinoid tumor. Axial CT at the level of the iliac crest after oral and intravenous contrast administration demonstrates a small soft tissue mass (*arrowheads*) with a sunburst pattern of radiating soft tissue density into the mesenteric fat. This is a characteristic appearance of a carcinoid tumor affecting the small bowel.

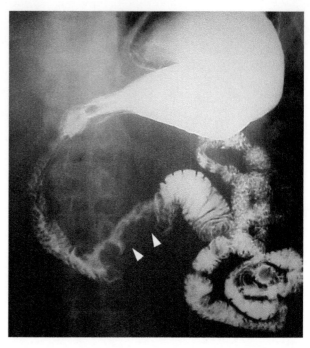

Figure 3–34 Duodenal adenocarcinoma. Single film after upper gastrointestinal contrast study demonstrating filling defect in the third portion of the duodenum (*arrowheads*). Biopsy showed duodenal adenocarcinoma.

include stricture, obstruction, and bowel infarction due to fibrosis of the mesenteric vessels. These tumors may be pedunculated and lead to intussusception. Luminal narrowing and fixation of bowel loops in the mesentery due to fibrosis may mimic Crohn's disease. Characteristic findings on CT include a small soft tissue mass, sometimes with central calcification, associated with a sunburst pattern of radiating soft tissue density in the mesenteric fat (Figure 3–33).

Adenocarcinoma occurs in the proximal portion of the small bowel, whereas carcinoid tends to occur in the distal ileum (Figure 3–34). The most common appearance of adenocarcinoma on barium studies is an "apple core" stricture of the small bowel. The extent of involvement can be appreciated on CT by demonstrating the irregular circumferential thickening of the bowel wall or eccentric focal mass.

The GI tract is the most common site for extranodal origin of lymphoma. The small bowel is the most commonly involved portion. There are a few different appearances of small bowel lymphoma. These include diffuse infiltration, exophytic mass, polypoid mass, or multiple nodules. Small bowel processes, including the remainder of the list in **Table 3–12**, are nicely evaluated with CT, which demonstrates extent of disease as well as characteristic findings for some lesions.

Diverticula can occur in the small bowel. Usually these are outpouchings of the mucosa through the bowel wall between the leaves of the mesentery and are incidental findings. They can become symptomatic if there is bacterial overgrowth due to stasis

of bowel content. The most common congenital anomaly of the GI tract is a Meckel's diverticulum. This is located in the antimesenteric border of the ileum up to 2 m from the ileocecal valve. Enteroclysis is the best method for evaluation in an adult. The diverticulum appears as a blind sac attached to the ileum.

Diffuse small bowel disease is associated with several pathologic conditions. The combination of clinical history plus imaging features helps determine the proper diagnosis. Conventional x-rays are a good place to start. In the evaluation of x-rays as described in this chapter, the thickness of the bowel wall, size and contour of the bowel lumen, and distribution of the mucosal folds are all key observations. Diseases that affect the small bowel are listed in **Table 3–13**.

An ileus is stasis of bowel contents. Peristalsis is absent or markedly decreased. Common causes are listed in **Table 3–14**. Diffuse, symmetric gaseous distention of the bowel is noted on conventional films (Figure 3–35). More loops of bowel are dilated with ileus than with obstruction. A sentinel loop is a short segment of an ileus (Figure 3–36). On serial x-rays, the loop does not change in appearance. This finding is seen in association with adjacent inflammatory processes such as acute cholecystitis or hepatitis (right upper quadrant loop).

Table 3-13 Differential Diagnosis of Diffuse Small Bowel Disease

Obstruction
Ileus
Adult celiac disease
Scleroderma
Lactase deficiency
Amyloidosis
Intramural hemorrhage
Edema
Ischemia
Radiation
Eosinophilic gastroenteritis
Mastocytosis
Whipple's disease
AIDS enteritis

Table 3-14 Causes of Ileus

Drugs
    Opiates
    Atropine
    Barbiturates
    Phenothiazines
Metabolic
    Diabetes mellitus
    Hypothyroidism
    Hypokalemia
    Hypocalcemia
Inflammation
    Pancreatitis
    Peritonitis
    Appendicitis
    Cholecystitis
    Abscess
Postoperative
Post-trauma
Postspinal injury

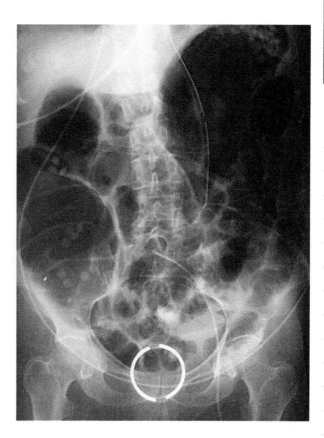

Figure 3–35 Ileus. KUB study demonstrates a marked dilation of large and small bowel. This finding is consistent with an ileus. A nasogastric tube and central venous catheter arising from the left femoral vein are also present. The round ring density in the lower portion of the pelvis is a pessary.

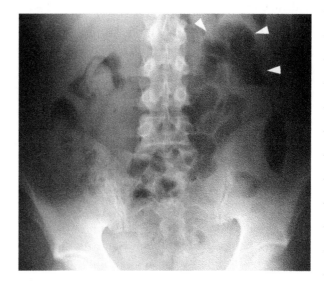

Figure 3–36 Sentinel loop. Focal dilated loop of small bowel is identified in the left upper quadrant (*arrowheads*) in a patient with pancreatitis. This finding represents the appearance of the sentinel loop. (Courtesy of William Thompson, MD.)

Small bowel obstruction (SBO) accounts for 80% of all intestinal tract obstruction. Adhesions account for more than half of SBO in Western society, whereas developing nations are more likely to see SBO as a result of incarcerated hernia. Conventional x-rays demonstrate dilated small bowel with air/fluid levels that exceed 2.5 cm in length. The level of the obstruction is determined by the dilated loops proximal to the obstruction and normal or empty bowel loops distal to the obstruction. Air/fluid levels at differing heights within the same

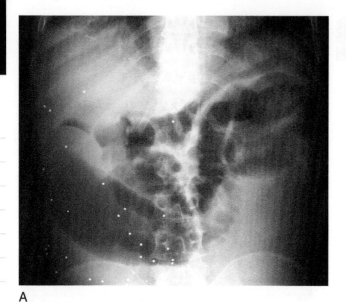

A

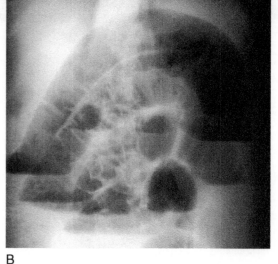

B

Figure 3–37 Small bowel obstruction. A, KUB study demonstrates dilated loops of small bowel. Note the valvulae conniventes indicating small bowel. No air is identified in the large bowel. Small white dots represent pellets from a BB gun.

B, Upright film in a different patient demonstrates multiple air/fluid levels in dilated small bowel. No air is identified in the large bowel. This appearance is compatible with a small bowel obstruction.

loop are strong evidence of obstruction (Figure 3–37). Evaluation with CT can confirm the obstruction and reveal the location and cause. Associated thickening of the bowel wall would suggest ischemia. If a hernia is present, it is generally well seen on CT. Additional causes of SBO include intussusception (especially in children) and polypoid tumor or gallstone ileus in adults. Gallstone ileus is a common cause of SBO in elderly patients. A large gallstone erodes through the gallbladder wall and passes into the intestine. This is usually accompanied by the development of a cholecystoduodenal fistula. The gallstone typically lodges in the distal ileum.

Lower Gastrointestinal Tract

The large bowel consists of the cecum (and appendix); the ascending, transverse, and descending colon; and the sigmoid, rectum, and anal canal. It is about 1.5 m in length from ileum to anus. Three longitudinal bands of muscle traverse the colon and function to shorten it, making the characteristic indentations called *haustra*. The cecum has the appendix hanging from its apex and the ileocecal valve projecting into it, forming a filling defect on contrast studies (Figure 3–38). The colon can be readily identified on CT by its haustral markings (small bowel has valvulae conniventes) and fecal content. The bowel wall is normally less than 5 mm in thickness.

Inflammatory disease can affect the colon. **Table 3–15** lists the inflammatory diseases of the large bowel. A few words about the imaging appearance will be mentioned here. Ulcerative colitis (UC) is an uncommon idiopathic inflammatory disease involving the mucosa and submucosa of the colon. The disease consists of superficial ulcerations, edema, and hyperemia. Barium adheres to the superficial ulcers, leaving a stippled appearance. Later, a coarse, granular pattern is produced by the replacement of ulcerated mucosa with granulation tissue (Figure 3–39). Late findings in UC include polypoid lesions and complications such as strictures, colorectal adenocarcinoma, toxic megacolon, and massive hemorrhage. **Table 3–16** lists the differences between UC and Crohn's disease.

Pseudomembranous colitis is an inflammatory disease of the colon characterized by the presence of a pseudomembrane of necrotic debris. Many causes of this inflammatory reaction exist. An irregular lumen is seen on barium enema, with "thumbprint" indentations resembling ischemic colitis. Superficial ulcers are common. The rectum is spared, and the pseudomembranes appear as plaque-like filling defects on barium studies. "Thumbprinting" is a result of blood and edema accumulation within the bowel wall. This finding can be seen in ischemic colitis as well as pseudomembranous colitis. The splenic flexure and descending colon are most susceptible to ischemic colitis, because this is a watershed area for circulation of the large bowel (Figure 3–40).

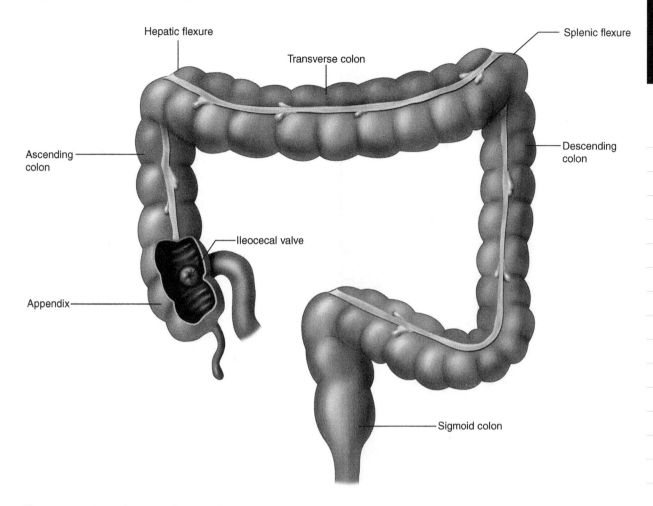

Figure 3–38   Normal anatomy. Drawing demonstrating the normal portions of the large bowel.

Commonly encountered filling defects in the colorectal area include adenocarcinoma, polyps, lymphoma, leiomyoma, leiomyosarcoma, and lipoma. Extrinsic masses can also mimic a filling defect. Colorectal cancer is the most common GI malignancy. Most of these cancers are annular constricting lesions and ulcerated mucosal lesions (Figure 3–41). The tumor spreads by lymphatic channels and hematogenously. Intraperitoneal

seeding is also seen if the tumor penetrates the colon wall. Obstruction is the most frequently encountered complication. Because of the ability of colorectal cancer to spread by lymphatic channels, direct extension, and hematogenously, CT of the abdomen is the examination of choice.

A polyp is defined as a mass that projects from the mucosa into the lumen. **Table 3–17** lists the different types of polyps in the large bowel. Polyps of less than 5 mm are thought to be hyperplastic polyps with a low risk of malignancy (0.5%). Polyps 5 to 10 mm in size are most often adenomas with a risk of malignancy of about 1%. Polyps measuring 10 to 20 mm are usually adenomas with a risk of malignancy of about 10%. Polyps larger than 20 mm are malignant about 50% of the time. Adenomatous polyps are premalignant and are a major risk for development of colorectal carcinoma. There are numerous syndromes, listed in **Table 3–18**, associated with colonic polyps.

Diverticula in the colon are an acquired condition in which the mucosa and the muscularis mucosa layer herniate through the muscularis

Table 3–15	Inflammatory Diseases of the Large Bowel

Ulcerative colitis
Crohn's disease
Pseudomembranous colitis
Amebiasis
Ischemic colitis
Radiation colitis
Cathartic colon

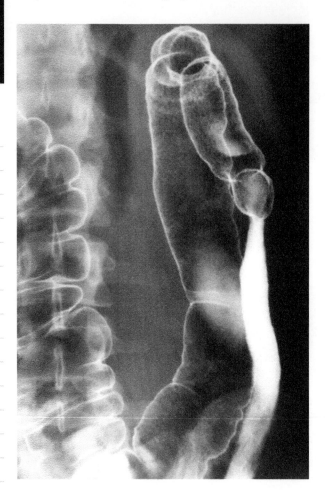

Figure 3–39 Ulcerative colitis. Coned-down view of air contrast barium enema demonstrating lack of haustra and "lead pipe" configuration. Mucosal appearance suggests tiny ulcers along the mucosa, consistent with ulcerative colitis.

Table 3-16 Characteristics of Ulcerative Colitis Versus Crohn's Disease

Ulcerative Colitis	Crohn's Disease
Continuous	Skip lesions
Terminal ileum usually normal	Terminal ileum usually diseased and narrowed
Rectum usually involved	Rectum normal in 50%
Shallow ulcers	Deep ulcers
No fistulae	Fistulae common
No pseudodiverticula	Pseudodiverticula
High risk of cancer	Low risk of cancer
Risk of toxic megacolon	No toxic megacolon

propria of the colon wall, leading to the formation of a sac. *Diverticulosis* (presence of sacs) is a cause of painless colonic bleeding that may be brisk and life-threatening. These sacs are most common in the sigmoid colon but can occur anywhere in the large bowel (Figure 3–42). *Diverticulitis* is inflammation of these diverticula, which may lead to perforation and intramural or pericolic abscess. It is safe to perform a barium enema in suspected diverticulitis, except when signs of bowel perforation or sepsis are present. Radiographic findings include diverticular sacs deformed by inflammation and perforation with extravasation of barium outside the lumen of the colon. Paracolic inflammation and abscess associated with diverticulitis, as well as the complication of fistula formation, are well imaged with CT (Figure 3–43).

Large bowel obstruction is generally seen in older adults. The cecum dilates to the greatest extent regardless of where the obstruction is located. When the cecum dilates to greater than 10 cm in diameter, it is at high risk for perforation with associated risks of peritonitis and septic shock. Common causes of large bowel obstruction are listed in **Table 3–19**. Conventional x-rays are often diagnostic in large bowel obstruction. The cecum and large bowel are distended, and bowel distal to the obstruction is devoid of gas.

A sigmoid volvulus is seen most often in the elderly and is a result of the sigmoid colon's twisting around its mesentery. On conventional x-rays, the sigmoid appears as a large gas-filled loop without haustral markings arising from low in the pelvis and extending high into the abdomen (Figure 3–44). Barium enema demonstrates an obstruction that tapers to a beak at the point of the twist (Figure 3–45). Another type of volvulus is a cecal volvulus. These are also much more commonly encountered in the elderly. Think about the level of obstruction here. Let's see if you've been paying attention. What would the conventional x-rays look like? If the colon distal to the obstruction is devoid of gas, then large bowel would not be seen on the x-ray, while the gaseous distention at the level of the cecum would likely lead to retrograde passage of gas through the ileocecal valve. Therefore, it would not be unusual to see distention of the distal small bowel (Figure 3–46). If this is your thought process, way to go! If I lost you, sorry, but read through this section again! The barium study would again identify a beak at the level of the obstruction. Neither sigmoid nor cecal volvulus is the most common cause of obstruction in the elderly. It is fecal impaction that leads to a large number of large bowel obstructions. After disimpaction, a cause for the obstruction should be sought.

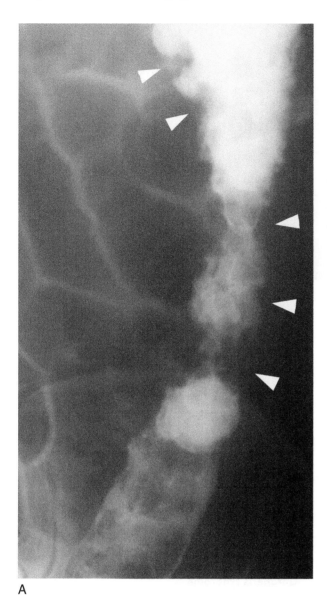

A

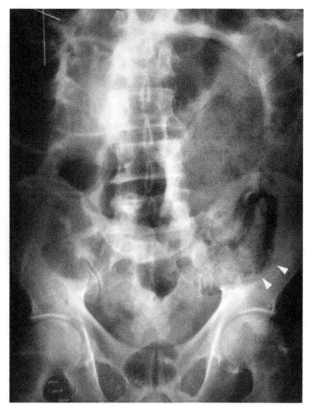

B

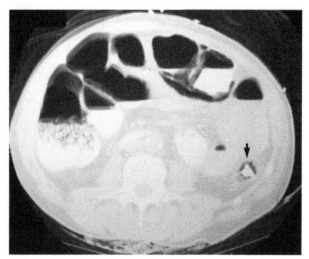

C

Figure 3–40 Pneumatosis intestinalis, a complication of ischemic colitis. A, Single-contrast barium enema in a patient with ischemic colitis demonstrating "thumbprinting," as indicated by indentations (*arrowheads*) along the descending colon. B, Patient with ischemic colitis demonstrating air within the bowel wall (*arrowheads*). This has a "soap bubble" configuration. If you compare the appearance of the bowel in the left lower quadrant with the bowel in the right lower quadrant, the air in the bowel wall becomes easier to appreciate. C, Axial CT using lung windows demonstrating air in the bowel wall (*arrow*). Lung windows are useful for evaluation of suspected pneumatosis intestinalis or pneumoperitoneum.

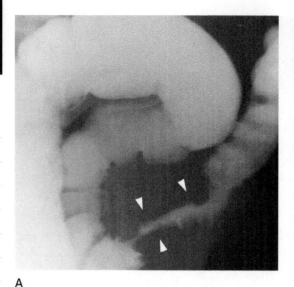

A

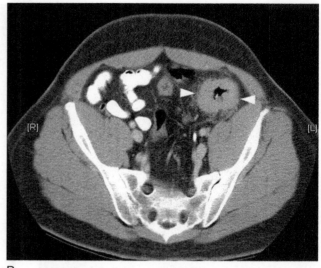

B

Figure 3–41   Colon cancer. A, Single-contrast barium enema demonstrates narrowing of the lumen of the bowel (*arrowheads*). B, Axial CT through the lower portion of the pelvis after administration of intravenous and oral contrast material shows marked thickening of the large bowel (*arrowheads*). This appearance is consistent with colon cancer.

Acute appendicitis is the most common cause of acute abdomen. Many times this is a straightforward presentation, and the patient quickly makes a trip to the operating room. However, when the diagnosis is not so straightforward, CT becomes a terrific way to evaluate the patient (Figure 3–47). Additional considerations for a patient who presents with abdominal pain include ruptured ovarian cyst, pelvic inflammatory disease, and diverticulitis. Acute appendicitis results from obstruction of the lumen of the appendix. An appendicolith may be seen on conventional films. Appendiceal abscess or inflammation may be seen as a soft tissue mass in the right lower quadrant on conventional x-ray. Complete filling of the appendix on barium enema precludes appendicitis. However, incomplete filling or lack of filling is not enough to be diagnostic of appendicitis. Barium enema is not performed for evaluation of acute appendicitis. Acute appendicitis can be evaluated with compression-ultrasound or CT. The advantage of CT is that a periappendiceal

Table 3–17   Large Bowel Polyps

Inflammatory
Hyperplastic
Adenomatous
Hamartomatous (juvenile)

Table 3–18   Syndromes Associated with Large Bowel Polyps

Familial multiple polyposis

Autosomal dominant
Multiple adenomatous polyps
Multifocal adenocarcinoma

Gardner's syndrome

Multiple adenomatous polyps
Bone and skin abnormalities

Turcot's syndrome

Autosomal recessive
Multiple adenomatous colon polyps
Central nervous system tumors

Cronkhite-Canada syndrome

Nonhereditary
Non-neoplastic polyps
Ectodermal changes
Protein-losing enteropathy
Rapidly fatal

Peutz-Jeghers syndrome

Hamartomatous polyps
Gastric or colon polyps
Small bowel polyps

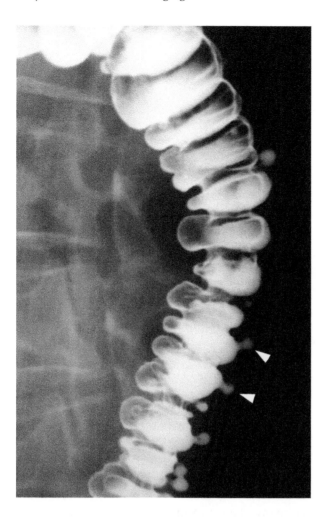

Figure 3–42 Diverticulosis. Air contrast barium enema demonstrating multiple outpouchings along the descending colon (*arrowheads*). These findings are consistent with multiple diverticula.

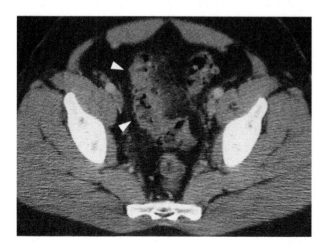

Figure 3–43 Diverticulitis. Axial CT after administration of intravenous contrast through the level of the acetabulum shows inflammatory change about the sigmoid colon (*arrowheads*) in a patient with multiple diverticula. This inflammatory change suggests diverticulitis.

Table 3–19 Causes of Large Bowel Obstruction
Colon carcinoma
Metastatic disease
Diverticulitis
Volvulus
Fecal impaction
Ischemia
Adhesions

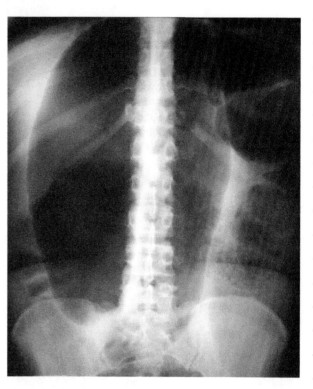

Figure 3–44 Sigmoid volvulus. KUB film demonstrates marked enlargement of the sigmoid colon. This is a characteristic finding of a sigmoid volvulus as it emanates from the pelvis and extends into the upper abdomen.

abscess can more readily be identified. This can be challenging on ultrasonography, given the artifact from surrounding bowel gas.

Liver, Biliary Tree, and Gallbladder

Cross-sectional imaging is used to evaluate the liver, biliary tree, and gallbladder as well as the pancreas and spleen. Ultrasonography provides a reasonable screening study for evaluation of these organs. Respiratory motion and peristalsis make it difficult to obtain reproducible magnetic resonance images, but CT is a wonderful modality due to its reproducibility, speed of examination, and ability to

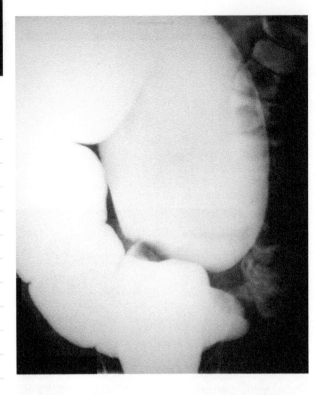

Figure 3–45   Sigmoid volvulus. Image from single-contrast barium enema shows marked distention of the contrast-filled sigmoid colon. Normal-caliber descending colon is present. The numerous filling defects in the descending colon are stool. (Courtesy of William Thompson, MD.)

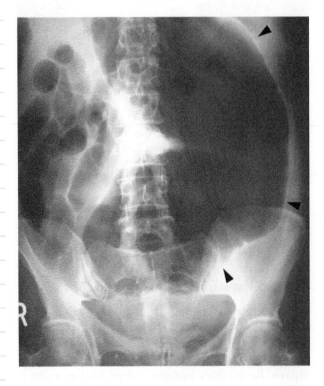

Figure 3–46   Cecal volvulus. Marked distention of the cecum (*arrowheads*). Distended air-filled cecum flops into left side of abdomen. (Courtesy of William Thompson, MD.)

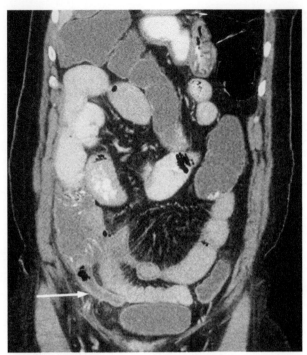

Figure 3–47   Appendicitis. Coronal reformation CT after oral and intravenous contrast in a patient presenting with right lower quadrant symptoms. Note distention of appendix (*arrow*) filled with fluid density.

see many shades of gray. Protocols have evolved that allow better visualization of intrahepatic abnormalities. These include imaging while contrast is in the arterial phase, CT angiography, and rapid injection coupled with rapid scanning. As equipment continues to improve, scans will be quicker and resolution of anatomy even more exquisite. The objective for this section of the chapter is to introduce pathologic processes affecting these organs. The reading list has additional texts that provide much more detail about the pathology. I will introduce the processes you are likely to encounter and the imaging modalities associated with the diagnosis.

Review of the anatomy of the liver is beyond the scope of this book, but refer to Figure 3–48 as a helpful orientation to the anatomy.

Processes that lead to diffuse liver disease include fatty infiltration, hepatomegaly, portal hypertension, cirrhosis, and hemochromatosis. A characteristic feature of fatty infiltration is the lack of both mass effect and displacement of hepatic blood vessels. Diffuse low density of the liver is seen on CT (Figure 3–49). Ultrasound demonstrates an echogenic liver (Figure 3–50). Hepatomegaly has many associated causes, including metabolic,

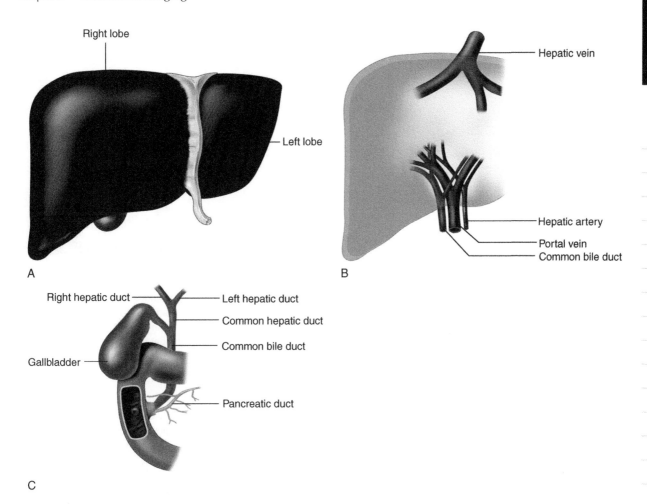

Right lobe

Left lobe

A

Hepatic vein

Hepatic artery

Portal vein

Common bile duct

B

Right hepatic duct

Left hepatic duct

Common hepatic duct

Common bile duct

Gallbladder

Pancreatic duct

C

Figure 3–48   A, Drawing of the lobes of the liver. B, Drawing of liver vascularity. Systemic arterial and venous flow and portal venous flow are indicated by three separate colors. C, Drawing of bile duct anatomy.

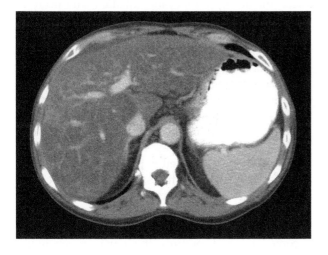

Figure 3–49   Fatty infiltration of the liver. Axial CT after the administration of intravenous and oral contrast material at the level of the midportion of the liver demonstrates low attenuation of the liver when compared with the spleen. This is characteristic of fatty liver. (Courtesy of William Brant, MD.)

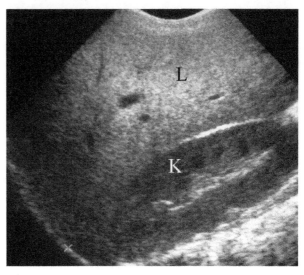

Figure 3–50   Fatty liver. Ultrasonogram of the liver (L) demonstrates increased echo texture when compared with the kidney (K). This is a finding seen with fatty infiltration of the liver. (Courtesy of William Brant, MD.)

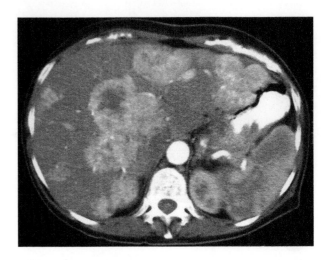

Figure 3–52   Liver metastases. Axial image through the liver after the administration of intravenous contrast material in the arterial phase demonstrates arterial blood flow in metastases in the liver. Patchy appearance of the spleen is characteristic of enhancement pattern in the arterial phase.

inflammatory, and infiltrative disorders, as well as passive congestion. Cirrhosis of the liver is diffuse parenchymal destruction and alteration of hepatic architecture. Nodular regeneration may also be seen as the liver's way of trying to repair itself. **Key Point 3–6** lists the associated findings of cirrhosis.

Portal hypertension is a result of the development of portosystemic collaterals due to an increase in portal venous pressure. Blood is shunted away from the liver rather than into the liver (Figure 3–51).

Hemochromatosis is the result of excessive iron intake from either parenteral or dietary sources, or it may be hereditary. It has interesting imaging features. On CT, a diffuse increase in liver density is noted. MRI shows signal loss (dark) on T2-weighted images. Long-standing hemochromatosis places the patient at risk for cirrhosis and hepatocellular carcinoma.

Masses can arise in the liver, and some are characteristic on CT and MRI. Ultrasonography is less useful in distinguishing benign from malignant processes. Solid masses that are commonly encountered include metastatic disease, hepatocellular carcinoma, cavernous hemangioma, focal nodular hyperplasia, and adenomas. Lymphoma also involves the liver as a diffusely infiltrative disorder that can be difficult to detect with imaging. Metastatic disease is 20 times more common than primary liver malignancies. Metastatic lesions have a variety of appearances, including solid, cystic, calcified, and necrotic (Figure 3–52).

Cystic lesions include simple hepatic cysts, abscesses, and necrotic tumors (Figures 3–53 and 3–54).

When imaging for blunt abdominal trauma, CT is the study of choice. The extent of liver injury can be classified as contusion, laceration, or intrahepatic or subcapsular hematoma. Contusions are seen as low-attenuation areas in the liver without associated hemoperitoneum. Jagged or stellate low-attenuation areas with associated intrahepatic hematoma and hemoperitoneum are considered lacerations. Subcapsular hematomas have blood trapped under the capsule of the liver. These can become large and compress the hepatic parenchyma (Figure 3–55).

Imaging of the biliary tree is done most often with CT and ultrasound. MRI can readily demonstrate biliary ductal dilatation as well as associated tumors. Refer to the schematic drawing (see Figure 3–48). The common bile duct enters the duodenum

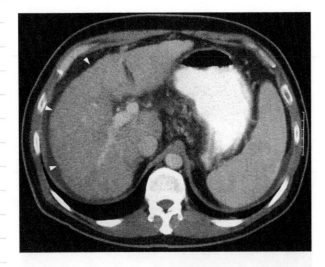

Figure 3–51   Cirrhosis. Axial image through the midportion of the liver after the administration of intravenous and oral contrast material demonstrates nodularity of the surface of the liver (*arrowheads*) and decreased size of the liver. These findings are seen in patients with cirrhosis. A small amount of fluid noted around the liver and spleen represents ascites.

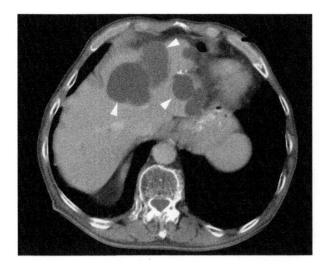

Figure 3–53   Liver cyst. Axial image through the upper portion of the liver after the administration of intravenous contrast material demonstrates multiple well-defined low-attenuation lesions compatible with hepatic cysts (*arrowheads*). (Courtesy of William Brant, MD.)

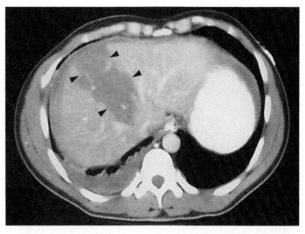

Figure 3–55   Liver laceration. Axial image through the upper portion of the liver after the administration of intravenous and oral contrast material demonstrates a wedge-shaped area of low attenuation representing a liver laceration (*arrowheads*) in this patient who was in a motor vehicle crash. A pleural effusion is also present.

and shares a common origin with the pancreatic duct in more than 50% of individuals. This common or close association of the ducts is why tumors of the ampulla obstruct both ducts. Signs of biliary dilatation include multiple branching tubular, round, or oval structures that course toward the porta hepatis. The common bile duct is dilated to greater than 6 mm. Causes of biliary dilatation and obstruction are listed in **Table 3–20** (Figure 3–56).

Imaging of the gallbladder is best performed with ultrasound. Although gallstones and cholecystitis may be demonstrated with CT, the

Table 3–20   Causes of Biliary Dilatation
Choledocholithiasis
Benign stricture
Pancreatitis
Sclerosing cholangitis
AIDS-associated cholangitis
Choledochal cysts
Pancreatic and ampullary carcinomas
Cholangiocarcinoma

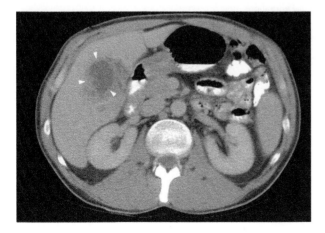

Figure 3–54   Hepatic abscess. Delayed axial image through the midportion of the liver after the administration of intravenous and oral contrast material demonstrates a thick-walled mass with a low-attenuation center in the liver (*arrowheads*). On biopsy, this was an intrahepatic abscess.

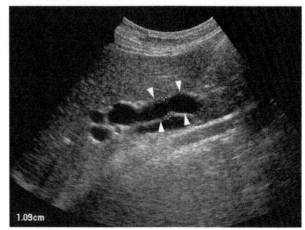

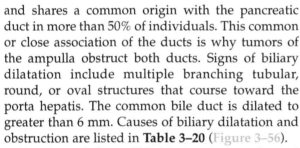

Figure 3–56   Common bile duct dilatation. Longitudinal image of the common bile duct demonstrates dilation (*arrowheads*). Note that the duct is normally anechoic. (Courtesy of Barbara Hertzberg, MD.)

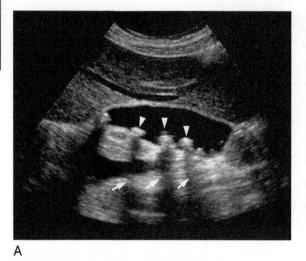

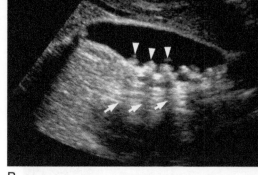

A

B

Figure 3–57 Gallstones. A, The gallbladder demonstrates multiple echogenic foci (*arrowheads*) with acoustic shadowing (*small arrows*), consistent with multiple gallstones that layer in a dependent fashion. B, After the patient changes position, the gallstones move to a dependent location again. (Courtesy of Barbara Hertzberg, MD.)

sensitivity is low. However, CT is useful in the diagnosis and staging of gallbladder carcinoma. Only 10% of gallstones are radiopaque and visible on conventional x-ray films (Figure 3–57). Gallstones are demonstrated by ultrasound as round, echogenic structures that cast acoustic shadows and move when the patient changes position. Differential considerations for lesions in the gallbladder that may be mistaken for gallstones include those listed in **Table 3–21**. *Acute cholecystitis* is readily diagnosed with ultrasonography and requires the presence of cholelithiasis, edema of the gallbladder wall, and a positive sonographic Murphy's sign (transducer pressure over the gallbladder causes pain). Complications of acute cholecystitis are listed in **Table 3–22**.

Chronic cholecystitis includes the presence of gallstones and chronic gallbladder inflammation. Imaging findings include gallstones, thickening of the gallbladder wall, contraction of the lumen, and occasionally a porcelain gallbladder (dystrophic calcifications in the wall of the gallbladder). Milk of calcium is a result of particulate matter with a high concentration of calcium in precipitated bile. This can be demonstrated on conventional x-rays.

Gallbladder wall thickening is defined as greater than 3 mm in patients who have fasted more than 8 hours. Conditions associated with wall thickening are included in **Table 3–23**.

Table 3–22 Complications of Acute Cholecystitis
Gangrenous cholecystitis
Perforation
Emphysematous cholecystitis
Mirizzi's syndrome (gallstone in cystic duct resulting in obstruction of cystic and common bile ducts)

Table 3–21 Differential Diagnosis of Gallbladder Lesions
Gallstones
Sludge balls
Cholesterol polyps
Adenomyomatosis
Adenomatous polyps
Gallbladder carcinoma

Table 3–23 Differential Diagnosis of Gallbladder Wall Thickening
Acute cholecystitis
Chronic cholecystitis
Hepatitis
Portal venous hypertension
Congestive heart failure
AIDS
Hypoalbuminemia
Gallbladder carcinoma
Adenomyomatosis

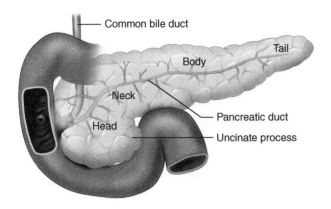

Figure 3–58   Drawing of the pancreas, pancreatic duct, and peripancreatic anatomy.

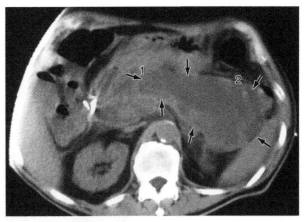

Figure 3–59   Pancreatitis with pseudocyst. Axial CT through the level of the pancreas without the administration of intravenous or oral contrast material. Low-attenuation focus is identified in the region of the pancreas (*arrows*). This pseudocyst replaces the normal appearance of the pancreas in this patient.

Pancreas

The normal appearance of the pancreas is demonstrated in Figure 3–58. *Acute pancreatitis* is generally diagnosed clinically. The role of imaging is to clarify the diagnosis when the clinical picture is unclear, assess the severity of the disease, determine prognosis, and detect complications. The best assessment is performed with cross-sectional CT imaging. Possible findings include enlargement of the pancreas, changes in density due to edema, and indistinctness of the margins due to inflammation. Complications that can be imaged with CT include fluid collections occurring in pancreatic and peripancreatic spaces and often widespread throughout the abdomen. Necrosis of portions of the pancreas (nonenhancing tissue) can be readily identified. Inflammatory masses as well as abscess formation, hemorrhage due to erosion of adjacent vessels, and pseudocyst formation are also possible complications that can be readily evaluated with CT (Figure 3–59).

Chronic pancreatitis is a result of recurrent and prolonged bouts of acute pancreatitis leading to parenchymal atrophy and fibrosis. Imaging findings associated with chronic pancreatitis include dilation and constriction of the pancreatic duct in a bead-like fashion, atrophy of the pancreas, calcifications in the pancreas (these can be seen on conventional x-rays) (see Figure 3–13), focal enlargement of the pancreas, and thickening of the fascia.

Pancreatic carcinoma is the second most common carcinoma of the GI tract and is rapidly fatal, with an average survival time of only 5 to 8 months. Surgical resection is the only hope for cure, although the surgery itself is associated with high morbidity. Surgery is not a viable option with extension beyond the pancreas.

Spleen

The parenchyma of the spleen is well evaluated with either ultrasonography or CT. Ultrasound normally demonstrates a homogeneous echo pattern, whereas CT reveals the density of the normal spleen to always be less than the density of the normal liver. Lobulations in splenic contour are commonly encountered and should not be interpreted as abnormal (Figure 3–60).

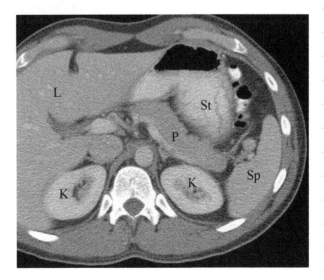

Figure 3–60   Normal spleen. Axial CT after the administration of intravenous and oral contrast material at the level of the spleen demonstrating normal anatomy. K, kidney; L, liver; P, pancreas; Sp, spleen; St, stomach.

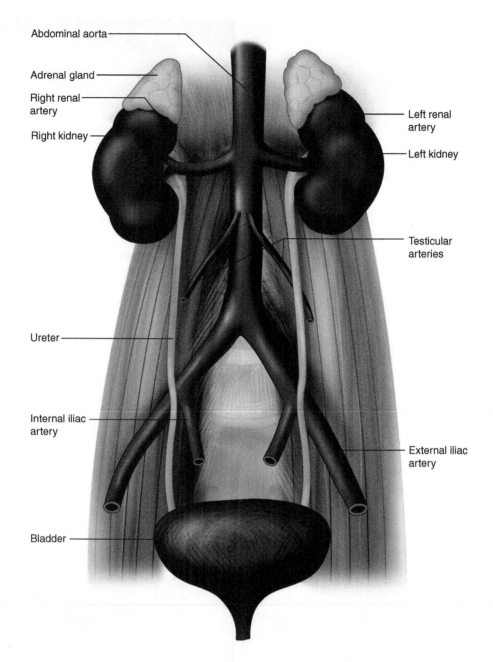

Figure 3–61   Sketch of the genitourinary anatomy that would be included on a KUB view.

Splenomegaly has many causes, including lymphoma, leukemia, infectious mononucleosis, hemolytic anemia, myelofibrosis, AIDS, portal hypertension, collagen vascular disease, storage diseases, and infection.

Lymphoma is the most common malignant tumor involving the spleen. Frequently there is associated adenopathy in the abdomen. The most common neoplasm in the spleen is hemangioma.

Contrast-enhanced CT is the best modality for evaluating splenic trauma. The spleen is the most commonly injured intra-abdominal organ in blunt trauma. A splenic laceration is seen as an irregular cleft through the splenic parenchyma with associated perisplenic or intra-abdominal blood. As in the liver, a subcapsular hematoma is seen as a lenticular-shaped density under the capsule that may have mass affect on the spleen and bow the capsule outward.

Genitourinary System

In this section, I will emphasize commonly encountered urinary tract pathology, including conditions affecting the kidneys, collecting system, ureters, and bladder. I will also emphasize

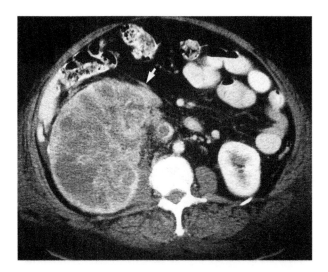

Figure 3–62 Renal cell carcinoma. Axial CT after the administration of intravenous contrast material demonstrates a large mass replacing the expected location of the right kidney (*arrow*). These lesions are typically highly vascular.

Table 3–24 **Cystic Renal Masses**
Simple cyst
Complicated cyst
Abscess
Renal cell carcinoma
Multilocular cystic nephroma

Table 3–25 **Renal Cystic Diseases**
Adult polycystic disease
Multiple simple cysts
von Hippel–Lindau syndrome
Tuberous sclerosis
Acquired cystic kidney disease

appropriate methods to best image these pathologic processes.

The anatomy of the collecting system is straightforward (Figure 3–61). The excretory urogram has traditionally been the method of imaging the collecting system. Cross-sectional imaging with ultrasonography, CT, or MRI provides a better and more complete evaluation of the renal parenchyma. When a renal mass is encountered, CT is the best method of evaluation to determine the type and extent of the lesion. In patients who cannot tolerate contrast, MRI is preferred over a noncontrast CT.

Masses affecting the kidneys can be solid or cystic in appearance. Renal cell carcinoma accounts for about 85% of all renal neoplasms. Therefore, any solid mass in the kidney should be considered suspicious for renal cell carcinoma. This tumor can spread through the capsule of the kidney as well as along the renal vein (Figure 3–62). Early diagnosis and staging can help determine whether the lesion is surgically amenable. This tumor metastasizes most commonly to the lung, bone, liver, adrenal glands, and the opposite kidney. These areas require additional evaluation for appropriate staging. When ultrasonography is performed, Doppler imaging must be used to assess patency of the renal veins and inferior vena cava. Echogenic thrombus suggests spread of carcinoma along the vessel.

Cystic lesions occur in the kidneys as well. **Table 3–24** lists cystic renal masses, and **Table 3–25** lists renal cystic diseases (Figures 3–63 and 3–64).

The discussion of renal masses is not complete without a discussion of renal infections. *Acute pyelonephritis* is due to ascending urinary tract infection, usually caused by gram-negative organisms, most often *Escherichia coli*. A swollen kidney with patchy areas of decreased density is seen on CT. An abscess is formed when necrosis of the renal parenchyma occurs, as demonstrated by a low-attenuation center with a surrounding thick wall. It is an ominous finding to see air in the renal parenchyma. This would imply that *emphysematous pyelonephritis* has developed, which is a life-threatening condition (Figure 3–65).

Trauma to the kidney can be from blunt or penetrating trauma. Contrast-enhanced CT is the

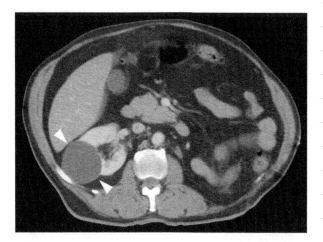

Figure 3–63 Simple renal cyst. Axial CT through the level of the inferior portion of the liver after the administration of intravenous contrast material. A well-defined low-attenuation lesion is noted that is exophytic from the midportion of the right kidney (*arrowheads*). The appearance is characteristic of a simple cyst. (Courtesy of William Brant, MD.)

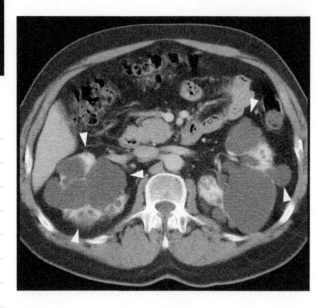

Figure 3–64   Adult polycystic kidney disease. Axial image through the inferior portion of the liver after the administration of intravenous contrast material. Multiple well-defined low-attenuation lesions are noted throughout both kidneys (*arrowheads*). These findings are seen in polycystic kidney disease. (Courtesy of William Brant, MD.)

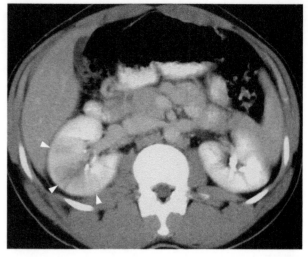

Figure 3–66   Renal contusion. Axial CT image through the level of the kidneys after the administration of intravenous and oral contrast material. Hypoattenuation (area of nonenhancement) in the right kidney (*arrowheads*) is noted in this patient who was involved in a motor vehicle crash. This appearance is consistent with a renal contusion. No blood is seen deep to the capsule around the kidney.

best technique to evaluate renal trauma. This allows for detection of injury to the renal artery by lack of enhancement of the kidney after contrast administration. A renal contusion is injury contained within the capsule. Patchy areas of nonenhancement are noted on CT (Figure 3–66). As with other abdominal organs, a subcapsular hematoma can cause compression on the kidney. In this case, compression of the renal parenchyma can lead to fibrosis and ultimately to hypertension. Fractures

and lacerations of the kidney will extend through the capsule into the perirenal space. The injured area will not perfuse normally after contrast-enhanced CT (Figure 3–67).

The capability of CT to evaluate renal masses has been clearly demonstrated with the above discussion. Its utility for evaluating the remainder of

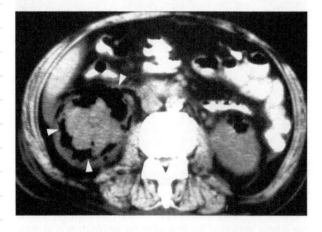

Figure 3–65   Emphysematous pyelonephritis. Axial CT after the administration of oral contrast material demonstrates air within the expected location of the right kidney (*arrowheads*). This is an ominous finding, and emergent treatment is indicated.

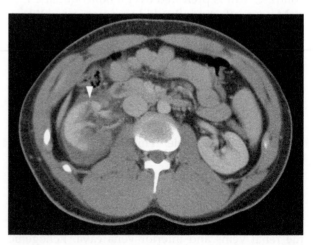

Figure 3–67   Renal laceration. Axial CT image through the level of the kidneys after the administration of intravenous contrast material. A focus of low attenuation is seen in the anterior portion of the right kidney (*arrowhead*), with surrounding density about the kidney compatible with blood in the perinephric location in this patient who sustained a renal laceration. (Courtesy of William Brant, MD.)

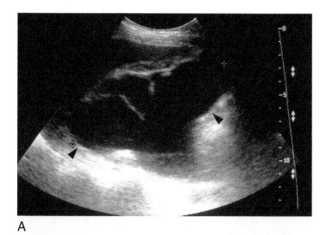

A

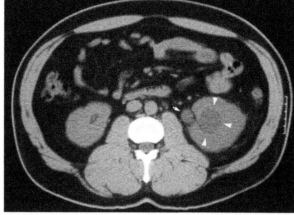

B

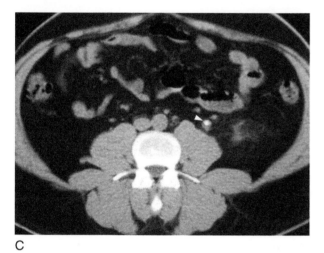

C

Figure 3–68 Hydronephrosis. A, Ultrasonogram through the kidney demonstrates marked enlargement of the collecting system, as evidenced by the enlarged pelvis (*arrowheads*). B, Axial CT image through the level of the kidneys without the administration of intravenous or oral contrast material demonstrates dilation of the collecting system (*arrowheads*) and proximal ureter (*arrow*). This finding is seen in hydronephrosis. C, CT obtained distal to the level in B demonstrates calcification in the midportion of the left ureter (*arrowhead*) compatible with a calculus leading to the development of hydronephrosis.

the urinary tract is equally excellent. It has the ability to distinguish tumor from stones or blood clots, all common causes of renal obstruction. This discussion will focus on the causes of ureteral obstruction.

Let's discuss the evaluation of renal stones. If you were concerned that your patient had a renal stone, how would you evaluate the patient? If you suggested a conventional x-ray (KUB), good answer. Remember that 85% of stones are radiopaque. But, the real concern is whether the stone is causing obstruction. How would you investigate that? If you answered with doing an ultrasound study, good idea. Ultrasound can demonstrate both radiopaque and radiolucent stones, because they will both demonstrate acoustic shadowing. Additionally, you will be able to determine hydronephrosis (dilation of the upper urinary tract) with ultrasonography. Small stones may blend with renal sinus fat and be a little more challenging to identify. If you answered with CT, how would you perform the CT? If you answered with contrast enhancement, you weren't thinking about the

density of the contrast material. What would you expect the stone to look like on CT? It should be white—coincidentally, the same shade as the contrast material in the ureter. Therefore, a noncontrast CT is suggested in the setting of evaluation for a renal stone. Hydronephrosis can still be appreciated with noncontrast CT examination (Figure 3–68).

Obstruction from a stone is only one cause of hydronephrosis. Additional causes include strictures, tumors, and extrinsic compression. Pyonephrosis refers to infection in an obstructed kidney. If you are seeing a patient who demonstrates obstruction and has fever, you must presume that the hydronephrosis is now the source of infection. Recognizing this process is essential, because it can result in rapid destruction of renal parenchyma. Relief of the obstruction must be performed promptly with ureteral stent or nephrostomy tube placement and antibiotics. Ultrasonography may show debris layering in the urine of the hydronephrosis, whereas CT may show the level of obstruction and the cause. Excretory urography

Table 3–26 **Abnormal Bladder Appearance**
Thickened bladder wall
Small capacity
Cystitis
Mass
Filling defect
Extrinsic mass (pear-shaped)
Outpouchings

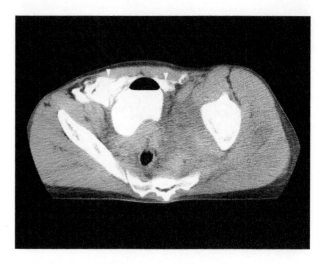

Figure 3–69   Extraperitoneal bladder rupture. Axial CT after contrast administration in a retrograde fashion through the bladder demonstrates leak of contrast outside the bladder into the extraperitoneal space (*arrowheads*). Air in the bladder is from contrast administered in a retrograde fashion.

has no role in this situation, because the kidney is likely to be functioning poorly, and therefore the important findings will not be demonstrated.

Causes of an abnormal-appearing bladder are listed in **Table 3–26**. Transitional cell carcinoma in the bladder is the most common urinary tract neoplasm. This carcinoma spreads by direct extension, via the lymphatics, and hematogenously. A common cause of bladder wall thickening is prostate enlargement. The enlarged prostate will have a mass effect on the inferior portion of the bladder. Chronic bladder outlet obstruction will lead to a thickened bladder wall. Imaging cannot reliably differentiate benign enlargement from carcinoma of the prostate.

Bladder diverticula are herniations of the bladder mucosa between muscle bundles. Most are located near the UVJ. These diverticula may contain stones or tumor.

Bladder rupture can be intraperitoneal or extraperitoneal, depending on whether the bladder was distended at the time of blunt trauma. Extraperitoneal rupture is generally a result of puncture of the bladder by a bone after pelvic trauma. Contrast will be identified in the extraperitoneal space and may track along the anterior abdominal wall and extend into the thigh. This injury cannot be identified on excretory urography. CT with distention of the bladder beyond 250 mL of contrast agent is necessary to make this diagnosis (Figure 3–69). Intraperitoneal rupture occurs when the bladder is distended at the time of trauma. Contrast will be seen in the peritoneal space, outlining bowel. Urine output is decreased, and urine will be absorbed by the peritoneal surface, increasing serum creatinine. Lack of urine output and elevated creatinine should make you think of something else, too—acute renal failure! Clinical history and CT will help make the distinction possible.

Emergencies

A number of emergency situations were presented in this chapter. Remember that you want not only to be able to identify free intraperitoneal air in the upright patient but also to be confident of the signs in the supine and decubitus views as well. Most patients with free air are going to be too sick to be upright. Allow time for the air to get there on the decubitus view. In the elderly patient, lower GI obstruction from sigmoid and cecal volvulus should be readily appreciated on the conventional x-ray and the distinction readily made.

The acute abdomen is often caused by appendicitis. However, it is not the only cause of an acute abdomen. Remember to assess the plain film for stones, air in abnormal locations, and soft tissue densities such as "thumbprinting." Perhaps the patient has an infarcted bowel. Remember that, when you are evaluating for renal stone, perform a noncontrast study in order to be able to identify the stone. Air in the renal parenchyma is a surgical emergency.

Finally, in the setting of trauma, look for evidence of visceral injury to all organs. It is imperative to look at each organ in the CT examination. Contrast-enhanced CT is very valuable in the setting of trauma, especially when evaluating for laceration and contusions.

Suggested Reading List

Brandt WE: The Core Curriculum: Ultrasound. Philadelphia, Lippincott, Williams, and Williams, 2001.

Federle MP, Jeffrey RB, Desser TS, et al.: Diagnostic Imaging: Abdomen. Philadelphia, WB Saunders, 2005.

Goldberg HI: Abdominal Imaging: Gastrointestinal Radiology. Philadelphia, Lippincott Williams & Wilkins, 1998.

Middleton WD, Kurtz AB, Hertzberg BS: Ultrasound, 2nd Edition: The Requisites. Philadelphia, Mosby, 2004.

Dunnick NR, Sandler CM, Newhouse JH, Amis ES Jr: Textbook of Uroradiology. Philadelphia, Lippincott Williams & Wilkins, 2001.

Zagoria RJ: Genitourinary Radiology, 2nd ed: The Requisites. Philadelphia, Mosby, 2004.

Musculoskeletal Imaging

Chapter outline

Musculoskeletal imaging as a specialty has become popular largely because of magnetic resonance imaging (MRI). However, for the needs of a student, MRI doesn't play an important role with the exception of a few situations which are described for you here. The emphasis of this chapter will be on the interpretation of conventional radiographs.

Imaging Techniques

Conventional x-rays are still the best way to evaluate many processes affecting the bones and joints. In the setting of trauma, conventional x-rays provide valuable information regarding the location and integrity of the bones. When evaluating bone tumors, proper assessment of benign versus malignant processes is assessed with the conventional x-ray. Arthritis is best characterized by the distribution and appearance on the conventional x-ray. At least two views taken 90 degrees to each other must be obtained for correct assessment of these abnormalities. In general, these views are anteroposterior (AP), lateral, and oblique. The joint that is an exception is the shoulder. It is not possible to get a "lateral" view. Additional views are obtained by changing the angle of the x-ray tube to try to evaluate the bones that comprise the shoulder joint.

MRI provides useful information in evaluating the musculoskeletal system, especially when attempting to evaluate structures that are not visible on conventional x-ray films, such as small structures in the joints (labrum, meniscus). Ultrasonography is used in musculoskeletal imaging, but with many limitations. As in the evaluation of abdominal and pelvic abnormalities, ultrasonography can provide a "yes" or "no" answer to the clinical question posed. It is not a good study for an overview of a joint. For instance, it may be able to determine whether the rotator cuff is torn, but it cannot determine if that is the only source of potential symptoms for the patient. When studying a joint with cross-sectional imaging, MRI is definitely the way to go. Because so much of musculoskeletal radiology involves evaluation of small intra-articular structures, high-quality MRI is imperative. Generally, strong magnets (≥ 1.0 T) are ideal. MRI is also particularly useful in evaluating occult fractures. This situation most often arises in evaluating the painful hip in an osteoporotic patient, or the painful wrist in a patient with suspected scaphoid fracture.

Anatomy

The bones are formed from various components that together yield the characteristic appearance we see on conventional radiographs. Bone comprises *periosteum,* a fibrous outer layer involved in intramembranous bone formation; *cortex,* the outer layer of bone that is dense and compact; *endosteum,* the inner layer of cortex; and *cancellous bone,* the medullary portion of spongy, trabecular bone. The *marrow cavity* is the central portion of the bone (Figure 4–1).

Various types of bones exist within the skeleton. *Long* bones are bones that have length greater than width (femur, tibia). *Small* bones are somewhat cuboidal in shape and are found in the carpus (wrist) and tarsus (midfoot). Flat bones are composed of two layers of compact bone separated by a thin marrow space. These bones are found in the sternum, ribs, pelvis, and scapula.

The skeleton is divided into an *appendicular* and an *axial* skeleton. Suffice it to say that the axial skeleton comprises the vertebral bodies and posterior elements (pedicles, transverse processes, facets, laminae, and spinous processes), sacrum, coccyx, bones of the skull, ribs, and sternum. The appendicular skeleton is the remainder of the bones. The bones of the skull are membranous bones and will not be discussed further.

The body would not work well if it were completely rigid. Therefore, *joints* are conveniently positioned throughout the skeleton to provide the ability to move (somewhat more gracefully!). There are three types of joints: *synovial, fibrous,* and *cartilaginous. Hyaline articular cartilage* covers the surface of the bone in the joint space in a synovial joint. In the knee, there is a fibrocartilage structure that is interposed between the tibia and femur (which are both covered by hyaline articular cartilage), called the *meniscus.* Usually, this is what the sports commentators are talking about when they say a player had "cartilage removed" or a "torn cartilage" at arthroscopic surgery. Examples of synovial joints are the shoulder, knee, hip, and ankle, as well as the small joints in the hands and feet. A fibrous joint is a union of two bones that eliminates a joint cavity. No motion occurs across these joints. Examples are syndesmoses and sutures. Cartilaginous joints have apposed bony surfaces united by cartilage. Examples are the diskovertebral joints and the pubic symphysis.

In addition to learning a little anatomy, you will learn new terms in this chapter that will come in handy as you are attempting to describe lesions in the bone. *Lucent* or *lytic* means that the appearance of the bone on conventional x-ray is more gray than surrounding bone. A process exists that has removed bone from that area (Figure 4–2). If the bone density is increased, the term *sclerotic* is used (Figure 4–3).

Trauma

Appendicular Skeleton

A fracture is defined as an interruption in the continuity of bone or cartilage. In order to be able to characterize the fracture, at least two orthogonal views (and if possible, three views) should be obtained (Figure 4–4). Remember, *one view is no view.* At a minimum, an AP and a lateral view are obtained. Oblique views are often added for further evaluation if possible. Some radiographic findings

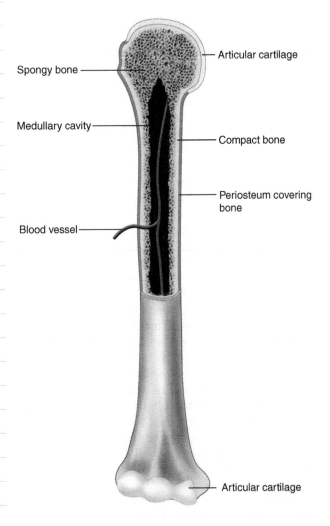

Spongy bone

Articular cartilage

Medullary cavity

Compact bone

Periosteum covering bone

Blood vessel

Articular cartilage

Figure 4–1. Longitudinal cross-section of a normal bone indicating components of the bone.

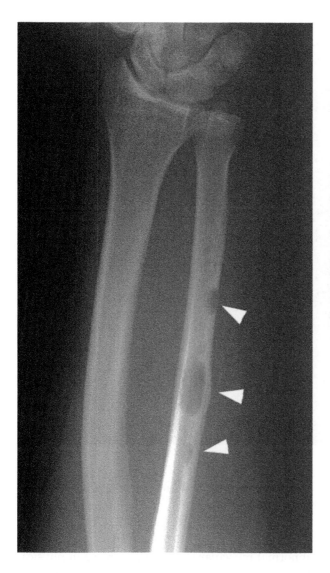

Figure 4–2. Lytic lesion. Multiple well-defined lytic lesions in the diaphysis of the ulna (*arrowheads*) in a patient with metastatic disease.

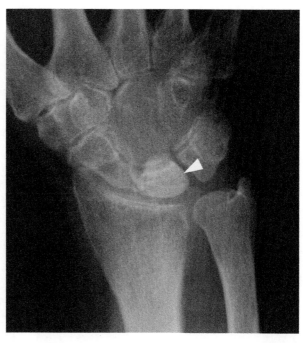

Figure 4–3. Sclerosis. Anteroposterior image of the wrist demonstrates increased sclerosis of the lunate (*arrowhead*) with respect to the remainder of the carpal bones. Increased white is sclerosis.

are helpful in identifying fractures. These include soft tissue swelling, which is often seen as increased density or size of the soft tissues in the region of the fracture. Obscuration or displacement of the fat pads or fat stripes around the fractured bone is another indication of fracture. *Lucency* is the term used to describe the interruption of the cortex and trabeculae. This is visualized as a black or gray line on the x-ray (Figure 4–5). Increased *density* can be seen with overlap of fracture fragments or with compression of the trabeculae. This is seen as an area that appears whiter on the x-ray (Figure 4–6).

Now that you can identify the fracture (by pointing to it), you will need to be able to verbally communicate this information to someone (such as an attending physician or a patient!). Therefore, you will need to become acquainted with the terms used

to describe fractures. First, it would be a good idea if you could name the bone that is involved. I am not going to review all bones in the skeleton, but I will label them for you in the figures as appropriate. Let's begin with the segments of the bone called the *epiphysis, metaphysis,* and *diaphysis* (Figure 4–7). The diaphysis can be further divided into proximal, middle, and distal thirds.

After noting the fracture and successfully identifying the bone involved, the orientation of the fracture must be described. The orientations of fractures are generally *transverse, oblique, spiral* (self-explanatory), *comminuted* (more than two fracture fragments), *open* (communicates with the outside world) or *closed* (overlying skin and soft tissues are intact). Now it is imperative to determine where the fracture fragments are relative to each other. By convention, fractures are described in terms of *position of the distal fragment relative to the proximal fragment.* The only way you can make this assessment is to have two orthogonal views. Commonly used terms for description of the displacement of fracture fragments include *overriding* of fracture fragments, which is a term used when the bone fragments are parallel to each other. *Distraction* is a separation of the apposing ends of fracture fragments (you can use "traction" as a way to remember this term). *Impaction* occurs when one fragment of bone is forcibly driven or telescoped into the

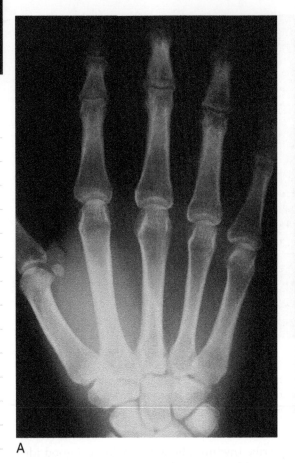

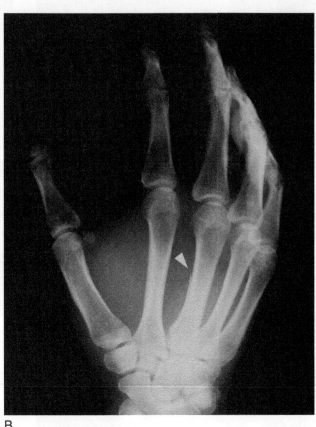

A   B

Figure 4–4.   A, No fracture is identified on this anteroposterior view. B, Oblique view of the same hand demonstrates a fracture of the base of the third metacarpal (*arrowhead*). This is a reminder that "One view is no view."

adjacent fragments (remember that this type of fracture will appear more white on an x-ray). Occasionally, a fracture may be angled toward or away from the midline of the body. If the bone fracture fragment distal to the fracture site points away from the midline of the body, the fracture is said to be laterally displaced (Figure 4–8). It is helpful when discussing a fracture (particularly if the information is being given over the telephone) to provide as accurate and detailed a description as possible. The above terms will help you to accomplish that.

A couple of additional types of fractures are worthy of mention. These include avulsion fractures, stress fractures, pathologic fractures, and insufficiency fractures. An *avulsion* fracture is a fragment of bone at an attachment site of muscle, ligament, or tendon that is pulled away from its original position by a force in the opposite direction (Figure 4–9).

Stress fractures result from abnormal stresses across normal bone. Several theories have been proposed for the development of these fractures, although they most likely are mediated through abnormal muscular stress. The increase in physical activity or repetitive trauma stresses normal bone beyond its capacity to maintain its form. Common physical activities associated with stress fractures include running, walking, and jumping. Radiographic signs to diagnose a stress fracture include a lucency and thick *periosteal reaction*, which is defined as solid or thick new bone formation around the fracture. If the area of bone affected is primarily cancellous, then a band of sclerosis (whiter bone) can be seen. Common locations for stress fractures are the tibia, femur, distal fibula, and metatarsals (Figure 4–10). If you are treating athletes and suspect a stress fracture, MRI is an excellent examination to identify this type of injury. The abnormality can be seen well on MRI before the changes are noted on conventional x-ray. In particular, stress fractures of the hip are potentially devastating injuries, and a diagnosis must be made in a timely fashion to prevent the horrible consequence of a complete fracture, which can result in avascular necrosis (AVN) (Figure 4–11). If MRI is not immediately available, the patient may be placed on crutch

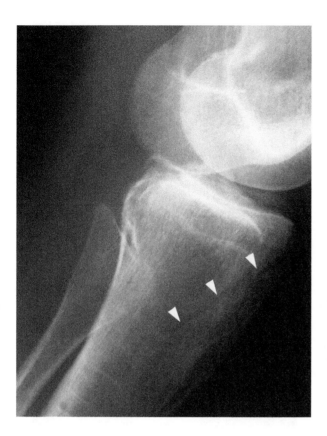

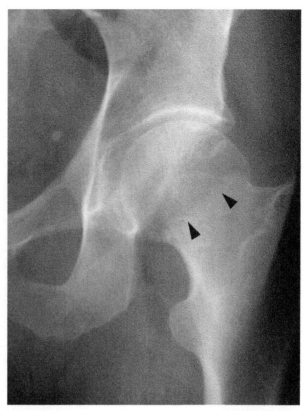

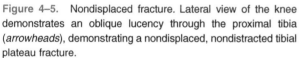

Figure 4–5.   Nondisplaced fracture. Lateral view of the knee demonstrates an oblique lucency through the proximal tibia (*arrowheads*), demonstrating a nondisplaced, nondistracted tibial plateau fracture.

Figure 4–6.   Impacted hip fracture. Anteroposterior view of the left hip shows a line of sclerosis (more white) (*arrowheads*) in the middle aspect of the femoral head in this older female patient who lost her balance and fell. The line of sclerosis is caused by overlapping bone from the "telescoping" of the fracture.

ambulation and referred to an MRI unit as soon as possible. Keep in mind that not only elite athletes can suffer stress fractures. The weekend warrior is also susceptible to this type of injury, through sudden increased duration of an activity, changes in training surface, or other factors that increase stresses across bones, including the use of new or poor running shoes.

Pathologic fractures occur in bone that has been weakened by a disease process, such as an underlying condition of osteoporosis, osteomalacia, primary tumor, or metastatic disease.

Insufficiency fractures occur when normal stress is placed upon bone that is deficient either in mineral or in elastic resistance. These types of fractures commonly occur in the femoral neck, sacrum, and pubic rami of patients with osteoporosis. When such a fracture results from osteoporosis and is nondisplaced, it can be very difficult to see on conventional radiographs. In the setting of a patient with osteoporosis and hip pain with an apparently normal x-ray, an MRI examination of the pelvis should be performed to exclude fracture. Imaging

with magnetic resonance allows for visualization of the fracture as it extends through the marrow cavity (Figure 4–12). Do not be dissuaded from thinking of the diagnosis of hip fracture because of the patient's inability to give a history of trauma or because the patient is able to bear weight at the time of examination. Neither of these clinical pieces of information is useful, and both are potentially misleading. The MRI should be performed while the patient is in the emergency room or clinic, before he or she is permitted to ambulate. Cases have occurred in which a patient has been allowed to walk to the bathroom while waiting for the MRI, causing an unrecognized fracture to displace. If the fracture is diagnosed on MRI before it is displaced on x-ray, the patient can be treated with percutaneous pinning through the hip (a less morbid procedure with a shorter hospital stay). However, once the fracture is displaced, the patient must undergo an internal fixation that may require a total hip arthroplasty and a longer hospitalization.

Children can sustain unique fractures. These fractures are addressed in Chapter 6.

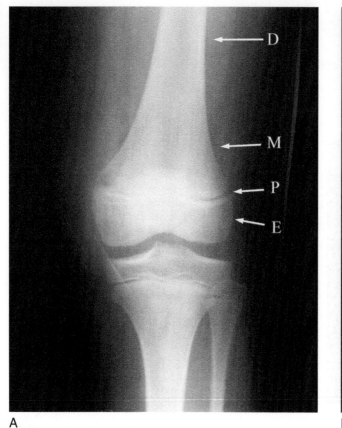

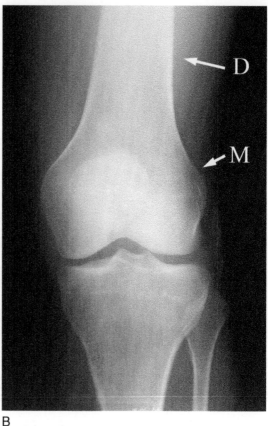

A   B

Figure 4–7. Pediatric bone. A, Anteroposterior view of the knee in a pediatric patient demonstrating open physis. D, diaphysis; E, epiphysis; M, metaphysis; P, physis. B, Same view in a skeletally mature patient.

Although a discussion of all possible fractures is beyond the scope of this textbook, some fractures are important to recognize. Intra-articular fractures are fractures that involve an articular surface of a joint. To recognize these important fractures, one can look for disruption of the normal architecture of the joint. *Fat/fluid levels* are an important indicator that there has been disruption of an articular surface. Marrow fat can leak into the joint and will float to the top of joint fluid. With a horizontal x-ray beam (cross-table lateral view), a fat/fluid level can be identified (Figure 4–13). When this is identified in the knee, the most likely fracture site is the tibial plateau. Generally, the fracture can be confirmed by obtaining oblique views of the knee, followed by either CT or MRI to assess the depression of the tibial plateau and possible associated injuries.

Intra-articular fluid may displace fat pads associated with the joint lining. This most commonly occurs in the elbow. Normally, the fat pads in the elbow hug the distal humerus. A small fat pad may be seen anteriorly, but posteriorly there is no visualization of a fat pad on the lateral x-ray (Figure 4–14). When intra-articular blood accumulates in

the elbow, the lateral x-ray will show migration of the fat pads away from the humerus, causing a characteristic appearance. Anteriorly, the fat pad resembles a "sail" from a sailboat, and posteriorly the fat pad becomes apparent (Figure 4–15). In the setting of trauma with fat pads visualized on a lateral x-ray, a fracture is presumed. In general, in the mature skeleton (physes closed) a radial head fracture is more typical, whereas children (open physes) would most likely have a fracture in the supracondylar region of the distal humerus.

Occult fractures may be encountered anywhere in the body. Previously, hip fractures were discussed. Another area where MRI plays an active role is in the evaluation of scaphoid fractures. Patients often complain of pain in the anatomic snuffbox. These fractures are a result of a *fall on outstretched hand* (FOOSH) injury. A scaphoid fracture is potentially devastating because it can result in AVN of the proximal fracture fragment (Figure 4–16). (Remember that the blood supply to the scaphoid is from distal to proximal.) A fracture across the waist will interrupt the blood supply. A timely diagnosis of this fracture must be made in

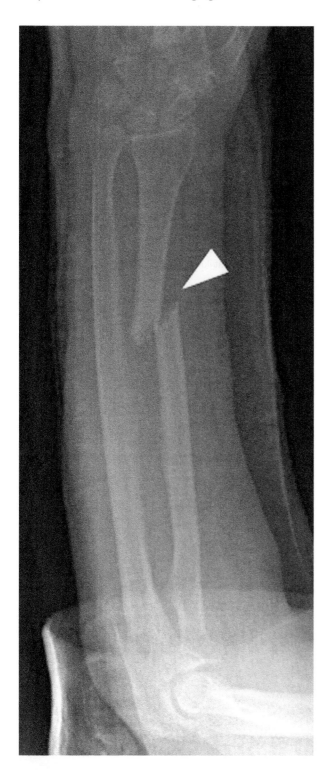

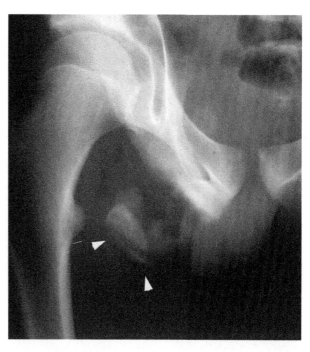

Figure 4–9.   Avulsion fracture. Large ossific density noted in the soft tissues adjacent to the lesser trochanter demonstrates avulsion of the hamstrings from the ischial tuberosity (*arrowheads*). Avulsion injuries are not uncommon in the pediatric population.

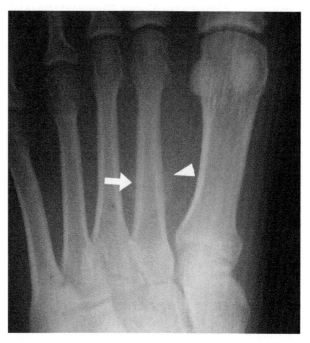

Figure 4–8.   Angulated fracture. Oblique fracture through the distal third of the radius with overriding of the fracture fragment (*arrowhead*). Patient is imaged in cast material. A lateral view should also be obtained in this setting to exclude the possibility of an ulnar dislocation.

Figure 4–10.   Stress fracture. Periosteal reaction is noted about the shaft of the second metatarsal (*arrowhead* and *arrow*). This finding is compatible with a stress fracture.

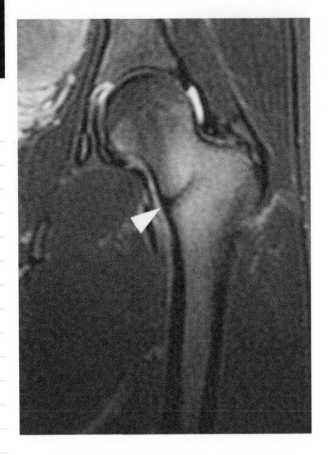

Figure 4–11. Stress fracture. Coronal T2-weighted MRI of the left hip demonstrates linear area of low signal (*arrowhead*), indicating a stress fracture of the femoral neck. High T2 signal around the fracture line represents bone marrow edema.

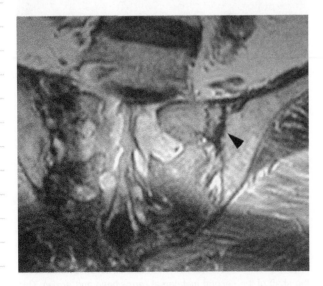

Figure 4–12. Sacral insufficiency fracture. Coronal T2-weighted image through the sacrum demonstrates a linear area of low signal through the sacral ala bilaterally (*arrowhead*). This finding is seen in osteoporotic patients or patients who have received radiation therapy to the pelvis.

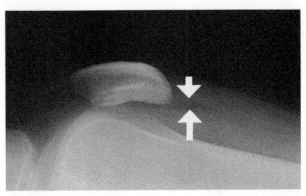

Figure 4–13. Fat/fluid level. Cross-table lateral view of the knee demonstrates well-defined lucency in the suprapatellar location, compatible with a fat/fluid level that indicates an intra-articular fracture.

order to avoid the complication of AVN. A previously accepted treatment plan was to cast the hand as though a fracture were present and repeat the conventional x-ray in 7 to 10 days, hoping to see better visualization of the fracture at the follow-up examination. This approach compromises the patient who needs to use the hand but does not have a fracture. A better (and more cost-effective)

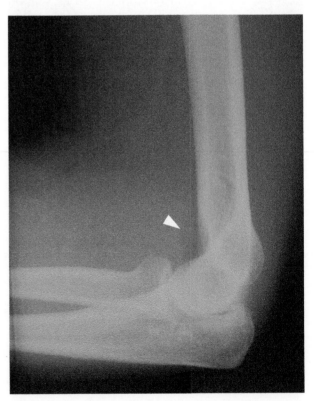

Figure 4–14. Normal lateral elbow. Anterior humeral fat pad without distention (*arrowhead*). There is no visualization of a posterior humeral fat pad.

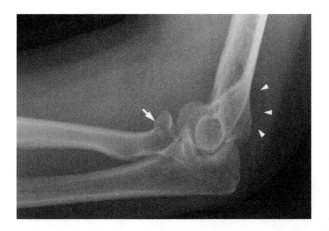

Figure 4–15. Radial head fracture. Oblique lateral film demonstrates presence of the posterior fat pad (*arrowheads*). This is distended due to an intra-articular fracture, as evidenced by the deformity of the radial head (*arrow*)

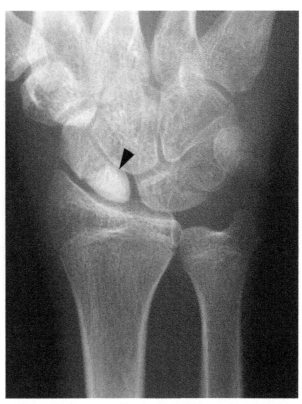

Figure 4–16. Avascular necrosis of the scaphoid. Anteroposterior view of the wrist in a skeletally immature patient demonstrating increased sclerosis of the proximal pole of the scaphoid (*arrowhead*). This finding is seen in patients with chronic scaphoid fracture due to inadequate blood supply to the proximal pole.

way to evaluate these patients is to perform MRI in the acute setting if no fracture is seen on the plain film but the patient has symptoms suggesting a fracture. An occult fracture will be readily identified with MRI (Figure 4–17). If MRI is not available to you at the time you are seeing the patient, the patient's wrist should be immobilized and an MRI should be performed at the earliest convenience.

A *dislocation* is complete disruption of the relationship of the two opposing bones in the joint (Figure 4–18). In order to address the direction of a dislocation, two views orthogonal to each other are imperative. (Has that point been emphasized enough?) A *subluxation* is diagnosed when there is displacement of one articular bone in the joint relative to the other, beyond the normal range of motion of the joint, but without complete dislocation. The convention of description of the subluxation or dislocation is the distal bone's displacement relative to the proximal bone.

Some encountered dislocations and joint abnormalities are worth special mention here, either because they occur often enough that you will need to be comfortable making the diagnosis or because a timely diagnosis can effect quick and appropriate treatment (usually surgical intervention). Anterior glenohumeral dislocations (shoulder) represent about 95% of all shoulder dislocations. This type of dislocation is easily recognized on an x-ray because the humeral head (on an AP radiograph) is positioned below the coracoid process (the round bony protuberance emanating from the anterior portion of the scapula). The humeral head moves inferior, medial, and anterior to the glenoid. If necessary, additional views that can be used to document this dislocation are the axillary view

and the scapula-Y or trauma-oblique view, which is obtained 45 degrees tangent to the joint (Figure 4–19).

Associated abnormalities of anterior dislocation are the *Hill-Sachs* and *Bankart lesions*. Hill-Sachs deformity is an impaction fracture of the posterolateral aspect of the humeral head. This portion of the humerus bangs into the anterior portion of the glenoid during the dislocation. A *Hill-Sachs* deformity is not identified on the conventional x-ray that shows the dislocation. Postreduction films are necessary to see this abnormality when it is present. It doesn't always occur, but it is present in severe, chronic, or recurrent dislocations. Views that best depict this deformity are the internal rotation, Stryker notch (arm raised over the head with x-ray beam focused in axilla), and trauma oblique views (Figure 4–20). The associated abnormality on the glenoid is the *Bankart* lesion. This is an injury to the anterior capsule, anterior labrum, or anterior bony glenoid rim. Capsular and labral injuries will not be appreciated on conventional x-ray. MRI best depicts these abnormalities

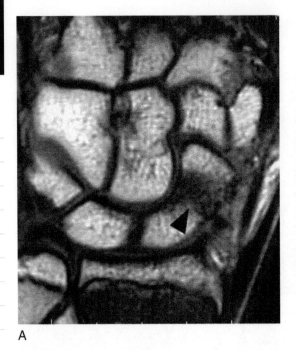

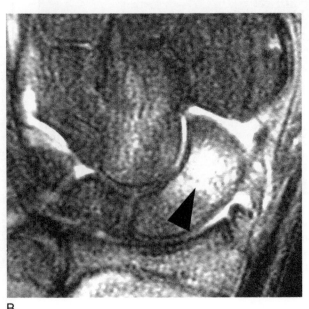

A   B

Figure 4–17. Scaphoid fracture. A, Coronal T1-weighted MRI of the wrist demonstrates linear low signal through the waist of the scaphoid (*arrowhead*). Note also low signal in the distal metaphysis of the radius. B, Coronal T2-weighted image demonstrates bone marrow edema in the scaphoid, as evidenced by the white or high T2 signal. Linear low signal through the area of edema represents the fracture line (*arrowhead*).

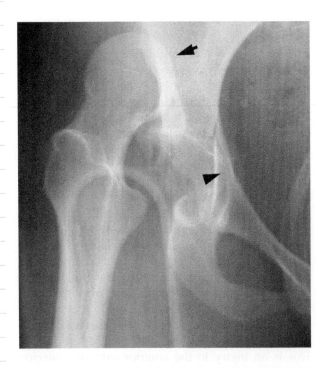

Figure 4–18. Hip dislocation. Coned-down anteroposterior view of the pelvis demonstrates superior location of the femoral head (*arrow*) with respect to the acetabulum (*arrowhead*).

(Figure 4–21). Current treatment for first-time dislocators has gone from conservative treatment in a sling to surgical intervention with capsular shrinkage and repair of the labrum. Timely reduction of this injury is necessary, because the longer the joint remains dislocated, the harder it is to reduce. The muscles about the shoulder begin to contract, making the reduction more difficult. Reduction requires countertraction while the arm is gently distracted to reduce the humeral head into the joint space.

Posterior dislocations account for a much smaller percentage of shoulder dislocations (2–4%). These dislocations can be very difficult to identify on a routine shoulder series. A degree of suspicion is necessary to identify this type of dislocation. A posterior dislocation can result from severe trauma, but a unique group of patients who can have this injury are those who have suffered a seizure or have received an electrical shock. Patients who have the potential to seize include patients with a wide range disorders, from idiopathic seizure disorders to metabolic abnormalities; alcoholics going through withdrawal; and patients receiving electroconvulsive therapy for severe depression. The conventional x-ray will demonstrate the humerus fixed in internal rotation. Many institutions perform only internal and external rotation of the shoulder as a

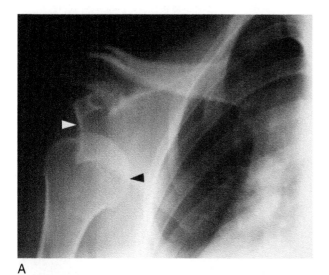

A

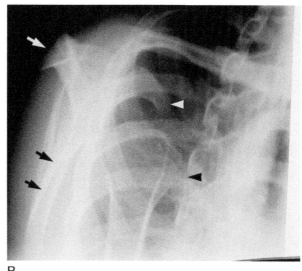

B

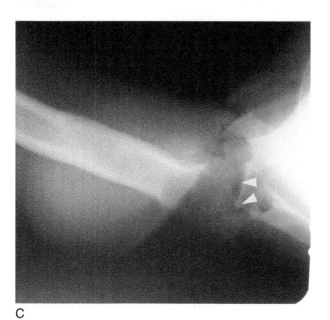

C

Figure 4–19.   Anterior shoulder dislocation. A, Anteroposterior view of the shoulder demonstrates inferior and medial location of the humeral head (*black arrowhead*) with respect to the glenoid (*white arrowhead*). This is characteristic of an anterior shoulder dislocation. B, Scapular Y view, showing the acromion (*white arrow*), coracoid process (*white arrowhead*), and body of the scapula (*black arrows*). The humeral head (*black arrowhead*) is sitting beneath the coracoid process, indicating an anterior shoulder dislocation. C, Axillary view, posterior dislocation. The x-ray plate is below the axilla, and the x-ray beam is perpendicular to the x-ray plate with arm extended to the side; this view demonstrates a *posterior* shoulder dislocation (*arrowheads*). The humeral head is hooked on the posterior portion of the glenoid.

"shoulder series." A key to recognizing posterior dislocation is that internal rotation, external rotation, and neutral views of the shoulder will demonstrate the humerus locked in internal rotation and will show the same round contour of the humeral head (Figure 4–22). The normal overlap between the humeral head and glenoid may be lost (absence of the crescent sign) (Figure 4–23). The impaction on the humeral head occurs at the anterior and medial aspect, because this area impacts the posterior portion of the glenoid. This abnormality is called a *reverse Hill-Sachs lesion* or *Trough sign.* The associated abnormality on the glenoid labrum is a *reverse Bankart lesion* (Figure 4–24).

Hip dislocations should be diagnosed in a timely fashion. If a dislocation is left unreduced for a period of time, the femoral head is left without its blood supply, rendering it at risk for bone death (AVN). Timely reduction and follow-up imaging with CT is recommended to ascertain whether any small bone fragments have been retained in the joint space. If small fragments are identified, surgery is indicated.

Combined fracture-dislocations can also occur. An important injury to identify in the wrist is the lunate or perilunate dislocation. The lateral radiograph is particularly useful in identifying this abnormality. This severe injury is a result of a FOOSH. On the lateral radiograph, the metacarpals align with the capitate, which sits inside the lunate, which in turn sits inside the curve of the distal radius (Figure 4–25). If the lunate is aligned with the distal radius and the remainder of the bones are malaligned, the injury is called a *perilunate*

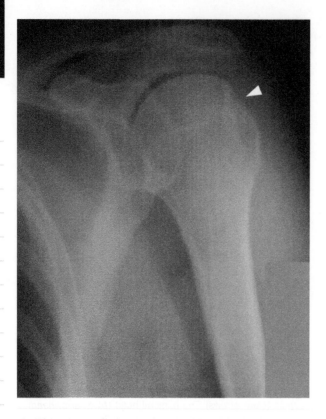

Figure 4–20. Hill-Sachs lesion. The defect is noted in the posterior portion of the humerus (*arrowhead*) seen on internal rotation. This defect can be seen after anterior shoulder dislocations.

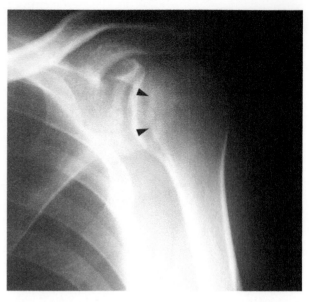

Figure 4–22. Posterior dislocation. Anteroposterior view of the shoulder in internal rotation demonstrates increased sclerosis in the humeral head (*arrowheads*), compatible with a reverse Hill-Sachs lesion.

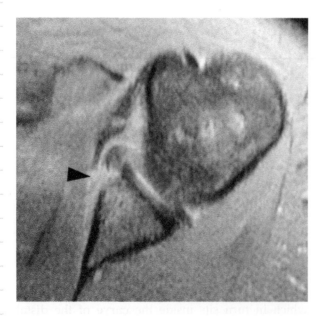

Figure 4–21. Bankart lesion. Axial MRI through the glenohumeral joint demonstrates a torn anterior labrum (*arrowhead*).

dislocation (around the lunate) (Figure 4–26). If the lunate is the only bone of the carpus that is malaligned, it is called a *lunate* dislocation (Figure 4–27). Recognizing the abnormality is imperative, because the neurovascular bundle that supplies the hand and wrist can be compromised with either of these types of injury. Prompt reduction with surgical intervention is the treatment of choice. Perilunate dislocation, more often than lunate dislocation, can be associated with a scaphoid fracture. It is very important to identify the associated injury. Up to 10% of x-rays with one abnormality have a second abnormality. So, don't stop your search pattern when you happen upon an abnormality. Look for additional abnormalities.

Another important fracture-dislocation to identify is in the foot. It is the *Lisfranc* injury. The *Lisfranc* joint is another accepted name for the tarsometatarsal joint space. Disruption along this joint space can lead to compromise of the neurovascular bundle in the foot. Identification of this abnormality is imperative and needs to be made in a timely fashion in order that appropriate surgical intervention be instituted to preserve sensation and circulation. Recognizing the abnormal alignment of the metatarsal bones with the tarsal bones identifies this injury. The medial aspect of the second metatarsal should align with the medial aspect of the second cuneiform, and, similarly, the medial aspect of the shaft of the fourth metatarsal should align with

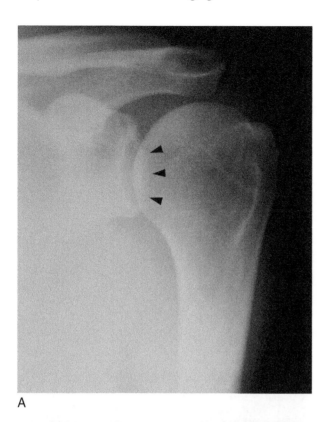

A

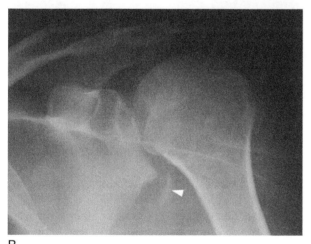

B

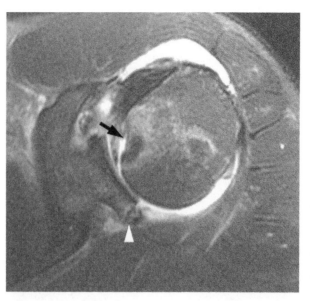

Figure 4–24.   Reverse Bankart lesion. Axial T2-weighted MRI through the glenohumeral joint demonstrates a reverse Hill-Sachs deformity (*black arrow*) in the humeral head, with a reverse Bankart deformity (*arrowhead*) of the posterior labrum. These findings suggest previous posterior shoulder dislocation.

Figure 4–23.   A, Normal. The normal overlap of the humeral head and glenoid is demonstrated (*arrowheads*) as a crescent-shaped area of sclerosis. B, Posterior dislocation. Antero-posterior view of the shoulder demonstrates slight superior migration of the humeral head with respect to the glenoid. An ossific density (*arrowhead*) is noted at the inferior portion of the joint space. This is a piece of glenoid that has been avulsed, representing a reverse bony Bankart injury.

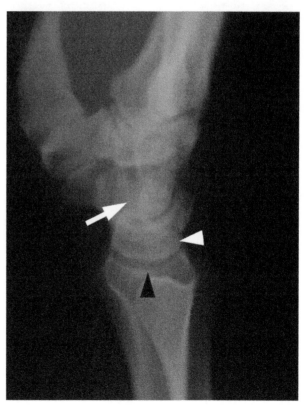

Figure 4–25.   Normal lateral wrist. Lateral view demonstrates normal alignment of the capitate (*arrow*), lunate (*white arrowhead*), and distal radius (*black arrowhead*).

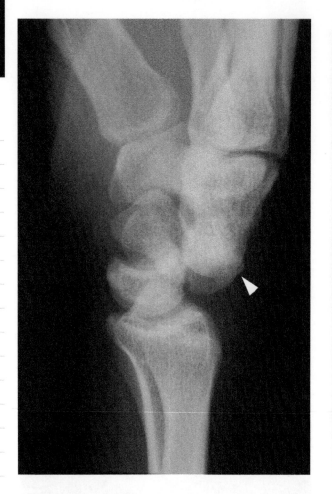

Figure 4–26. Perilunate dislocation. Lateral wrist view demonstrates normal alignment of the lunate with the distal radius, but the remainder of the carpus is dorsally located (*arrowhead*). This is the appearance of a perilunate dislocation.

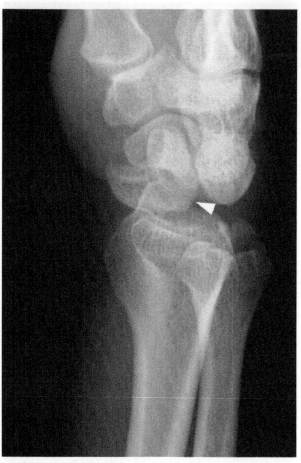

Figure 4–27. Lunate dislocation. Oblique lateral view of the wrist demonstrates malalignment of the lunate with respect to the distal radius (*arrowhead*). This is the pattern seen in lunate dislocation.

the medial aspect of the cuboid (Figures 4–28 and 4–29).

Axial Skeleton

Entire textbooks are dedicated to the topic of the axial skeleton. I will address a proper search pattern, and some of the more commonly encountered injuries will be discussed.

An organized search pattern is necessary for evaluating spine injury. There are important structures needing evaluation. First the cervical spine (C-spine) will be discussed. Most importantly, start the search pattern with the lateral film. If you can count to seven, you are in good shape! That is, you should see all seven cervical vertebral bodies. Many emergency room physicians like to visualize through the first thoracic vertebra (T1). Now you will want to make sure all the "lines" are intact (Figure 4–30). Assess the anterior vertebral line, the

posterior vertebral line, the spinolaminar line, the prevertebral soft tissues, and finally, a line that I find particularly useful in assessing abnormalities at C1 and C2. Draw a short line assessing the spinolaminal line of C1 to C3. The spinolaminal line of C2 should fall within 2 mm of this line. Disruption of this line can be a subtle finding for a hangman's (C2) fracture or a C1 ring fracture (Jefferson's fracture). Key Point 4–1 lists the search pattern of the cervical spine. If the spinolaminar line is breached by a fracture, this is an ominous finding, suggesting posterior element involvement and impending instability (Figures 4–31 and 4–32). This is to be distinguished from a clay shoveler's fracture, which is typically a vertically oriented, isolated spinous process fracture affecting only C6 or C7 (Figure 4–33). After assessing these lines, the disc spaces should be evaluated, as well as the distance between the anterior arch of C1 and the odontoid process or dens of C2 (predental space).

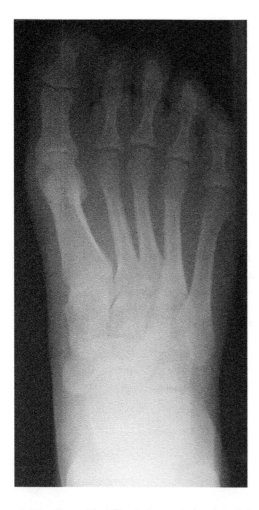

Figure 4–28.   Normal foot film. Anteroposterior view of the foot demonstrates normal metatarsal phalangeal joints and tarsometatarsal joint spaces.

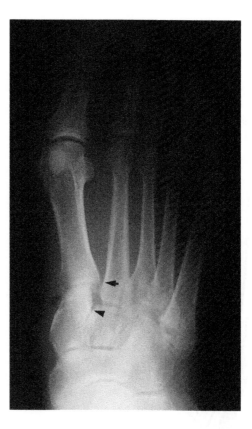

Figure 4–29.   Lisfranc fracture-dislocation. Widening of the first and second tarsometatarsal joint space (*arrowhead* and *arrow*), compatible with disruption of the Lisfranc ligament. Malalignment between the second metatarsal and middle cuneiform suggests disruption.

This is best assessed on the lateral view. The normal distance in an adult measures less than 2.5 mm. The lateral view should also show the alignment of the facet joints. These should look like shingles on a house and should line up symmetrically. The open-mouth view can be viewed next. The open-mouth or odontoid view allows assessment of the relationship of the lateral masses of C1 with the dens. These spaces should be symmetric bilaterally (Figure 4–34). The AP view should be checked for alignment of the lateral aspects of the C-spine. The oblique views allow for assessment of the pedicles, neural foramina, and lamina.

Currently, CT of the cervical spine is not recommended as a routine screening examination. Conventional x-rays are still obtained and are used as a screening examination for a patient with cervical trauma. If the spine cannot be completely evaluated with plain films (you can't see to C7 level), then a CT should be performed if the patient

has neck pain. The clinical history is very important in evaluating a patient with cervical spine trauma. If the patient is unable to give a history (altered mental status or distracting injuries), a thorough radiographic workup is recommended. If a fracture has been identified on conventional films, CT examination is performed to evaluate the extent of the fracture.

Specific injuries that occur to the cervical spine include *hyperflexion, hyperextension,* and *vertical compression fractures.* The mechanism of injury is not important, quite frankly. Recognizing the abnormality on x-rays is. A *flexion teardrop* fracture usually affects the lower cervical spine and results in a wedge-shaped vertebral body. Ligamentous injury and facet malalignment can also occur. Assessing the lines as instructed above will help you recognize these diagnoses. That is, you will assess the spine the same way regardless of whether the injury was caused by hyperextension or flexion. A burst fracture is a compression fracture of the vertebral body resulting from an axial load that extends into the posterior elements, rendering the

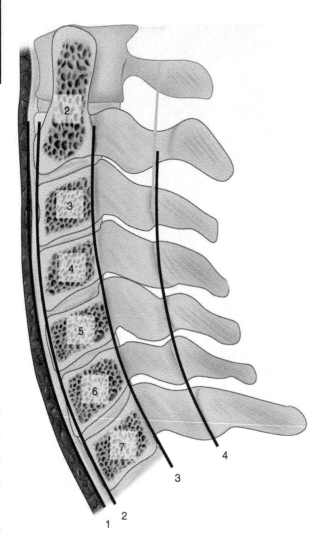

Figure 4–30. Normal lateral cervical spine. Sketch indicating normal lines for evaluation of the cervical spine. 1, Prevertebral soft tissues; 2, anterior vertebral line; 3, posterior vertebral line; 4, spinolaminal line; blue line, short spinolaminal line of C1 to C3. This latter line is useful for evaluating injuries to C1 or C2. If the spinolaminal line of C2 is located more than 2 mm beyond the line extending from C1 to C3, then a fracture in C1 or C2 is present.

fracture unstable. Dens fractures are classified into types I, II, and III. Type I is a fracture of the tip of the dens, type II is a fracture through the base of the dens, and type III is a fracture through the body (below the base of the dens). Fractures can further be divided into whether they are stable or unstable. In short, if two of the three columns that comprise the spine are involved with a fracture, then it is unstable (Figure 4–35). Jefferson's and hangman's fractures result from cervical trauma and are demonstrated in Figures 4–36 and 4–37.

Key   Point 4–1

Search Pattern for Cervical Spine Radiographs

Lateral view
Vertebral bodies
Lines
    Prevertebral soft tissues
    Anterior vertebral line
    Posterior vertebral line
    Spinolaminar line
Disc spaces
Predental space
Facet joints
Odontoid view
Space between dens and lateral masses of CI
Anteroposterior (AP) view
Lateral aspects of vertebral bodies
Oblique view
Pedicles
Neural foramina
Lamina

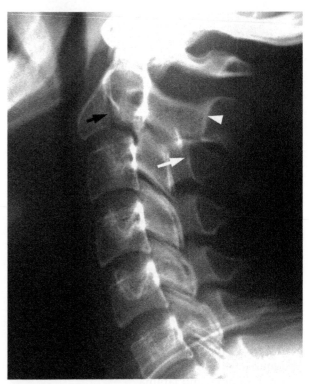

Figure 4–31. Breech of spinolaminal line C1 to C3. Note the posterior location of C2 (*arrowhead*) with respect to the spinolaminal line of C3 (*white arrow*). The fracture is noted through the body of C2 (*black arrow*). Note the lack of prevertebral soft tissue swelling. Lack of prevertebral soft tissue swelling should not dissuade you from concluding that a fracture is present.

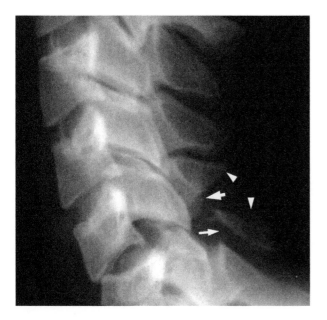

Figure 4–32. Breach of spinolaminal line. Limited lateral cervical spine view demonstrates interruption of the spinolaminal line (*arrow*). An oblique fracture through the spinous process of C5 is noted (*arrowhead*). Note also the widening of the space between the spinous processes of C5 and C6 (*arrows*). The C5 vertebral body and C6 vertebral body are malaligned compared with the levels above C5. This fracture should not be confused with a clay shoveler's fracture, which would not involve the spinolaminal line or lead to an unstable fracture as is the case in this example. Clay shoveler's fractures are vertically oriented and are generally seen in the C7 spinous process. Clay shoveler's fractures do not affect C5 or above.

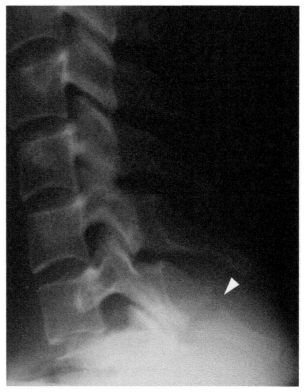

Figure 4–33. Clay shoveler's fracture. Vertical fracture through the spinous process of C7 (*arrowhead*). This appearance and location are characteristic of a clay shoveler's fracture. This fracture can also occur at C6. Note that these fractures are always vertically oriented.

In the thoracic and lumbar spine, anterior wedge configurations of the vertebral body can be a result of compression fractures (Figure 4–38). A burst fracture will have a retropulsed fragment associated with the compression deformity as well as posterior element involvement, rendering it unstable. This can be appreciated by looking at the interpedicular distance on the AP film, measuring the distance on the vertebral body in question, and comparing that with the interpedicular distance of the vertebral body more caudal (Figure 4–39). The normal interpedicular distance increases with caudal progression through the lumbar spine. A deviation from this progression suggests a burst fracture of the vertebral body in question.

Spondylolysis is a fracture through the pars interarticularis (pars defect) and can be unilateral or bilateral. The oblique film resembles a "Scottie dog" (Figure 4–40). If the dog is wearing a "collar," a spondylolysis is present. If the pars defect is bilateral, it can be seen on the lateral film (Figure 4–41). Most often, the lumbar levels are affected (L5–S1 followed by L4–L5). *Spondylolisthesis* is anterior subluxation of a vertebral body relative to the inferiorly located vertebral body. It is graded by the severity of the subluxation. Grade 1 is less than 25% subluxation relative to the lower vertebral body, grade 2 is 25% to 50% subluxation, grade 3 is 50% to 75% subluxation, and grade 4 is slip of the entire vertebral body relative to the lower level (Figure 4–42).

Infection

There are several routes of infection into the bone: direct implantation from a penetrating wound, contiguous spread from soft tissue or cellulitis, and hematogenous spread. The area of the bone in the joint involved with infection from hematogenous spread depends on the age of the patient. In the infant, metaphyseal vessels penetrate to the epiphysis, so a metaphyseal infection may involve the epiphysis and the joint. In the child, terminal vessels in metaphyses do not cross into the epiphyses, so epiphyses are not commonly involved in childhood metaphyseal infections (**Table 4–1**).

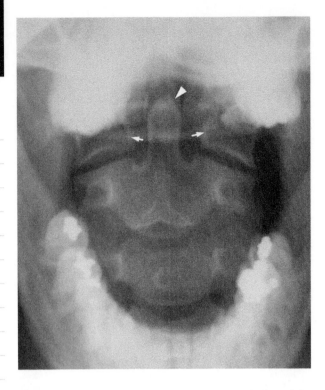

Figure 4–34.   Odontoid view. Normal open-mouth view of the dens showing the lateral masses of C1 (*arrows*) and the dens (*arrowhead*).

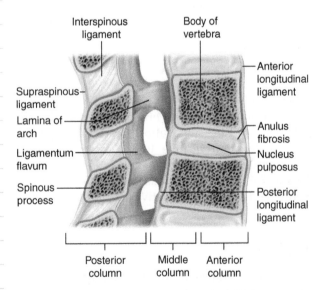

Figure 4–35.   Normal columns of the spine, sagittal view (Denis classification). This is a helpful classification when trauma has occurred.

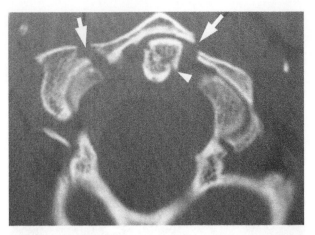

Figure 4–36.   Jefferson's fracture. Axial CT with bone algorithm demonstrating a comminuted fracture of the ring of C1 (*arrows*) as well as a fracture through the tip of the dens (*arrowhead*).

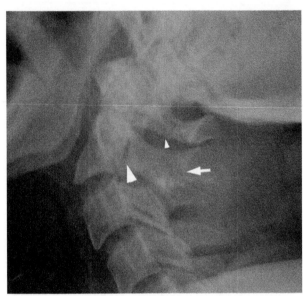

Figure 4–37.   Hangman's fracture. Lateral cervical spine view demonstrates a fracture of C2 (*large arrowhead*) as well as a nondisplaced fracture of the posterior ring of C1 (*small arrowhead*). The spinolaminal line is offset at C2 (*arrow*).

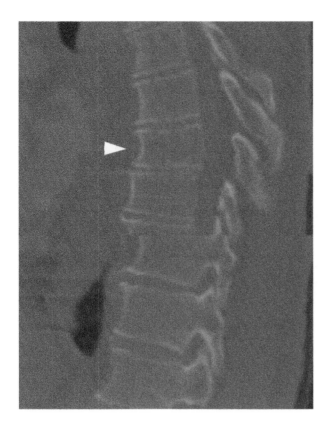

Figure 4–38. Anterior wedge deformity. Sagittal CT reformation of the thoracic and lumbar spine in a patient who sustained trauma shows anterior height loss of a lower thoracic vertebral body (*arrowhead*). Evaluation of the posterior elements is necessary to exclude an unstable fracture. Note the misregistration artifact just distal to the wedge compression.

Acute osteomyelitis is not appreciated on conventional x-rays until 1 to 2 weeks after symptoms have developed. Bone destruction is seen only after 30% to 50% of the bone is lysed. The initial bone changes may appear aggressive and difficult to differentiate from a malignant tumor. Findings on conventional films suggestive of osteomyelitis are soft tissue swelling, periosteal reaction, lytic foci, reactive sclerosis, sequestrum or involucrum formation (chronic), and soft tissue abscess or sinus tract formation (Key Point 4–2). A sequestrum is necrotic bone isolated from the rest of the bone, and an involucrum is reactive new bone that surrounds the sequestrum. These are more commonly seen in children (Figure 4–43).

Osteomyelitis has a variable appearance and can occur at any age in any bone. It may or may not be expansile, have a border, or be associated with periosteal reaction. This is why infection appears on many differential diagnoses when a lytic lesion is present in the bone. When infection is a clinical consideration and the conventional x-rays are insensitive, which study (or studies) are available

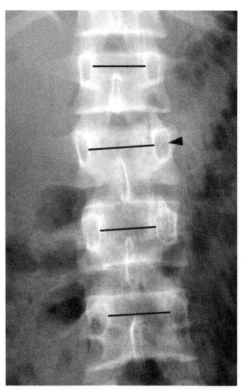

A

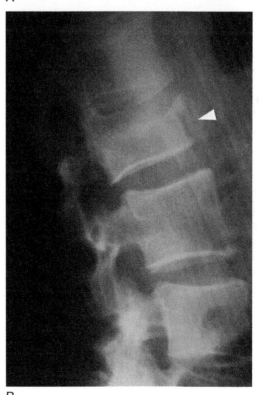

B

Figure 4–39. Abnormal interpedicular widening. A, Anteroposterior view demonstrates widening of the interpedicular distance of L1 (*arrowhead*), which suggests involvement of the posterior elements and an unstable fracture. B, Burst fracture of L1 with anterior displaced fragment and curved posterior vertebral line (*arrowhead*).

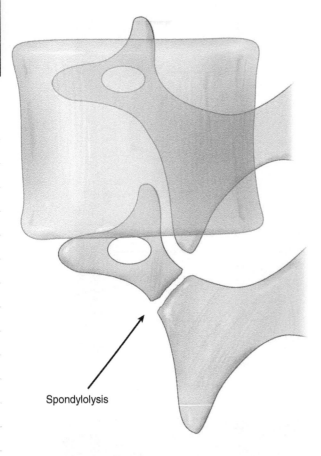

Figure 4–40.   Spondylolysis. Sketch of an oblique film showing a pars interarticularis defect.

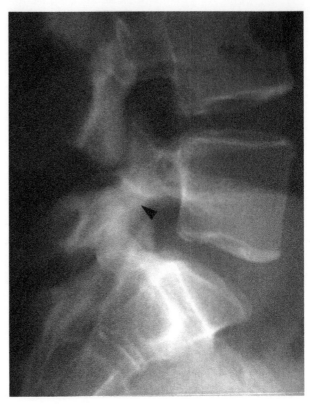

Figure 4–41.   Spondylolysis. Oblique x-ray shows a lucency through the L5–S1 level which represents a spondylolysis.

for further evaluation? Radionuclide bone scan imaging is more sensitive than conventional radiography, but it is not specific. It can become positive hours to days after the onset of symptoms. This imaging modality is helpful to evaluate additional sites of involvement, and it can support the diagnosis, but it is not specific for the diagnosis when positive. Gallium and indium-111 white blood cell scans are more specific for inflammation and infection but take up to 24 hours to make a diagnosis. MRI is very sensitive, especially when associated fluid collections or abscess are identified. There are many causes of abnormal bone marrow signal on MRI, however. Osteomyelitis is just one of those causes. If cortical destruction is seen with MRI, or if a fluid collection is noted in the bone, those findings would be virtually diagnostic of osteomyelitis. MRI is particularly helpful when the bone marrow signal is totally normal. In that case, you can be sure there is *no* osteomyelitis.

A very important finding on conventional x-ray is identifying gas in the soft tissues. If the patient has not had a recent surgical procedure or open wound to explain the presence of the gas, you should be concerned that the patient has a severe

ascending infection such as gangrene, which is a surgical emergency (Figure 4–44).

Subacute osteomyelitis is also referred to as a Brodie's abscess. Conventional x-rays demonstrate a well-defined lytic lesion that may have a rim of sclerosis and or periosteal reaction (Figure 4–45). Brodie's abscesses are often metaphyseal in children. Chronic osteomyelitis will demonstrate a thick sclerotic periosteal reaction resulting in thickened bony cortex with variable sites of lucency. A sequestrum can be present. Chronic osteomyelitis is most often encountered in the tibia and femur (Figure 4–46).

Discitis typically affects children but certainly can be seen in adults. Conventional x-rays demonstrate decreased disc height and vertebral end-plate irregularities with loss of the cortical margin. Patients with discitis have back pain, elevated C-reactive protein, and an increased sedimentation rate. A paraspinal mass or inflammatory collection is usually seen in discitis or vertebral osteomyelitis. This is seen best with MRI. One organism that spares the disc space until late in the infection is tuberculosis. Tuberculosis infection of the spine is referred to as Pott's disease. This infection typically occurs near the thoracolumbar junction and can

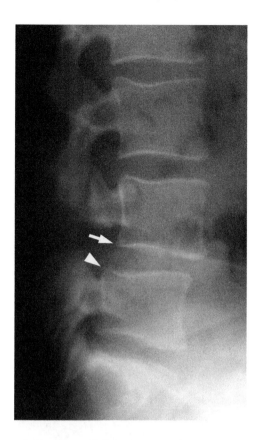

Figure 4–42. Spondylolisthesis. Lateral conventional x-ray demonstrates slip of cephalad vertebral body more anterior (*arrow* at L4) with respect to L5 (*arrowhead*). Spondylolisthesis can be caused by facet disease, pars interarticularis defect, or trauma.

Table 4–1 Patterns of Bone Involvement in Pediatric Osteomyelitis
Infant
Metaphysis
Epiphysis
Joint space
Child
Metaphyses only

lead to acute angular kyphosis (gibbus deformity). A paraspinous abscess may develop with associated calcifications.

Arthritis

Many students (and even radiology residents) find the topic of arthritis confusing, and even boring! I intend to present this in a way that is easy to

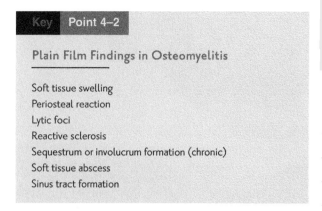

Key	Point 4–2

Plain Film Findings in Osteomyelitis

Soft tissue swelling
Periosteal reaction
Lytic foci
Reactive sclerosis
Sequestrum or involucrum formation (chronic)
Soft tissue abscess
Sinus tract formation

remember. First, understand that there is more to arthritis than degenerative disease and rheumatoid arthritis. Arthritis is best determined by the distribution of the process. So, all you really need to do is recognize a pattern of distribution and then remember the few arthritides that are associated with that distribution. It's pretty easy! The tables in

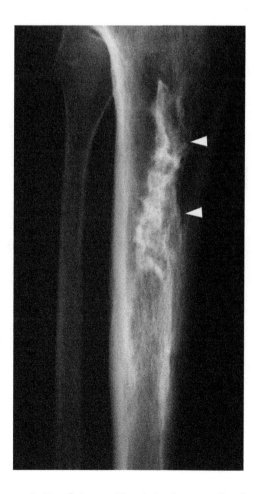

Figure 4–43. Osteomyelitis. Lateral conventional x-ray demonstrates an area of sclerosis within the diaphysis of the tibia (*arrowheads*), consistent with a sequestrum in this patient with osteomyelitis.

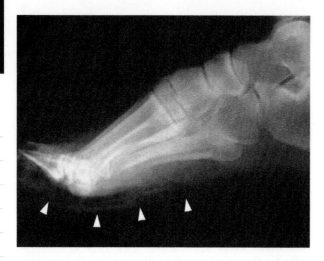

Figure 4–44. Gas gangrene. Lateral conventional x-ray demonstrates air density within the soft tissues (*arrowheads*). Recognition of air in the soft tissues is an ominous finding and a surgical emergency. Correlation should be made to exclude recent debridement to account for the air.

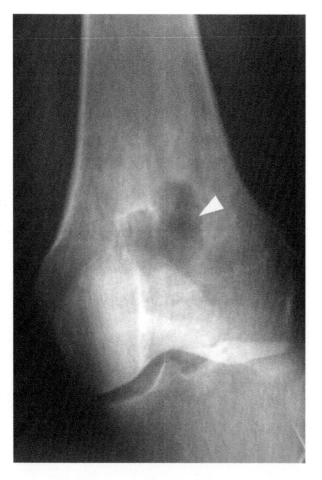

Figure 4–45. Brodie's abscess. Conventional anteroposterior radiograph of the knee demonstrates a lucency in the metaphysis. The lesion was biopsied because it resembles numerous pathologic processes and was shown to be an abscess.

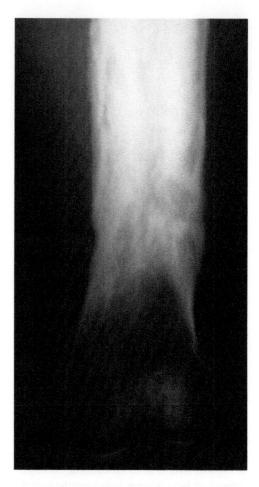

Figure 4–46. Chronic osteomyelitis. Conventional anteroposterior radiograph of the femur shows benign thickening of the cortex in this patient with chronic osteomyelitis.

this section should help you to remember the important features. When attempting to determine the type of arthritis, look at the distribution, the symmetry (bilateral), bone density, and erosions (**Key Point 4–3**).

The distribution is either proximal or distal. The arthritides associated with proximal distribution are rheumatoid arthritis and calcium pyrophosphate deposition disease (CPPD). Distal distribution are either psoriasis, Reiter's syndrome, or osteoarthritis (OA) (**Table 4–2**). To be clear, osteoarthritis (or osteoarthrosis) in the hands is referred to as primary OA. The osteoarthritis that is noted in other joints is a secondary type (generally from wear and tear or trauma).

When the distribution appears relatively symmetric from one hand to the other, it is typical of OA or rheumatoid arthritis. The only arthritis associated with abnormal bone density (osteoporosis) is rheumatoid arthritis. All the others mentioned above are associated with normal bone density. OA

Characterization of Arthritis

Distribution
Symmetry
Bone density
Erosions

Table 4–3   Arthritides with Subchondral Cyst Formation
Osteoarthritis
Rheumatoid arthritis
Calcium pyrophosphate deposition disease (CPPD)
Avascular necrosis

is often seen in older individuals; they might be osteoporotic, but the process of the arthritis is not what caused the abnormal bone density, as would be the case for rheumatoid arthritis.

Subchondral cysts are well-defined lytic lesions at the articular surface seen in a few of these entities. Identifying subchondral cysts (also referred to as geodes) can narrow the differential diagnosis of the suspected arthritis. The diagnoses include OA, rheumatoid arthritis, CPPD, and AVN (**Table 4–3**).

OA (osteoarthrosis is the more technically correct term, since there is little in the way of an inflammatory component) is also referred to as degenerative joint disease (DJD). When it occurs in the hands, it is thought to be primary and affects middle-aged women (Figure 4–47). There is a hereditary component to primary OA. Secondary OA is thought to be caused by trauma or overuse. The hallmarks of OA are sclerosis, osteophytes, and joint-space narrowing (Figure 4–48) (**Key Point 4–4**). If the three hallmarks are not present on the radiograph, another diagnosis should be considered. There is only one entity that can cause osteophytes without joint-space (or disc-space) narrowing or sclerosis. This is *diffuse idiopathic skeletal hyperostosis* (DISH). There are just a few joints in which OA may manifest with erosions instead of the usual osteophytes. These are the acromioclavicular joint, sacroiliac joint, temporomandibular joint, and pubic symphysis.

Table 4–2   Differential Diagnosis of Arthritis by Distribution
Proximal
Rheumatoid arthritis
Calcium pyrophosphate deposition disease (CPPD)
Distal
Psoriasis
Reactive arthritis
Osteoarthritis

Rheumatoid arthritis can affect any synovial joint in the body. As mentioned, the distribution in the hands is proximal (meaning that the wrist is affected before the fingers). Soft tissue swelling is a prominent feature and often affects the region of the ulnar styloid process. Osteoporosis is part of the disease process. This is defined in the hands as the added width of the cortices being less than two-thirds the width of the medullary space. Joint-space narrowing that occurs with rheumatoid arthritis is symmetric. For example, when OA affects the hip, it leads to narrowing in the superolateral aspect of the joint space. Rheumatoid arthritis, by contrast, narrows the joint symmetrically (Figure 4–49). Rheumatoid arthritis is also associated with erosions (Figure 4–50) (**Key Point 4–5**).

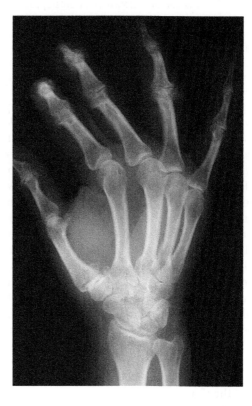

Figure 4–47.   Primary osteoarthritis. Conventional oblique view of the hand shows osteophytes at the distal interphalangeal joints and the first carpal metacarpal joint space. These are findings seen in primary osteoarthritis.

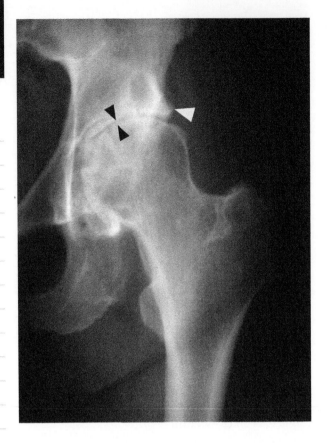

Figure 4–48.   Osteoarthritis. Conventional anteroposterior view of the hip shows superolateral migration with joint space narrowing (*black arrowheads*), sclerosis, and small osteophyte formation (*white arrowhead*).

Seronegative spondyloarthropathies are HLA-B27–positive disorders linked to the histocompatability antigen. These arthritides include *ankylosing spondylitis* (AS), *inflammatory bowel disease* (IBD), *psoriasis*, and *Reiter's syndrome* (also known as *reactive arthritis*). Some researchers believe that AS and IBD represent a spectrum of a disease in which some individuals present with bowel manifestations while others demonstrate the bone findings. These two disorders have generally symmetric involvement in the spine; when the large joints are involved, the joints resemble ones affected by rheumatoid arthritis. Psoriasis and Reiter's syndrome are very similar in their appearance, and these should be mentioned together in the differential diagnosis. Psoriasis often has skin manifestations, and Reiter's syndrome has a predilection for the feet. When the spine and sacroiliac joints are involved, a symmetric distribution is noted about 50% of the time.

Hallmarks of psoriasis (and reactive arthritis) include distal distribution (it is unusual for reactive arthritis to affect the hands), soft tissue swelling ("sausage" digits), and proliferative erosions (new

bone formation in addition to erosion), periostitis, and asymmetric syndesmophytes (Figure 4–51) (Key Point 4–6). Syndesmophytes are vertically oriented bony protuberances from the vertebral body seen in the spondyloarthropathies. These are to be distinguished from osteophytes by their orientation. Osteophytes are horizontal before they become vertical and are seen in OA and DISH. Syndesmophytes are seen in AS, IBD, psoriasis, and reactive arthritis.

Recognition of sacroiliac (SI) joint involvement with erosions, sclerosis, or ankylosis (bony fusion)

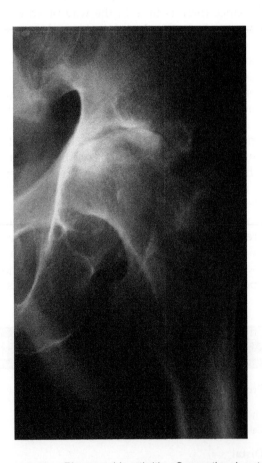

Figure 4–49.   Rheumatoid arthritis. Conventional anteroposterior radiograph of the left hip demonstrates circumferential narrowing of the joint space characteristic of rheumatoid arthritis. The bones are osteopenic, a finding also seen with rheumatoid arthritis.

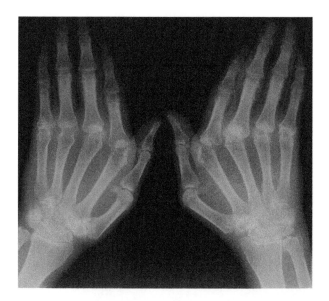

Figure 4–50. Rheumatoid arthritis. Conventional antero-posterior radiograph of bilateral hands demonstrates erosions of the metacarpal heads, ulnar subluxation of the proximal phalanges, and carpal crowding. The findings are bilateral and symmetric.

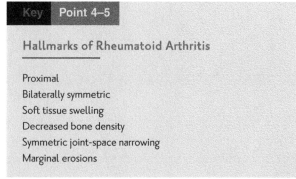

Key   Point 4–5

Hallmarks of Rheumatoid Arthritis

Proximal
Bilaterally symmetric
Soft tissue swelling
Decreased bone density
Symmetric joint-space narrowing
Marginal erosions

should prompt a short differential diagnosis that includes the spondyloarthropathies, OA (remember the discussion about OA having erosions in the SI joint?), infection (which can cause bone destruction), and gout (**Table 4–4**).

There are only two arthritides associated with crystals that you need know. These are gout and CPPD. The hallmarks of gout include normal mineralization, sharply marginated erosions (sclerotic margins), and soft tissue nodules (which may calcify in the setting of renal failure) (Figure 4–52) (**Key Point 4–7**). CPPD (pseudogout) has chondrocalcinosis (stippled calcification seen along the cartilage) and resembles OA but occurs in an atypical location for OA. That is, CPPD has osteophytes, joint-space narrowing, and sclerosis, but the joint affected is usually in the upper extremity (shoulder, radiocarpal joint, elbow) or isolated to the patellofemoral joint (**Key Point 4–8**). The typical locations of chondrocalcinosis in an individual with CPPD are the triangulofibrocartilage complex (TFCC) in the wrist, the meniscus in the knee, and the pubic symphysis. Other conditions associated with CPPD include primary hyperparathyroidism, hemochromatosis, and gout.

A destructive process that is often considered to be a type of arthritis is sarcoid. At first glance, it would appear to be an arthritis; however, on closer inspection, bone destruction without an organized distribution is noted (Figure 4–53).

AVN is bone death resulting from trauma, sickle cell disease, alcoholism, renal failure, pancreatitis, marrow-packing disorders, and idiopathic causes, to name just a few etiologies. In the early stages of AVN, the conventional x-rays are normal. Then increased sclerosis is noted along the joint line, followed by a subchondral lucency and then collapse (Figure 4–54). The earlier the diagnosis can be made, the earlier surgical intervention can be instituted. Secondary OA can be seen in patients with collapse who have not had surgical intervention. Because early diagnosis is imperative for timely surgery, MRI plays a key role when the conventional x-rays are normal (Figure 4–55).

Bone Tumors

The goal for this section is not to make you a bone radiologist, but to make you aware of some helpful clues for benign versus aggressive lesions using information available in this section and your application of logic. Notice that I have carefully chosen my words—"benign" and "aggressive" rather than benign versus malignant. This will become important as you read through this discussion.

The best way to make the distinction between benign versus aggressive processes is the "zone of transition." This is defined as the border between the lesion and the surrounding bone. If you can draw with a fine line the edge of the lesion, then that represents a narrow zone of transition or a benign process (Figure 4–56). If you feel that you can't really tell where the abnormal bone ends and the normal bone begins, you are probably looking at a wide zone of transition or an aggressive lesion (Figure 4–57). *Permeative process* is a term often used to describe an aggressive lesion with a wide zone of transition.

Periosteal reaction is characterized as benign or aggressive. Benign periosteal reaction is smooth, thick, homogeneous, and undulating, similar to the callus formation seen around a fracture (Figure 4–58). Aggressive periosteal reaction is described with terms such as *lamellated, sunburst,* and *Codman's*

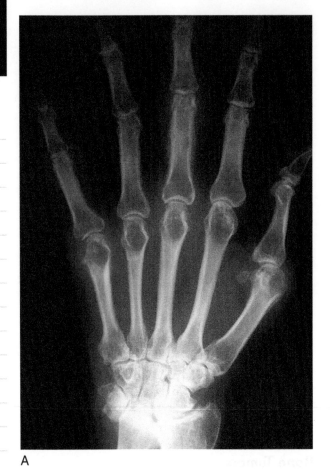

A

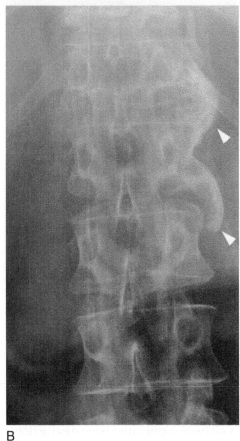

B

Figure 4–51. Psoriasis. A, Conventional anteroposterior (AP) radiograph of the hand demonstrates a sausage digit of the third finger of the right hand with proliferative changes along the third proximal phalanx. These findings are characteristic of psoriasis.

B, Coned-down conventional AP x-ray of the spine shows large syndesmophytes (*arrowheads*) emanating from the lateral aspect of T12 and L1. Syndesmophytes are present in the spondyloarthropathies.

triangle (Figure 4–59). Benign disease processes such as infection can have aggressive periosteal reaction. Therefore, using periosteal reaction as a discriminator for benign versus malignant processes is not recommended.

Despite the fact that you might see cortical destruction around a lesion, it is not an indication that the process is malignant. Don't be fooled by

the fact that some benign lesions can thin the cortex of the bone such that it is imperceptible on conventional x-rays.

Many appropriate differential diagnoses are based on the patient's age. Aggressive lesions in a young individual (<30 years of age) would include two malignant tumors and two benign processes. The most common malignant tumors in this age

---

Key Point 4–6

Hallmarks of Psoriasis and Reactive Arthritis

Distal distribution
Soft tissue swelling
Proliferative erosions
Periostitis
Asymmetric syndesmophytes

Table 4–4 Arthritides with Sacroiliac Joint Involvement

Ankylosing spondylitis
Inflammatory bowel disease
Psoriasis
Reactive arthritis
Osteoarthritis
Infection
Gout

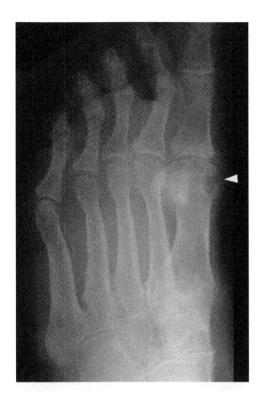

Figure 4–52.   Gout. Conventional oblique x-ray demonstrates a large erosion with a sclerotic margin and overhanging edge, characteristic of gout (*arrowhead*).

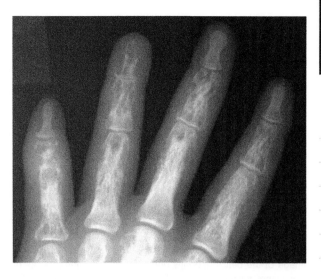

Figure 4–53.   Sarcoid. Conventional anteroposterior radiograph of the fingers demonstrates a "lace-like" pattern of all the phalanges. Note that this is not a joint process. This is pathognomonic for sarcoid involvement.

| Key | Point 4–7 |

Hallmarks of Gout

Normal mineralization
Sharply marginated erosions
Soft tissue nodules

| Key | Point 4–8 |

Hallmarks of Calcium Pyrophosphate Deposition Disease (CPPD)

Identical to osteoarthritis (OA)
Atypical location for OA
Chondrocalcinosis

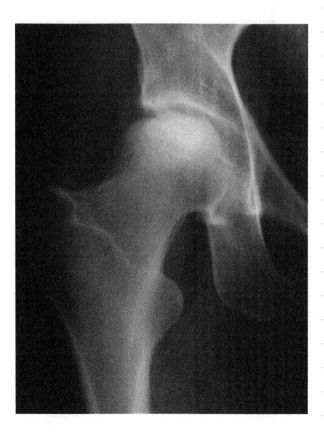

Figure 4–54.   Avascular necrosis (AVN). Conventional anteroposterior radiograph of the right hip demonstrates sclerosis and irregularity along the femoral head. The findings are characteristic of AVN.

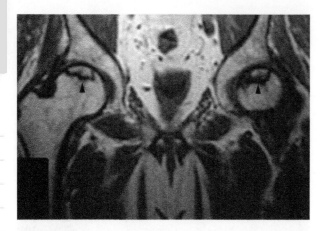

Figure 4–55.   Avascular necrosis (AVN). T1-weighted coronal image of the pelvis and hips demonstrates curvilinear areas of low signal within the femoral heads bilaterally (*arrowheads*), diagnostic of AVN.

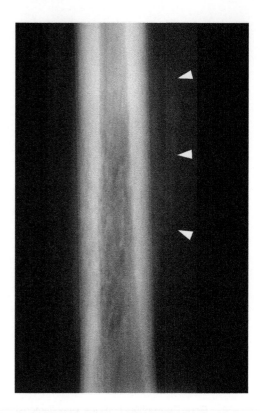

Figure 4–57.   Wide zone of transition. Coned-down view of the femur demonstrates a wide zone of transition, suggesting an aggressive process. The associated benign periosteal reaction (*arrowheads*) indicates that the lesion cannot be a malignant process. This was osteomyelitis due to *Streptococcus* viridans.

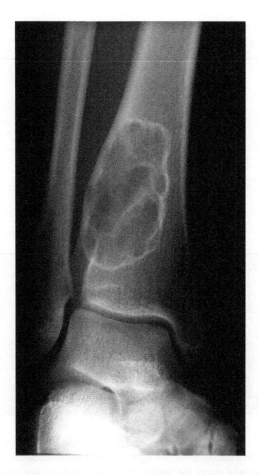

Figure 4–56.   Narrow zone of transition. Conventional antero-posterior x-ray demonstrates a well-defined lesion with a thin sclerotic border. You can draw an edge around the lesion with a pencil. That is a good indicator that it is a narrow zone of transition and therefore a benign process. This is a nonossifying fibroma.

group are osteogenic sarcoma and Ewing's sarcoma. The two benign processes that can mimic the appearance of these malignant tumors are infection and an entity called *eosinophilic granuloma* (histiocytosis). These latter two entities get mentioned in just about every differential diagnosis in someone younger than 30 years of age who has a bone lesion, because these lesions can look like anything (aggressive, benign, lytic, large, small) (**Table 4–5**). Osteosarcoma is a bone-forming tumor. If you identify a tumor that is making osteoid in a disorganized fashion, it will be an osteosarcoma. However, one of the imaging appearances of an osteosarcoma is to resemble Ewing's sarcoma. That is why these sarcomas are mentioned together when looking at an aggressive lytic lesion. Contrary to many books and written board examinations, osteosarcoma is a tumor found in patients younger than 30 years of age. There is no "bimodal distribution." The only time this occurs in older individuals is in malignant degeneration of a previously irradiated bone or in Paget's disease that has undergone malignant degeneration.

Multiple myeloma and metastatic disease have protean appearances and should appear on all

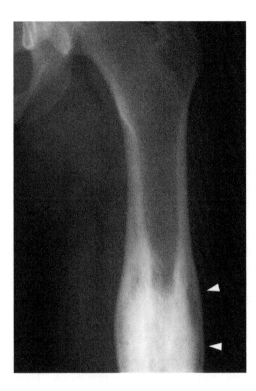

Figure 4–58.   Benign periosteal reaction. Conventional antero-posterior radiograph demonstrates thick cortical reaction along the midshaft of the femur, characteristic of benign periosteal reaction in this patient with chronic infection.

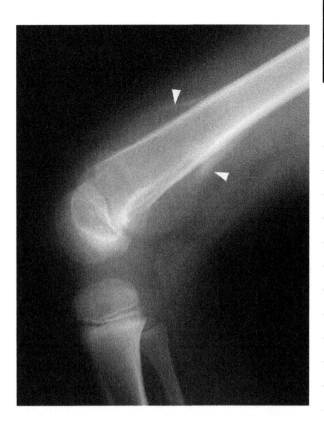

Figure 4–59.   Aggressive periosteal reaction. Conventional lateral x-ray in a child shows a Codman's triangle (*arrowheads*) with a soft tissue mass. Pathologic analysis identified this lesion as an osteosarcoma.

differential diagnoses in patients older than 50 years of age. If you always think of them together, you will never forget to mention these lesions. Another entity that was previously mentioned that has no respect for age or appearance is infection (**Table 4–6**).

Multiple myeloma is almost always a lytic process, whereas metastatic disease can be lytic, blastic, or mixed. Renal cell carcinoma and thyroid carcinoma metastases are always lytic in appearance.

Chondroid matrix can be seen in both benign and malignant processes. Chondroid matrix has calcifications in a characteristic shape of arcs and circles. The presence of matrix is not helpful as a discriminator for benign or malignant processes. Similarly, fibrous matrix can be seen in lytic lesions but has no implication in distinguishing benign from aggressive processes.

Metabolic Bone Disease

This topic likely rivals arthritis in level of excitement! Here it will be discussed in a logical way appropriate for your level of training. *Osteoporosis* is defined as diminished bone quantity in which the bone is otherwise normal. This contrasts with *osteomalacia*, in which the bone quantity is normal but the quality of the bone is abnormal due to lack of normal

mineralization. The main radiographic finding of osteoporosis is thinning of the cortex. Senile osteoporosis affects the older patient population. Disuse osteoporosis can be seen in a patient of any age as a result of immobilization from a variety of causes. Occasionally, aggressive osteoporosis from

Table 4–5	Aggressive Lesions in a Patient Younger Than 30 Years of Age
Osteosarcoma	
Ewing's sarcoma	
Eosinophilic granuloma	
Infection	

Table 4–6	Lesions Affecting Patients Older Than 50 Years of Age
Metastatic disease	
Multiple myeloma	
Infection	

disuse can mimic a permeative lesion (pseudo-permeative) such as Ewing's sarcoma (young patient) or metastatic disease and multiple myeloma (older patient) because the multiple cortical holes that project over the medullary space mimic a permeative process. Recognizing the holes within the cortex makes the distinction between the permeative process (no cortical holes) and that of pseudopermeative process (cortical holes) (Figures 4–60 and 4–61).

Osteomalacia is the result of too much nonmineralized osteoid. The most common cause is renal osteodystrophy. In children this is called rickets. Hyperparathyroidism is also associated with osteomalacia. In addition, subperiosteal bone resorption and osteosclerosis can also be seen on conventional radiographs. Subperiosteal bone resorption is best identified on the radial aspect of the middle phalanges. Additional locations include the sacroiliac joint and proximal tibia. Brown tumors are lytic lesions that are often expansile, can be aggressive in appearance, and are seen in hyperparathyroidism (primary and secondary) (Figures 4–62 through 4–64).

There are a few abnormalities that are associated with dense bones. The entities you are most likely to encounter are *sickle cell disease*, *myelofibrosis*, *metastatic disease*, and *Paget's disease*. In *sickle cell disease*, there would also be other findings, such as H-shaped vertebral bodies, as well as evidence of AVN (bone death), usually seen in the femoral head and humeral head (Figure 4–65). *Myelofibrosis* is associated with splenomegaly and evidence of extramedullary hematopoiesis. *Metastatic disease* can present as diffuse or focal lesions. Clinical history and multiplicity of lesions is helpful in suggesting this diagnosis. *Paget's disease* has three phases: a purely lytic phase, a sclerotic phase, and a mixed lytic-sclerotic phase. Generally, Paget's disease starts at one end of the bone and goes toward the other. The bone is usually overgrown and associated with thickening of the trabecula as well as cortices. The other entities described here associated with dense bones will not demonstrate this property.

Films NOT to Order

This section could be one of the most significant that you will encounter in this book. That is, a consideration of films that should NOT be ordered. Let me introduce this to you in an organized

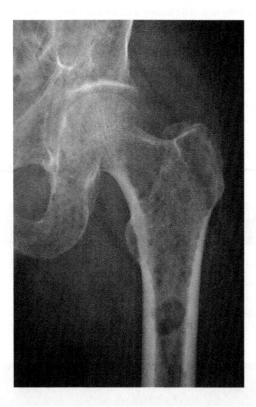

Figure 4–60.   Permeative process. Conventional x-ray of the hip and femur demonstrates multiple lucencies and a permeative process, suggesting an aggressive lesion. In patients older than 50 years of age, the differential diagnosis must include multiple myeloma and metastatic disease. This was multiple myeloma.

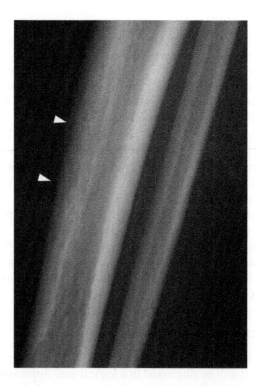

Figure 4–61.   Pseudopermeative process. Coned-down lateral film of the tibia demonstrates a pseudopermeative process. This lesion demonstrates holes in the cortex in the distal aspect of the tibia (*arrowheads*) in this patient with a hemangioma.

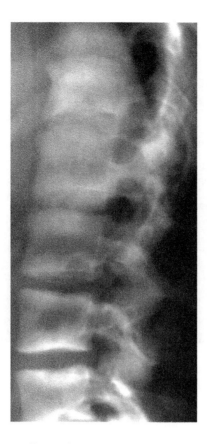

Figure 4–62.   Rugger jersey spine. Conventional lateral x-ray shows bands of sclerosis at the end plates, consistent with a rugger jersey spine in a patient with hyperparathyroidism.

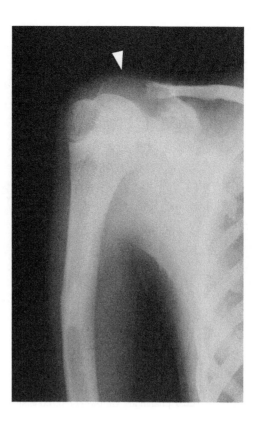

Figure 4–63.   Brown tumor. Conventional anteroposterior radiograph of the humerus and shoulder demonstrating an expansile lytic lesion of the acromion (*arrowhead*) along with bowing of the humerus and a sclerotic focus in the humerus. The constellation of findings suggests hyperparathyroidism, and the expansile lytic lesion is a brown tumor.

progression. Think about the utility of skull films. In the setting of trauma, what is to be gained by doing a skull series? Follow the thought process all the way through. If your patient has a fracture, what is it you are concerned with? Are you going to put a metal plate or cast on the skull to treat the fracture? You are most interested in the consequence of the fracture, which is an intracranial bleed. The patient may have suffered an epidural, subdural, or subarachnoid hemorrhage. Therefore, a noncontrast head CT is the radiology examination of choice. A noncontrast head CT will allow visualization of acute blood that is the same attenuation as the contrast material. Using bone windows, fractures can be seen as lucencies which appear more sharply defined than sutures. Is there ever a time when skull films are necessary? The answer is yes, but not in the setting of trauma (except child abuse, when you are looking for previous episodes of trauma). Skull films are valuable in assessing patients who have multiple myeloma or metastatic disease to the skull, and in children for assessing involvement of the skull with eosinophilic granuloma and child abuse.

A facial bones series is a different examination from a sinus series, which in turn is different from a nasal bone series. So which, if any, of these examinations is useful? As it turns out, a facial bone series is a good screening examination for facial trauma. Examinations that are positive or equivocal will get follow-up CT examinations through the facial bones. Let's say that you are seeing a patient who complains of "sinus" headaches. What is the yield of a sinus series? Perhaps the sinus series will show air/fluid levels in the sinuses suggesting acute sinusitis. But what if it doesn't? Do you not treat your patient? You don't want to treat the x-ray. You treat the patient. Bone destruction, which can occur with chronic sinusitis, is a very late finding on conventional x-rays. It can be more readily appreciated and seen earlier on CT examination. In addition, CT can reveal the presence of a mass and allows evaluation of the structures that make up the sinuses and osteomeatal complex. A CT of the paranasal sinuses would be a much better consideration for evaluation of suspected sinus disease. The radiation dose to the lens of the eye can be

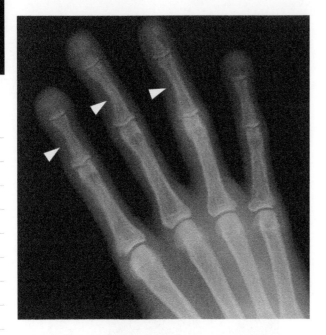

Figure 4–64.   Subperiosteal bone resorption. Conventional x-ray of the hand demonstrates distal tuft resorption as well as osteopenia and subperiosteal bone resorption of the radial aspect of the middle phalanges (*arrowheads*), consistent with hyperparathyroidism.

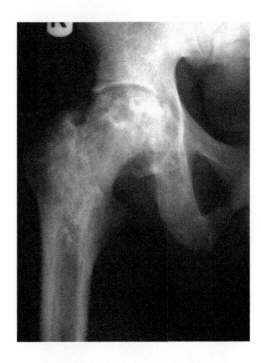

Figure 4–65.   Sickle cell disease. Conventional x-ray of the right hip demonstrates dense bones as well as increased sclerosis of the femoral head representing avascular necrosis.

minimized using CT, and the cost is nearly the same as for conventional imaging.

When is it appropriate to get images of the nasal bones? In the setting of acute trauma, will you cast the nose if a fracture is present? Patients are treated with supportive measures. Should the fracture lead to a cosmetic problem, CT is performed in the preoperative setting for repair. There really is little utility for nasal bone films. The lens of the eye also gets exposed to unnecessary radiation during this conventional film examination.

When is it appropriate to order rib films? If you answered "trauma," you are missing the point of this section. What is the treatment for a rib fracture? Will you not treat the patient for the pain even if you don't see a fracture? You should be appropriately concerned about the potential complication of rib fractures, and that would be the injury to the pleura. The best way to assess for that injury is a chest x-ray to evaluate for a pneumothorax or a hemothorax (hydrothorax). Good detailed rib films may not reveal nondisplaced rib fractures. Many times rib fractures are identified on follow-up films after callus has formed around the fracture. So why is it that rib films are still listed on hospital billing sheets? Well, think about the patient with a rib lesion such as metastatic disease, multiple myeloma, or other tumors that can affect the rib. In these

patients, rib films can be useful. Trauma, however, is not the time to perform a rib series. In the setting of nonaccidental trauma, rib films can be helpful in identifying previous episodes of abuse.

Consideration must be given to evaluation of the lumbar spine. Suffice it to say that patients who have sustained trauma to the lumbar spine deserve conventional x-rays of the spine for further evaluation. But what if the patient doesn't have trauma but has back pain? Clinical history is very important in this setting. If the patient is older than 50 years of age, diseases other than disc disease and degenerative disease can occur. These include metastatic disease, multiple myeloma, and osteoporotic collapse. So all patients older than 50 years of age deserve conventional radiography of the lumbar spine when presenting with back pain. If you are examining a young patient with possible disc disease or paraspinous pain, conventional x-rays are not going to help you with that diagnosis. Therefore, why risk the radiation exposure to the gonads (particularly in females whose gonads cannot be shielded for this examination)?

Children can have a couple of entities in the spine that are unique to them. For instance, a pars interarticularis defect often presents in teenagers, as do early findings of spondyloarthropathies. Additionally, a painful scoliosis can be the result of an osteoid osteoma, a small tumor that can be found in the posterior elements in children. Careful history and physical examination will help you determine the utility of conventional x-rays when evaluating patients complaining of back pain.

It really goes without saying, though I'll say it anyway, that x-rays should be ordered if you are going to alter the treatment of the patient based upon the findings. In keeping with this theory, ankle films are an often-requested examination in emergency departments and clinics around the country. Ankle sprains occur with alarming frequency. It is likely that many of you reading this book have turned an ankle. But, how many of you went to the emergency room for it? I suspect few. Perhaps some of you have learned of the Ottawa rules. These rules are essentially criteria that should be met before considering ordering an ankle series. The criteria are a result of a study performed in Ottawa, Canada (thus the name) to more clearly define the appropriate indication for ankle films. The Ottawa ankle rules can significantly reduce the number of unnecessary ankle radiographs. The rules are not a substitute for sound clinical judgment, but they augment findings in the history and physical examination to help the clinician determine the appropriateness of ankle films. If the rules are met and radiographs are avoided, it is unlikely, especially with good communication and follow-up, that a patient will turn out to have a significant fracture. Assess for tenderness over the inferior pole of medial, lateral, and posterior malleolus. Assess the patient's ability to bear weight. If the patient cannot take four steps at the time of injury and at the time of examination, x-rays are recommended. If the patient has tenderness along the base of the fifth metatarsal or navicular bone, x-rays should be obtained. Inversion injuries can lead to base of the fifth metatarsal fractures, and this bone should be carefully evaluated on all ankle images. Similarly, the anterior process of the calcaneus can be fractured, and this can be easily overlooked. Therefore, this area of the bone should be carefully inspected on the lateral x-ray. Applying the aforementioned criteria and evaluating the x-rays that are obtained should yield a high positive predictive value for an ankle series.

Emergencies

There are just a few emergencies in musculoskeletal radiology. Air identified in the soft tissues is a surgical emergency once inquiry has excluded surgical or traumatic reasons for the presence of air. These infections ascend quickly and can lead to serious consequences, such as amputation or even death if the infection disseminates quickly.

Dislocations should be reduced in a timely fashion. Hip dislocations can lead to the development of AVN if left in a nonreduced position. Follow-up CT after reduction is helpful to exclude shear fractures with fragments retained in the joint space. Other dislocations that require timely diagnosis and reduction include lunate, perilunate, and Lisfranc dislocations.

Certainly, careful evaluation of the spine is imperative in excluding fractures and dislocations. Follow-up examination with CT is necessary in all cases with fractures. A careful evaluation of the lines in cervical spine films and assessment of the interpedicular distance on AP radiographs will determine involvement of the posterior elements.

Suggested Reading List

Greenspan A: Orthopedic Imaging: A Practical Approach. Philadelphia, Lippincott Williams & Wilkins, 2004.

Helms CA: Fundamentals of Skeletal Radiology, 3rd ed. Philadelphia, WB Saunders, 2005.

Resnick D, Kransdorf MJ: Bone and Joint Imaging, 3rd ed. Philadelphia, WB Saunders, 2005.

Chapter 5

Neuroimaging

Chapter outline

Technique

Anatomy

Evaluation

Trauma

Stroke

Tumors

Infection

Disc Disease

Emergencies

In many general radiology textbooks, the neuroimaging chapter is the largest chapter in the book. There is a tremendous amount of anatomy to be learned and a great number of disease processes that can affect the brain and spine. Additionally, there are a number of neurologic disorders that are unique to the pediatric population. In keeping with the approach to this book, the disorders that are more commonly encountered and are likely to cause acute decompensation will be discussed. I have included a brief discussion of disc disease, because you may have to review magnetic resonance imaging (MRI) examinations of this problem with your patients. For a detailed review of anatomy as well as a discussion of additional topics mentioned in the tables, the reading list is helpful.

Technique

A variety of modalities are used to evaluate the brain and the spine. In emergency situations, computed tomography (CT) is most often used. There is great utility of MRI in the evaluation of diseases affecting the brain and the spinal cord, and more and more often sophisticated imaging is being performed with mapping techniques, functional imaging, and spectroscopy to identify subtle areas of disease and the affect on behavior and function. These techniques make for fascinating reading, just not in this chapter! Ultrasonography is used in neonates for evaluation of bleeds and hydrocephalus. The open sutures allow easier access to the brain, because the transducer does not have to penetrate bone in order to see brain matter. Angiography (conventional as well as magnetic resonance [MR] angiography and CT angiography) allows for diagnostic capability of vascular diseases in the brain as well as the vessels leading to the brain.

CT is the study of choice for evaluating hemorrhage. Hemorrhage can occur in the setting of acute trauma as well as stroke. In the patient suffering "the worst headache of her life," hemorrhage in the subarachnoid space certainly must be a consideration. It is imperative that intravenous contrast material NOT be administered in the setting of evaluation for hemorrhage. Think about this for a moment. Why would you not want a contrast agent to be administered? The answer is rather basic.

What attenuation is blood? What attenuation is contrast? Since they are both high attenuation, blood can be overlooked with contrast administration. The CT can be performed using bone and neurologic algorithms (Figure 5–1). Detail in the skull and spine is well delineated with bone windows. This allows for identification of fractures. The implication of a skull fracture is to look at the brain parenchyma deep to the fracture for associated collection of fluid or hemorrhage. It is often difficult to identify skull fractures, especially when trying to distinguish them from sutures. A fracture often will demonstrate crisp margins, whereas a suture line is more irregular in its appearance. As mentioned in Chapter 4, when a fracture in the spine has been identified or is suspected on conventional x-ray, CT examination is performed. The ability to acquire thin slices and render reformations is very useful in identifying the extent of the fracture.

Another utility for CT is in the evaluation of masses. Whereas MRI can often very precisely identify a mass and the associated edema, CT is an excellent tool for making the initial diagnosis. Intravenous contrast is helpful when identifying a mass or abscess. Sometimes the presence of a mass within the brain parenchyma (intra-axial) can lead to a shift of brain parenchyma (herniation) (Figure 5–2). This is an important observation, and it is readily evaluated with CT. Herniation of vital structures can lead to acute decompensation and death if not recognized.

MRI is an excellent modality for the evaluation of both benign and malignant masses. Often the signal intensity of the lesion and the pattern of enhancement can narrow the differential diagnosis. When evaluating a patient with a stroke, MRI is more sensitive. It shows the edema in the brain parenchyma to better advantage than CT does. The ability to visualize the posterior fossa is made much easier with MRI than with CT. The posterior fossa is seen on just a few images with CT and has some artifact associated with the skull base. When evaluating a patient who has had a history of brain trauma, MRI in the delayed setting can be helpful by identifying blood products at different stages. Because blood in the subarachnoid space, particularly in the acute setting, is similar in signal intensity to cerebrospinal fluid (CSF), MRI is not recommended. Suspected cases of subarachnoid hemorrhage should be evaluated with CT. Although bone marrow is well seen with MRI, skull fractures and even the small bones of the posterior elements can be difficult to evaluate on MRI. Therefore, for evaluation of bone detail in the setting of fracture, CT is recommended as the study of choice. For associated injuries to the spinal cord or nerve roots, MRI is the way to go.

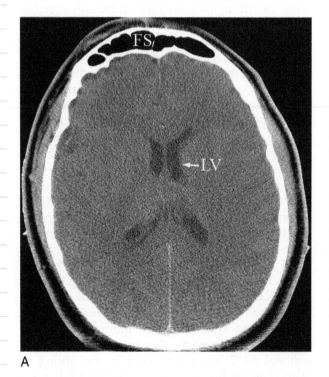

A

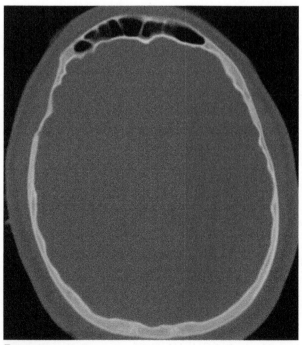

B

Figure 5–1. Normal brain. A, CT at the level of the frontal horns, a part of the ventricular system viewed in brain windows. These are normal in appearance. FS, frontal sinus; LV, lateral ventricles. B, CT at the same level as A viewed with bone algorithm.

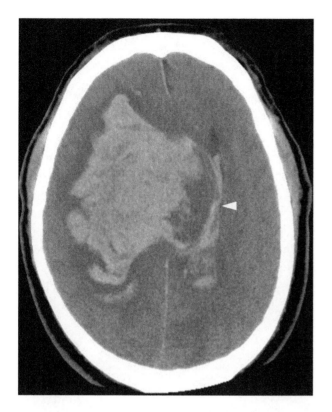

Figure 5–2. Intraparenchymal hemorrhage. CT without the administration of intravenous contrast material. High attenuation with marked mass effect is blood in the brain. Note the shift of the midline structures to the left hemisphere of the brain with blood in the lateral ventricle (*arrowhead*).

Table 5–1 Use of CT Versus MRI
Neurologic CT
Hemorrhage (no intravenous contrast)
Fracture (skull, spine)
Mass (abscess, tumor) with intravenous contrast (generally less sensitive than MRI)
Neurologic MRI
Mass (benign or malignant)
Stroke (more sensitive than CT)
Posterior fossa lesion
Later in course of cranial trauma
NOT for fracture or subarachnoid hemorrhage
Spine
Neuroangiography (conventional angiography, MR angiography, CT angiography)
Intracranial circulation (vasculitis, thrombus, dissection)

When you are trying to determine which study is best for your patient, sometimes it is both studies. Each technique excels in different areas. Because the soft tissues in the spinal canal are so well seen with MRI, this technique should be performed if there is concern for disc disease or cord abnormalities. If, however, you are caring for a patient who is not MRI compatible, a CT may be warranted. Some centers still perform CT myelography to assess mass effect on the thecal sac and cord. This is not a benign procedure, and strong consideration should be given to performing CT myelography versus conventional CT imaging alone. In general, CT of the brain is performed if the onset of neurologic symptoms is within 48 hours. If the problem has persisted longer than 3 days, an MRI is recommended. The MRI can accurately depict the region of the brain involved and the compartment of a localized extra-axial fluid collection, and it is extremely sensitive in assessing the extent of parenchymal injury to the brain.

If the imaging study suggests a vascular lesion (aneurysm or arteriovenous malformation), angiography is recommended. MR angiography is being utilized more frequently in place of catheter angiography. If the initial study suggests a tumor, intravenous contrast material should be administered. A carotid ultrasound examination would be indicated for a patient who does not demonstrate an abnormality on CT or MRI but has symptoms of a stroke or transient ischemic attack. Intravenous contrast is not recommended in the acute setting of neurologic abnormality unless abscess or tumor is being considered. MRI with gadolinium administration is recommended in the setting of seizures in adults, history of cancer (looking for mass lesion), or infectious disease (looking for abscess or abnormal enhancement) (**Table 5–1**).

A number of disease processes can affect the vessels in and leading to the brain, including vasculitis, thrombus, and dissection. These processes can be assessed with conventional angiography as well as MR angiography and CT angiography (**Table 5–2**).

Anatomy

There is much anatomy to know in the brain and spine. However, when assessing a CT in the middle of the night, you won't need to know all of the anatomy. For reference, a few images of the brain have been included for review of anatomy. Figures 5–3 through 5–6 show basic anatomy at the level of the posterior fossa as well as at the level of the circle of Willis. Figure 5–7 demonstrates the spaces in the brain.

Table 5–2 **Neuroimaging Modalities**

CT
MRI
Ultrasonography (infants)
Angiography

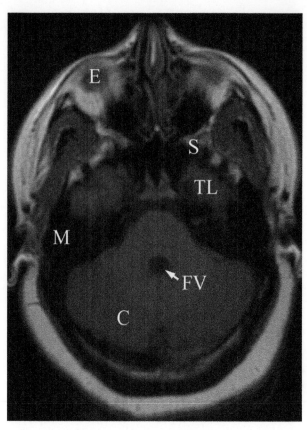

Figure 5–4. MRI showing normal anatomy at the level of the posterior fossa. T1-weighted axial image (fluid is dark). C, cerebellum; E, eye; FV, fourth ventricle; M, mastoid air cells; S, sphenoid sinus; TL, temporal lobe.

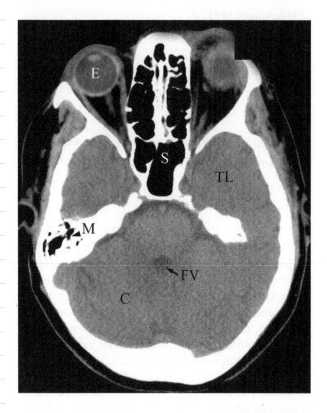

Figure 5–3. CT showing normal anatomy at the level of the posterior fossa. C, cerebellum; E, eye; FV, fourth ventricle; M, mastoid air cells; S, sphenoid sinus; TL, temporal lobe.

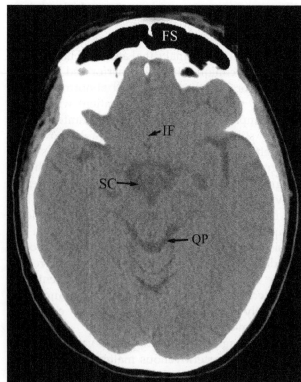

Figure 5–5. CT showing normal anatomy at the circle of Willis. Brain windows. FS, frontal sinus; IF, interhemispheric fissure; QP, quadrigeminal plate cistern; SC, suprasellar cistern.

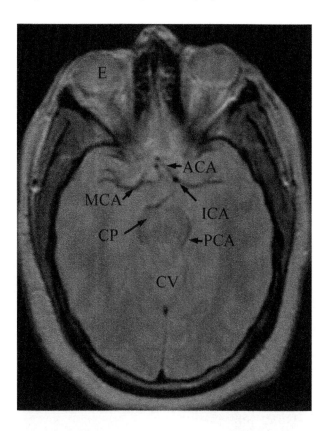

Figure 5–6.   MRI showing normal anatomy at the level of the middle cerebral artery. T1-weighted axial image. ACA, anterior cerebral artery; CP, cerebral peduncle; CV, cerebellar vermis; E, eye; ICA, internal carotid artery; MCA, middle cerebral artery; PCA, posterior cerebral artery.

Evaluation

Clearly there is more anatomy to know, but my editors would have killed me if I had included all of it in this book. There is so much anatomy in such a small space. I will review a few principles that will help you to avoid overlooking a neurosurgical emergency. A review of basic concepts is in order. A *mass* is a space-occupying lesion. The brain is confined within the calvarium. Therefore, the mass will displace normal cerebral structures away from it. The normal midline structures will be shifted away from the mass. The sulci adjacent to the mass may be effaced, because the CSF occupying the sulci is displaced by the mass. Ipsilateral ventricular structures can be compressed by a mass, rendering them smaller than the contralateral ventricle. If a mass is identified, the first assessment is whether the mass is *intra-axial*, within the brain and causing expansion, or *extra-axial*, outside the brain and compressing it. Usually, this is an easy distinction, but sometimes it is not. Intra-axial masses are less easily treated and are dangerous to the patient. Some examples include intracranial hemorrhage, primary intracranial tumors, metastatic lesions, and brain abscesses. Extra-axial masses are more readily treated and include subdural or epidural hematomas, meningiomas, dermoid or epidermoid cysts, and arachnoid cysts (**Key Points 5–1 and 5–2**).

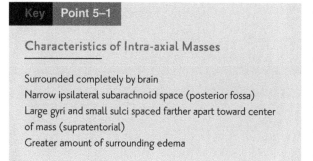

Key   Point 5–1

Characteristics of Intra-axial Masses

Surrounded completely by brain
Narrow ipsilateral subarachnoid space (posterior fossa)
Large gyri and small sulci spaced farther apart toward center of mass (supratentorial)
Greater amount of surrounding edema

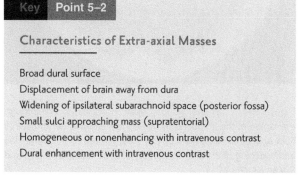

Key   Point 5–2

Characteristics of Extra-axial Masses

Broad dural surface
Displacement of brain away from dura
Widening of ipsilateral subarachnoid space (posterior fossa)
Small sulci approaching mass (supratentorial)
Homogeneous or nonenhancing with intravenous contrast
Dural enhancement with intravenous contrast

Figure 5–7.   Sketch demonstrating subarachnoid, epidural, and subdural spaces.

Once you have determined the intra-axial or extra-axial location, check out the density of the mass. Is it white? Are you dealing with hemorrhage? More about that later.

Atrophy is a result of too little brain tissue. Findings include widening of ipsilateral sulci or enlargement of the ventricle adjacent to the lesion. The brain doesn't experience midline shift toward the side of the atrophy (unless it is congenital hemiatrophy). A pattern of diffuse atrophy should prompt inquiry as to the patient's age. Patients older than 65 years of age with normal cognitive function can have findings of atrophy on CT (Figure 5–8). If the patient is younger than 65 years of age, white matter diseases should be considered. However, three common causes of reversible atrophy are related to dehydration and starvation. Addison's disease, eating disorders such as anorexia and bulimia, and alcoholism are associated with correctable forms of atrophy. Although the neurotoxic effects of alcohol are not reversible, the nutritional deficiencies may be corrected, resulting in a more normal-appearing brain on imaging studies (**Table 5–3**).

Table 5–3 **Reversible Causes of Cerebral Atrophy**
Addison's disease
Eating disorders (bulimia, anorexia nervosa)
Alcoholism

It is important to understand the concept of *herniation.* Herniation refers to a shift of the midline structures. Symmetry is important when evaluating a CT or MRI of the brain. The middle of the brain should be in the middle of the skull, and the two hemispheres should resemble each other. Shift of the midline structures represents mass effect on the side away from which the midline is displaced. There are no lesions in the brain, as there are in the chest, that will cause "shift" to the side that is collapsed (Figure 5–9). As you noticed in Figures 5–3 through 5–6, the interventricular septum (septum pellucidum) and the third ventricle are located in the midline. Therefore, no subfalcine

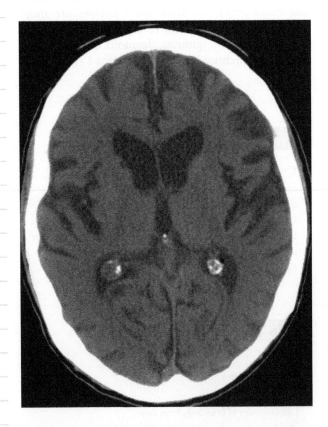

Figure 5–8. Cerebral atrophy. Axial noncontrast CT through the region of the frontal horns. Note the increased cerebrospinal fluid space, as illustrated by the enlargement of the ventricles and widening of the sulci. (Courtesy of Srini Mukundan, MD, and Susan Kealey, MD.)

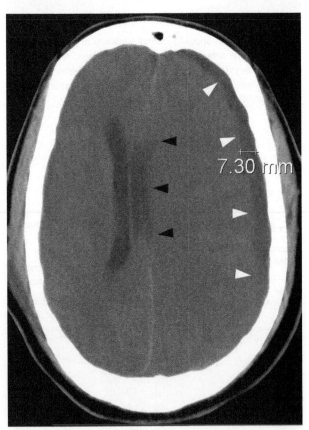

Figure 5–9. Subfalcine herniation. CT with brain windows showing a low-attenuation collection in the subdural space that (*white arrowheads*) that has caused a midline shift to the right with compression of the lateral ventricle (*black arrowheads*).

herniation is present. Herniation can occur through the falx cerebri (subfalcine) as well as through the tentorium cerebellum (ascending or descending transtentorial herniation), and cerebellar tonsil herniation can occur through the foramen magnum.

In addition to evaluating the midline, symmetry should be assessed. The pattern of sulci and gyri should be symmetric from one hemisphere to the other. The sulci should extend to the inner table of the skull. In older patients, this may not be the case due to atrophy that can occur. However, care should be taken not to assume that atrophy has caused the appearance of sulci to not extend to the inner table. Other causes include opacification of the subarachnoid space with blood or the presence of an extracerebral fluid collection. These fluid collections may resemble the same density as brain parenchyma. So, when evaluating the periphery of the brain, exercise caution and exclude the aforementioned causes if the sulci do not appear to extend to the inner table. Subtle but important signs of an intracranial mass include distortion of the CSF spaces of the posterior fossa. This area is often difficult to see on CT, and therefore careful scrutiny of this area of the brain is strongly encouraged. Key structures to evaluate in the posterior fossa and at the base of the brain include the quadrigeminal plate and the suprasellar cistern (see Figure 5–5). The quadrigeminal plate has the appearance of a smile on axial images. The smile should be symmetric. Causes of asymmetry include a mass in the cerebellum or brain stem, subarachnoid hemorrhage, and transtentorial herniation resulting in rotation of the brain stem and thus deformity of the smile. The suprasellar cistern should resemble a pentagon and have the attenuation of CSF. Asymmetry may be due to uncal herniation; opacification of the cistern may be due to subarachnoid hemorrhage or meningitis; and a central mass may be a result of a sellar or suprasellar tumor.

Evaluate the ventricular system. The lateral ventricles and CSF spaces are of low attenuation. The fourth ventricle in the posterior fossa is the most difficult to see on CT. Asymmetry of the fourth ventricle may be the only sign of a significant intracranial mass. Assess the size of the ventricular system. Enlarged lateral ventricles and third ventricle in the clinical setting of headache or signs of intracranial mass may represent hydrocephalus. This can be fatal if not treated, and it should be distinguished from enlarged ventricles in a patient who has atrophy. Signs suggesting atrophy include frontal and temporal horn enlargement, round appearance to the anterior portion of the third ventricle, and appearance of the sulci (as mentioned previously) (Key Point 5–3).

Key Point 5–3

Search Pattern for Neurosurgical Emergencies

Presence of white (blood)
Middle of brain in middle of skull
Symmetry of hemispheres
Quadrigeminal plate (smile) and suprasellar cistern
    (pentagon) are of cerebrospinal fluid (CSF) density and
    symmetric
Fourth ventricle midline and symmetric
Size of lateral ventricles
Appearance of sulci
Gray-white distinction

Once a mass is identified and its intra-axial or extra-axial location determined, a count of the number of lesions should be made. Multiple lesions are likely the result of widespread or systemic disease. A single infarct is likely the result of ipsilateral carotid artery disease, whereas multiple infarcts are likely the result of cardiac emboli.

If the lesion is within the brain, the next determination is whether gray matter, white matter, or both are involved. The gray and white matter components of the brain should be visible as two distinct densities. Obliteration of the distinction between gray and white matter indicates edema in this region. Disorders that affect the gray matter are most often infarct, trauma, or encephalitis. Acute lesions are associated with mass effect, whereas chronic lesions are associated with tissue loss.

An expansile lesion involving just the white matter has associated *vasogenic* edema. This pattern of edema is frond-like and is lower density on CT but demonstrates increased signal on T2-weighted images on MRI (Figure 5–10). It is caused by disturbances in capillary junctions that occur with tumors, abscesses, or hematomas. More edema is typically seen with abscesses or tumors than with hematomas. White matter expansion associated with gray matter involvement and low density on CT or high T2 signal on MRI is *cytotoxic* edema. This edema is caused by increased tissue water content due to the neuropathologic response to cell death. When this constellation of findings is present, infarct, trauma, and encephalitis should be considered (Figure 5–11).

Trauma

Noncontrast CT is the imaging modality of choice in head trauma. As mentioned in Chapter 4, skull films aren't useful and do not correlate with the

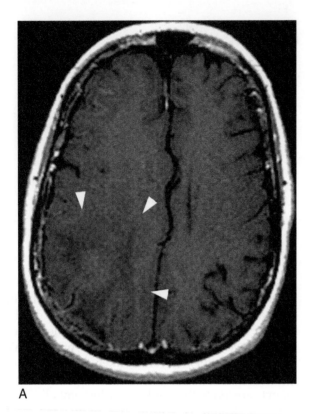

A

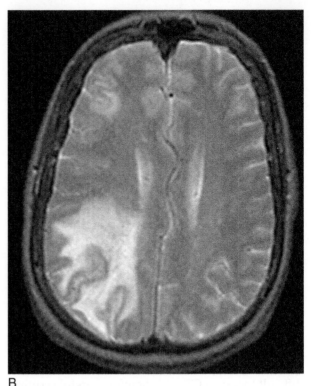

B

Figure 5–10. Vasogenic edema. A, T1-weighted image through the upper portion of the brain demonstrates low signal in the posterior white matter (*arrowheads*). B, T2-weighted image at the same level as A shows the increased signal of the vasogenic edema that is "frond-like" in appearance, involving only the white matter. (Courtesy of Srini Mukundan, MD, and Susan Kealey, MD.)

severity of intracranial injury. MRI is best used to evaluate subacute and chronic trauma as well as suspected child abuse. Your task is to identify abnormal increased attenuation (white) that would suggest blood in the acute stage on CT.

Skull fractures can be linear (most common), depressed, or sutural diastasis. A depressed skull fracture requires surgical elevation if a fragment is displaced beneath the inner table to a depth greater than the skull thickness. Complications of skull fractures are listed in **Table 5–4**.

Traumatic lesions have characteristic locations. They tend to occur at the orbital frontal and frontal polar regions, the temporal poles, and the occipital poles in acceleration/deceleration injuries. A direct blow in a closed-head injury produces an injury directly beneath the site of the blow (coup injury) and a lesion opposite the site of the blow (contrecoup injury). A penetrating object has a track that is usually easy to identify.

Intracranial bleeds are determined to be intra-axial or extra-axial in location (**Key Point 5–4**). Extra-axial collections have characteristic shapes that can assist in localizing the hemorrhage. CT will show fluid in the *epidural* space (between the skull and dura) as a biconvex or lenticular-shaped mass in the brain (Figure 5–12). Ninety percent are caused by arterial injury, usually to the middle meningeal artery. The remaining epidural hematomas, caused by venous bleeds, are more commonly seen in children. *Epidural* hematomas (EDH) are most common in the temporoparietal region. These hematomas do not cross sutures but can traverse dural attachments, meaning that they can cross the midline.

Subdural hemorrhage (SDH) occurs in the potential space between dura and arachnoid membrane as a result of injury to cortical veins. CT demonstrates subdural hematomas as crescent-shaped masses paralleling the surface of the skull that will cross sutures but not the dural attachments (Figure 5–13). That is, these collections won't cross midline. The falx or the tentorium can be involved, and blood will be seen to layer on these structures. The most common location for this hemorrhage is the frontoparietal location. The CT and MRI findings of the appearance of blood are listed in **Table 5–5**. Isodense fluid on CT can be very subtle, and secondary signs should be sought, such as examining the ventricles and cortex for displacement. As mentioned earlier, the sulci may not extend to the calvarium. Contrast can be used in the subacute

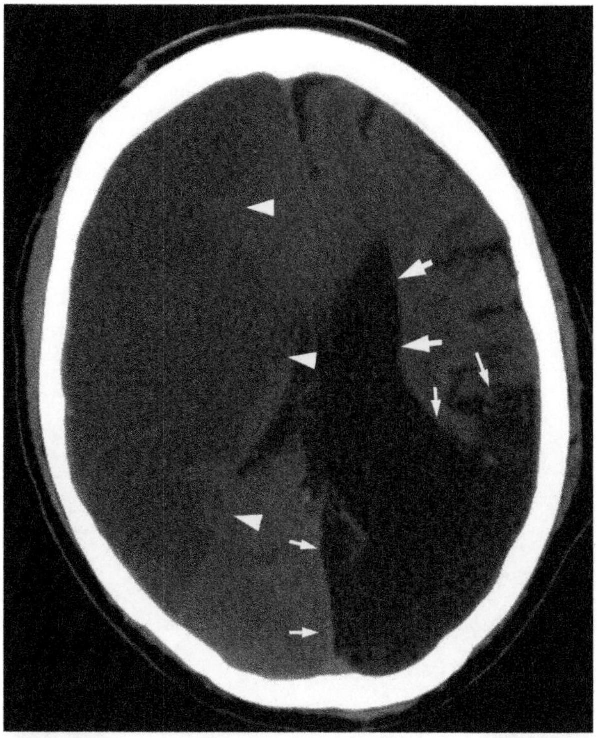

Figure 5–11. Cytotoxic edema. Noncontrast axial CT through the level of the frontal horns illustrates cerebral edema with involvement of the gray and white matter of the right hemisphere (*arrowheads*) in this patient who had symptoms of a stroke. Note the cerebral atrophy in the left hemisphere as demonstrated by enlargement of the ventricles (*large arrows*) and low attenuation from a previous stroke in the posterior parietal region (*small arrows*). (Courtesy of Srini Mukundan, MD, and Susan Kealey, MD.)

Table 5–4 Complications of Skull Fracture

Epidural hematoma
Cortical laceration of parenchyma as a result of a depressed
    fracture fragment
Carotid artery dissection
Pseudoaneurysm with carotid canal fracture
Infection
Leak of cerebrospinal fluid
Pneumocephalus
Leptomeningeal cyst (growing fracture)
Hearing loss or facial nerve injury with temporal bone fracture

Key Point 5–4

Locations of Intracranial Hematomas

Epidural
Subdural
Subarachnoid
Intracerebral
Contusion

cause. Nontraumatic causes of SAH include aneurysms and, rarely, arteriovenous malformation. CT is the imaging study of choice.

Intracerebral hematomas (ICH) most often are identified in the frontotemporal white matter and basal ganglia. The hematoma expands between relatively normal neurons. This is in contradistinction to a contusion, where the blood is mixed with edematous, contused parenchyma. There are other causes of parenchymal hematomas not associated with trauma. These are listed for you in **Table 5–6**.

setting. In this situation, cortical vessels may show displacement, and the subdural membranes will enhance.

Subarachnoid hemorrhage (SAH) occurs beneath the arachnoid and diffuses over the surface of the gyri distributed throughout cisterns, sulci, and fissures (Figure 5–14). Trauma is the most common

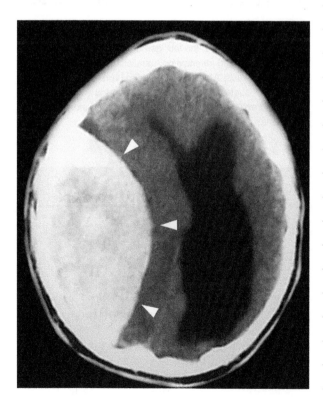

Figure 5–12. Epidural hematoma. Axial CT with brain windows demonstrating a lenticular-shaped, high-attenuation lesion (*arrowheads*) with marked mass effect and midline shift with dilated ventricles. This is a large epidural hematoma. These lesions do not cross sutures. The brain is under significant pressure, and loss of gray-white distinction is noted adjacent to the hematoma in the right hemisphere.

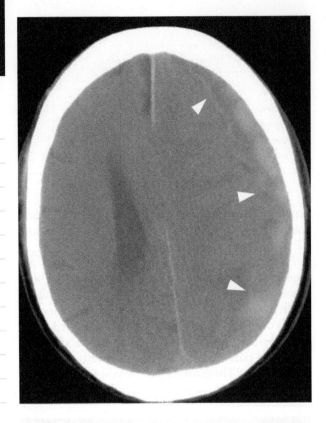

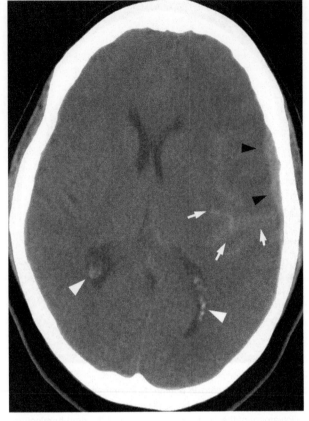

Figure 5–13. Subdural hematoma. Axial CT with brain windows at the level of the falx demonstrates a crescentic fluid collection with high attenuation paralleling the surface of the brain (*arrowheads*). The high attenuation represents blood in this patient who sustained head trauma. Subdural hematomas will cross sutures, but not dural attachments, Therefore, subdural hematomas do not cross the midline.

Figure 5–14. Subarachnoid hemorrhage. Axial CT with brain windows shows a small extra-axial fluid collection (*black arrowheads*) and high attenuation around the sulci and gyri in the left hemisphere (*small white arrows*). This is diagnostic of blood in the subarachnoid space. Calcified choroid plexus (a normal finding) is noted in the ventricles (*arrowheads*).

Table 5–5	CT and MRI Appearance of Blood Products	
Age	**Appearance**	
CT		
Acute (0–4 days)	High-attenuation fluid	
Subacute (4–20 days)	Gradual decrease in attenuation:	
	Isodense to brain at 1–2 wk	
	Hypodense to brain at 2–3 wk	
Chronic (>20 days)	Low attenuation	
MRI		
Immediate	T1: black	T2: black
Acute	T1: white	T2: black
Subacute	T1: white	T2: white

Table 5–6	Causes of Intracerebral Hematoma
Trauma	
Hypertension (basal ganglia, pons, cerebellum)	
Vascular malformation	
Aneurysm (subarachnoid hematoma)	
Hemorrhagic tumor	
Bleeding diathesis	
Hemorrhagic infarct	
Amyloid angiopathy	

Finally, *intraventricular* hemorrhage (IVH) is an uncommon finding as an isolated post-traumatic entity. It is commonly seen with diffuse axonal injury of the corpus callosum and brainstem due to rupture of subependymal veins.

Trauma can result in primary neuronal injury as well. This is seen as *cortical contusion* or *diffuse axonal injury*. *Cortical contusion* is a superficial injury to the cortex that contacts the bone. This injury tends to become more evident days after trauma, and it is most commonly seen involving the temporal lobes and frontal lobes. Initial imaging findings with CT are subtle and will evolve with time, leading to edema, mass effect, and petechial hemorrhage. Delayed hemorrhage may develop. *Diffuse axonal injury* or shearing injury is an indirect white matter injury caused by shear-strain forces. Patients initially have severe neurologic impairment, often with poor clinical outcome. The most common locations for this injury are lobar white matter, the corpus callosum, and the midbrain/pons region. For evaluation of this entity, MRI is the imaging study of choice. These are small lesions that will demonstrate increased T2 signal.

Unilateral or bilateral hemispheric swelling and edema can occur with severe trauma. Cerebral swelling can occur within hours due to increased cerebral blood volume. It is usually associated with other intracranial injuries. On imaging, there is sulcal and cisternal effacement with small ventricles and loss of gray-white matter interface (Figure 5–15).

Blunt trauma can lead to vascular intracranial injuries as well. Blunt intracranial injury can result in a carotid-cavernous fistula (usually seen with fractures of the skull base), pseudoaneurysm (which usually occurs at points of vessel transition between mobile and fixed segments), and meningeal artery lacerations.

The above discussion focused on intracranial injuries. However extracranial (outside of the brain) blunt trauma can lead to life-threatening vascular injuries also. Carotid arteries are injured slightly more often than vertebral arteries. Dissections and intimal tears of the vessels can result and can lead to stenosis, occlusion, pseudoaneurysm, and distal embolization of the affected vessel. Angiography will demonstrate a smooth tapering of the vessel, whereas MRI may show no flow, slow flow, or crescentic hemorrhage within the vessel wall.

No discussion of trauma is complete without a reminder to consider child abuse when assessing a patient with unexplained (or poorly explained) injuries. In the head, the most common injury is a subdural hematoma. On CT or MRI examination, you might see hemorrhage of varying ages. Shaking injuries are identified by patterns of acceleration/

deceleration injuries such as shear injuries, contusions, and hypoxic injuries as a result of damage to the cerebral circulation or events leading to hypoxia. Skull fractures are an additional indication. Because the carotid artery is relatively easy to compress, strangulation may result in carotid artery territory infarct.

Stroke

Stroke is the clinical term used to describe an abrupt nontraumatic brain insult. Strokes are caused most of the time by brain infarction (75%) and less often by hemorrhage (25%). Infarction is a permanent injury that occurs when tissue perfusion is decreased long enough to lead to necrosis. Transient ischemic attacks (TIAs) are characterized by symptoms lasting less than 24 hours. Hemorrhage can occur as a result of blood rupturing through the arterial wall, with resultant spilling of blood into the subarachnoid space or surrounding parenchyma. The patient with hemorrhage may have an associated aneurysm or arteriovenous malformation. These patients have different treatment options than a patient with a stroke. Therefore, the radiologist plays a key role in triaging these patients.

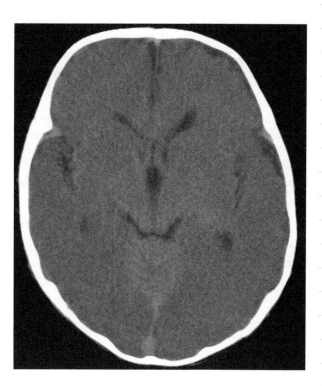

Figure 5–15. Cerebral edema. Noncontrast axial CT through the level of the third ventricle. Note the sulcal and cisternal effacement. These zones, being of the same attenuation, illustrate the loss of gray-white interface. (Courtesy of Srini Mukundan, MD, and Susan Kealey, MD.)

Table 5–7   Types of Acute Stroke

Thrombotic
Embolic
Watershed
Lacunar
Hemorrhagic
Hypertensive
Amyloid angiopathy

CT is often used as the first examination. However, CT can miss early strokes, and therefore MRI is being emphasized for early diagnosis in acute stroke. Early diagnosis is important, because treatment options can be instituted much earlier in this setting. MR diffusion imaging allows detection of cerebral ischemia within minutes of onset, and temporal evolution of diffusion characteristics enables differentiation of acute from chronic stroke. Diffusion imaging has tremendous potential for helping direct the treatment of acute ischemic stroke and is therefore routinely performed for evaluation of acute cerebrovascular accident (CVA). Diffusion is discussed in more detail in the included reference list at the end of this chapter. The types of acute strokes are listed in **Table 5–7**. Findings on CT for an acute stroke (0–24 hr) are listed in **Key Point 5–5**. Figure 5–16 demonstrates some of the findings. Findings of an acute stroke on MRI are included in **Key Point 5–6** and are illustrated in Figure 5–17.

Subacute strokes are seen on CT as swelling of the sulci/gyri with mass effect and shift. The area of involved territory demonstrates increased hypodensity and becomes more sharply defined. A subacute stroke on MRI demonstrates decreased

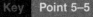

Key   Point 5–5

CT Findings of Acute Stroke

Effacement of sulci and gyri
Loss of gray-white differentiation
Hyperdense vessel supplying vascular territory
Loss of insular cortex (middle cerebral artery)

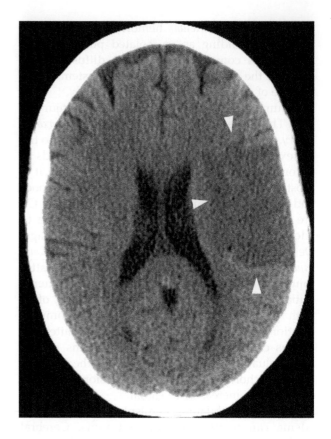

Figure 5–16. Acute cerebrovascular accident. Noncontrast axial CT through the lateral ventricles demonstrates presence of cytotoxic edema in the left middle cerebral artery distribution (*arrowheads*). The hyperdense vessel is not seen in this image, but the loss of gray-white differentiation and effacement of sulci and gyri are nicely demonstrated. Loss of the insular cortex is best appreciated when comparing the affected left middle cerebral artery distribution with the normal right side. (Courtesy of Srini Mukundan, MD, and Susan Kealey, MD.)

Figure 5–17. Acute cerebrovascular accident. A, T1-weighted axial noncontrast image through the region of the upper margin of the ventricles demonstrates a subtle decrease in signal of gray-white matter in the left hemisphere in the distribution of the left middle cerebral artery (*arrowheads*). Subtle mass effect is present involving the sulci. B, T2-weighted image in the same location as A shows a subtle increase in signal of gray-white matter. C, T1-weighted image after intravenous contrast administration at the same level as A and B demonstrates no significant contrast enhancement. After contrast enhancement, slow flow of arterial blood can be seen in the affected area. D, Diffusion-weighted image through the same area shows marked increase in signal (*arrowheads*) diagnostic of a stroke. (Courtesy of Srini Mukundan, MD, and Susan Kealey, MD.)

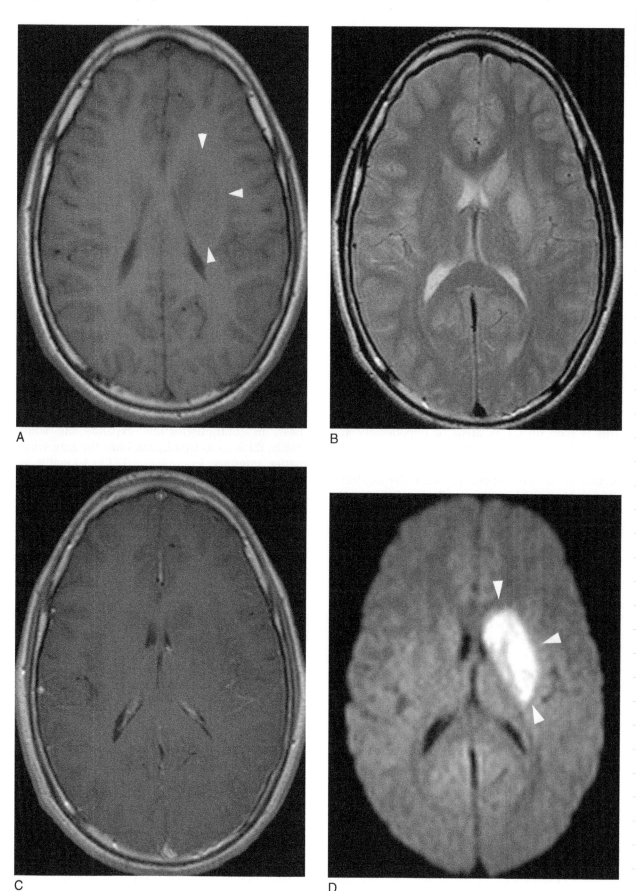

A

B

C

D

MRI Findings of Acute Stroke

T1: subtle decrease in signal of gray and white matter and subtle mass effect on sulci

T2: subtle increase in signal of gray and white matter (may also be normal)

MRI with intravenous contrast: slow flow of arterial blood to affected area

Diffusion: "light bulb" appearance of affected area

Spectroscopy: decreased N-acetyl aspartate (NAA) and increased lactate

signal intensity on the T1-weighted images due to the cytotoxic edema and may demonstrate swelling. This area is high in signal on the corresponding T2-weighted images. After contrast administration, there is leptomeningeal enhancement (Figure 5–18).

Chronic strokes result in atrophy of brain tissue. This is seen on CT as areas of hypodensity and encephalomalacia and dilation of adjacent CSF spaces (sulci and ventricles). No shift or mass effect occurs. A chronic stroke on MRI demonstrates decreased signal intensity on T1-weighted images with atrophy of the affected area and encephalomalacia. These areas correspond to high T2 signal. Contrast enhancement diminishes at approximately 6 weeks to 2 months. Spectroscopy shows that N-acetyl aspartate (NAA) remains low, and previously elevated lactate normalizes.

Venous infarctions occur as a result of occlusion of superficial or deep cerebral veins or dural sinuses and can be seen in pregnancy, hypercoagulable states, infection, mastoiditis, meningitis, and tumors. These infarcts can be distinguished radiographically from arterial infarcts because venous infarcts can be bilateral and subcortical in location. The area affected by a venous infarct overlaps arterial-supplied territories (Figure 5–19). Venous infarcts are associated with hemorrhage. Clot can be seen in the dural sinuses or superficial veins with MRI and CT.

Tumors

Neoplasms of the central nervous system (CNS) are rare. In patients younger than 15 years of age, the majority of lesions are located in the posterior fossa and metastatic lesions are rare. CNS tumors trail leukemias as the most common type of cancer in this age group. In patients older than 15 years, most CNS neoplasms will be supratentorial, and metastatic lesions are the most common lesions. Imaging evaluation is for tumors is similar to evaluation for trauma. Many institutions will begin with CT examination. Often a precontrast and postcontrast study is performed. This is done in order to see if there is hemorrhage associated with the tumor; also, if there are intrinsic calcifications, this will be apparent on a nonenhanced CT. MRI details the tumor and adjacent anatomy to much greater efficacy. It has essentially replaced CT in the evaluation of CNS masses. Research is underway to use contrast enhancement with perfusion and diffusion for assessing and delivering treatment for tumor neovascularity.

Just as with trauma, the assessment of intra-axial versus extra-axial location is imperative for the correct treatment. In general, extra-axial tumors tend to have a wide base and arise either from the meninges or the bones of the skull. These lesions have smooth indentation on the brain with thinning of the white matter fronds. The gray-white matter interface is maintained (Figure 5–20). An intra-axial mass, in contradistinction, expands the white matter, thickens its fronds, and blurs the gray-white matter interface (Figure 5–21). Occasionally an intra-axial lesion will arise from the surface of the brain, making distinction from an extra-axial lesion difficult. The multiplanar capability of MRI makes identification of intra-axial from extra-axial masses easier. Assessment of associated mass effect and shift or herniation is imperative. These must be acted upon expeditiously.

The imaging appearance of tumors varies with the cellular composition of the tumor as well as association of hemorrhage and internal matrix. On CT, the tumor will be hypodense. On MRI, the mass is usually low in signal on T1 and bright on the T2-weighted images with surrounding edema. Blood products can cause heterogeneous signal intensity, and occasionally calcification will image as hyperintense on T1-weighted imaging, although it usually images as a signal void (black). Lesions that contain fat will image as high signal on the T1-weighted images and will follow the signal characteristics of subcutaneous fat on the T2-weighted images. Melanin (as seen in melanoma) can also be high in signal on the T1-weighted images.

Contrast enhancement in CT and MRI works by the same principle. The molecules in the contrast agent are too large to penetrate the blood–brain barrier under normal circumstances. The fact that a lesion enhances after contrast administration means

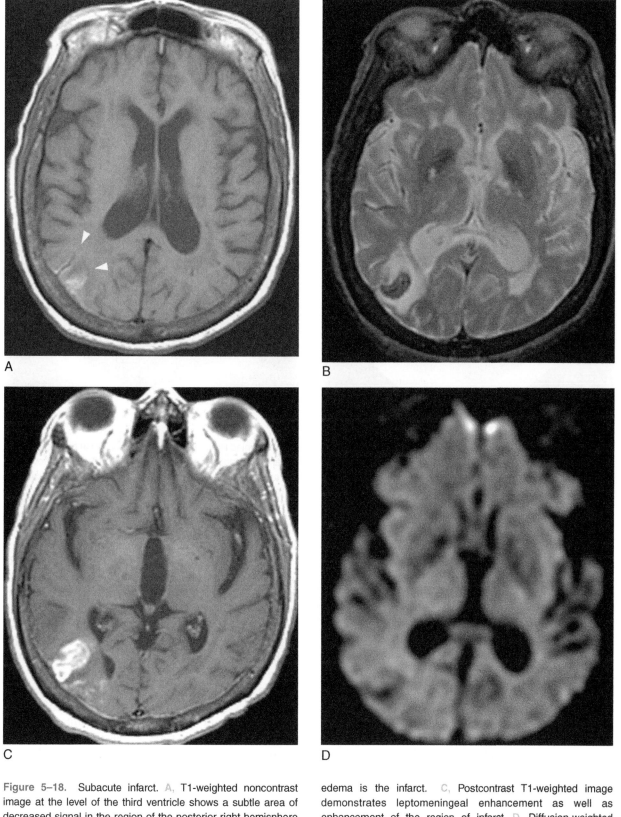

A

B

C

D

Figure 5–18.   Subacute infarct.   A, T1-weighted noncontrast image at the level of the third ventricle shows a subtle area of decreased signal in the region of the posterior right hemisphere (*arrowheads*). High signal along the leptomeningeal area may represent blood products.   B, T2-weighted image at the same level as A illustrates increased signal at the gray-white matter resembling cytotoxic edema. The area of low signal within the edema is the infarct.   C, Postcontrast T1-weighted image demonstrates leptomeningeal enhancement as well as enhancement of the region of infarct.   D, Diffusion-weighted image demonstrates no evidence of "light bulb" high signal that is seen with diffusion imaging for acute stroke. (Courtesy of Srini Mukundan, MD, and Susan Kealey, MD.)

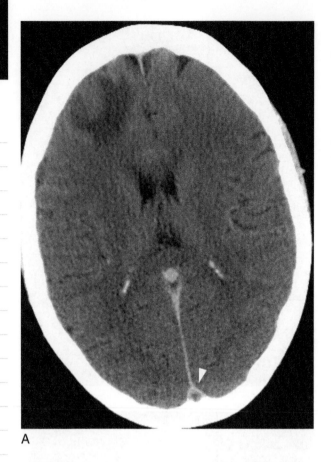

A

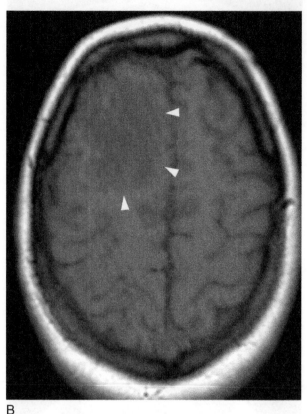

B

Figure 5–19.   Venous infarct. A, Axial CT after administration of intravenous contrast material shows the "empty delta" sign. Contrast is seen in the region of the transverse dural sinus. The nonenhancing center is a result of clot in the sinus (*arrowhead*).

B, T1-weighted image in the upper portion of the brain shows low signal in the subcortical white matter (*arrowheads*) that overlaps the arterial circulation from the anterior and middle cerebral arteries.

only that it does not have an intact blood–brain barrier. There is no significance to the enhancement pattern in terms of malignancy. Additionally, there are areas of the brain that normally enhance after contrast administration. These are listed for you in **Table 5–8**.

Infection

The ability to image CNS infections with CT and MRI has decreased the mortality associated with these conditions. Infections in the brain may occur as a result of direct extension after trauma (mean-spirited or postsurgical), sinusitis, dental infections, or mastoiditis. Hematogenous spread is usually via endocarditis, congenital heart disease, or lung infections. The frontal and parietal lobes are most affected. Pathologically, there are four stages of evolution of a brain abscess that correlate with imaging findings.

Early cerebritis occurs within the first few days of the infection. The infected portion of the brain is swollen and edematous. CT may show an area of low density, but more likely it will be normal. MRI will show an area of low T1 signal and corresponding high T2 signal intensity. After contrast enhancement, a ring is *not* identified at this stage. Enhancement is irregular and patchy. These imaging features are nonspecific and can be seen with tumors or infarcts. The distinction is often made with the clinical history.

Late cerebritis occurs by 1 or 2 weeks of infection. Central necrosis is increased. Vascular proliferation and recruitment of abundant inflammatory cells occurs at the periphery of the lesion as the brain's effort to contain the infection. Contrast enhancement at this point is thick and irregular at the edge of the lesion. Vasogenic edema is noted beyond this rim. At this point, there still is no discrete capsule on the T2-weighted images.

Early capsule formation occurs with time. A necrotic center is present, and contrast enhancement shows a well-defined rim. The rim images as low signal on T2-weighted images. The central area of

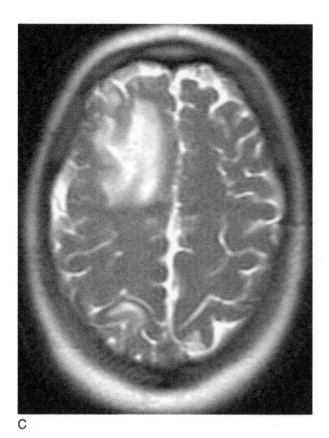

C

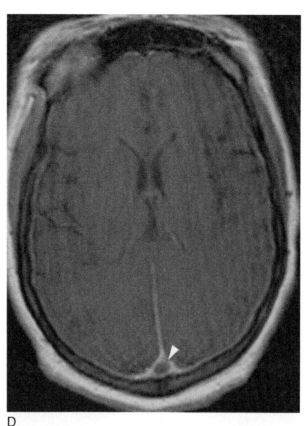

D

Figure 5–19. *Continued.* C, T2-weighted image at the corresponding location shows high signal. D, The postcontrast T1-weighted image shows no enhancement of the clot in the transverse sinus (*arrowhead*). (Courtesy of Srini Mukundan, MD, and Susan Kealey, MD.)

necrosis is low in signal on T1- and high in signal on T2-weighted images. Prominent surrounding vasogenic edema (which will also be low on T1- and high on T2-weighted images) is also present at this stage.

Finally, the late capsule stage can be seen. The rim of enhancement becomes even more well defined and thin, reflecting more complete collagen in the abscess wall. CT will demonstrate vasogenic edema with a well-defined rim after contrast enhancement (Figure 5–22). Multiloculation is common. Characteristic findings of the capsule make the diagnosis easier at this stage. The capsule is isointense or hyperintense to white matter on the T1-weighted image, and it is hypointense to the white matter on the T2-weighted images. The appearance is characteristic for an abscess, because capsules are not typically seen in tumors. Rupture of the capsule can lead to ventriculitis and ependymitis.

Disc Disease

The focus of this section is disc disease in the lumbar spine. The reason I think this section will be useful to you is that many of you will be seeing patients with low back pain and ordering an MRI (see Chapter 4 regarding ordering of conventional x-rays). It is a common ailment. Many times the patient has pain with no apparent findings on MRI, and at other times there are numerous disc bulges that don't correspond to the patient's symptoms. So the radiologist's responsibility is just to report the findings, and it is up to the physician caring for the patient to determine the significance of the findings.

By and large, disc disease is evaluated with MRI. MRI has essentially replaced CT, with the exception of patients who are not compatible with MRI, such as those with a pacemaker or implant. In the postoperative setting, MRI with contrast enhancement has improved the ability to distinguish postoperative fibrosis from recurrent or persistent disc protrusion.

Terminology plays a role for the radiologist in evaluating disc disease. It is important to understand what the surgeons at your institution prefer to call disc abnormalities (Figure 5–23). A disc bulge is protrusion of the disc material beyond the posterior margin of the vertebral body (Figure 5–24). A disc extrusion is a sequestration or free fragment

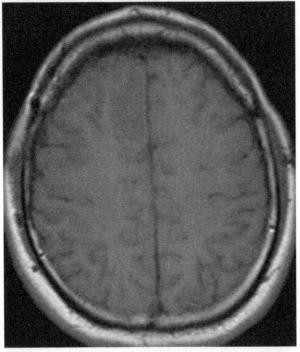

A

B

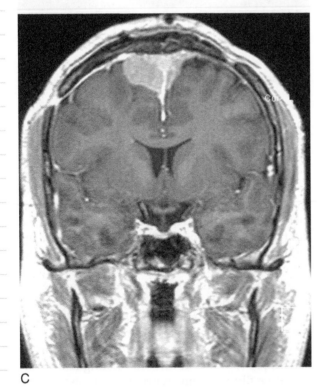

C

Figure 5–20. Extra-axial mass. A, T1-weighted image through the upper portion of the brain demonstrates vague low signal along the region of the falx. B, Postcontrast axial T1-weighted image shows smooth indentation on the brain. The gray-white matter interface is maintained. C, The coronal T1-weighted image after contrast enhancement shows the well-marginated mass and clear distinction between the gray-white matter interface characteristic of an extra-axial mass. (Courtesy of Srini Mukundan, MD, and Susan Kealey, MD.)

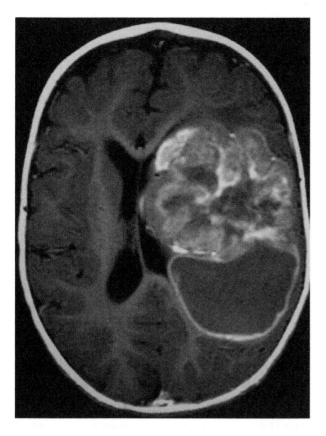

Figure 5–21. Intra-axial mass. T1-weighted axial MRI after contrast enhancement of a glioblastoma in a child demonstrates marked mass effect with compression of the left lateral ventricle as well as inability to distinguish gray-white matter in this location. The peripheral enhancement of the posterior portion of the lesion is an associated area of necrosis in the tumor.

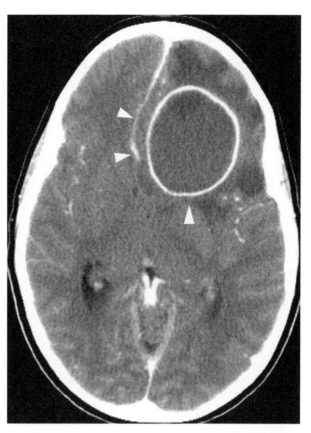

Figure 5–22. Intracerebral abscess. Axial CT after the administration of intravenous contrast material. The vasogenic edema is seen as the low-attenuation area. A well-defined ring of contrast is noted in this patient with an intracerebral abscess (*arrowheads*).

of disc material that has migrated away from the parent disc space. These are important for the radiologist to recognize. Failure to do so can lead to failed back surgery as this piece of disc material is left behind, likely to cause continued symptoms (Figure 5–25).

In addition to disc disease, *spinal stenosis* is a cause of back pain or radicular symptoms. Spinal stenosis is encroachment of the bony or soft tissue structures in the spine on one or more of the neural elements. Stenosis can be classified as central canal, neuroforaminal, or lateral recess. The most common

cause of central canal stenosis is degenerative disease of the facet joints with bony hypertrophy (Figure 5–26). Similarly, bony hypertrophy can lead to neuroforaminal stenosis. Additional causes of neuroforaminal stenosis include free disc fragments and lateral disc protrusions. Lateral recess stenosis can result from hypertrophy of the superior articular facet from degenerative disease. The lateral recess is the anatomic location of the nerve roots after they leave the thecal sac. Degenerative disease of the facet is the most common cause of encroachment. Certainly, a migrated free fragment can cause encroachment as well. Identification of the abnormality at the proper anatomic site is imperative, because surgery can take place at the wrong disc level if the identification is overlooked.

Emergencies

There are a number of entities discussed in this chapter that would be considered emergencies. Mass effect leading to herniation needs to be acted

Table 5–8   Structures That Normally Enhance after Contrast Administration
Choroid plexus
Pituitary and pineal glands
Tuber cinereum
Area postrema

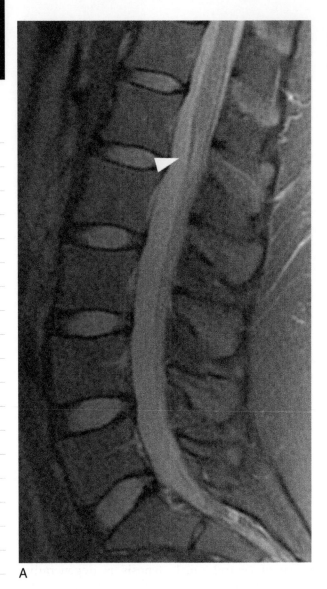

A

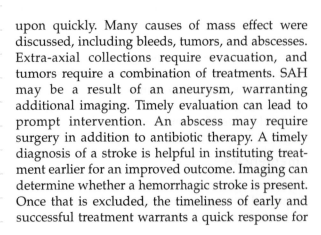

B

Figure 5–23.   Normal lumbar spine. A, Sagittal T2-weighted image with fat suppression demonstrates a normal location of the conus (*arrowhead*) and well-hydrated discs, as evidenced by the higher signal intensity in the discs. There is no evidence of disc protrusion on this particular image. B, Axial T2-weighted image at the L5–S1 level shows the normal appearance of the thecal sac. No disc bulge (protrusion) is noted at this level.

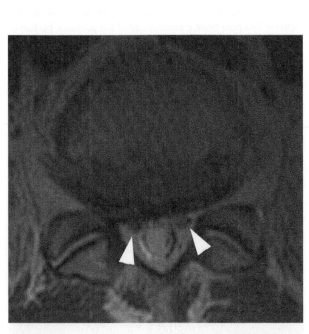

Figure 5–24.   Broad-based disc bulge. Axial T2-weighted image through the L5–S1 level demonstrates a disc bulge that approaches the S1 nerve roots (*arrowheads*). It cannot be determined by MRI whether this is responsible for the patient's symptoms, and the MRI examination should always be compared to the clinical findings.

upon quickly. Many causes of mass effect were discussed, including bleeds, tumors, and abscesses. Extra-axial collections require evacuation, and tumors require a combination of treatments. SAH may be a result of an aneurysm, warranting additional imaging. Timely evaluation can lead to prompt intervention. An abscess may require surgery in addition to antibiotic therapy. A timely diagnosis of a stroke is helpful in instituting treatment earlier for an improved outcome. Imaging can determine whether a hemorrhagic stroke is present. Once that is excluded, the timeliness of early and successful treatment warrants a quick response for

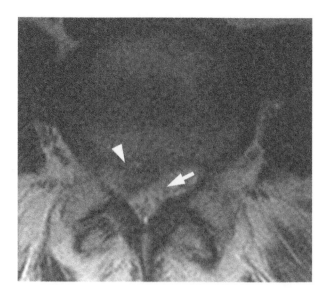

Figure 5–25. Lateral recess stenosis. Axial T2-weighted MRI shows a "free fragment," a migrated disc from the level above, in the right lateral recess (*arrowhead*). Mass effect is noted on the thecal sac (*arrow*).

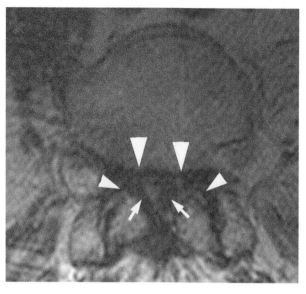

Figure 5–26. Central canal stenosis. Axial T2-weighted image shows marked narrowing of the thecal sac due to degenerative changes of the facet joints (*small arrowheads*), buckling of the ligamentum flavum (*arrows*), and a small, broad-based disc bulge (*large arrowheads*).

expeditious imaging and interpretation. In evaluating intra-axial masses, assessment for herniation is imperative to prevent additional injury of vital structures.

Suggested Reading List

Osborn G, Blaser S, Salzman KL: Diagnostic Imaging: Brain. Philadelphia, Elsevier, 2004.

Ross JS, Brant-Zawadzki M, Chen MZ, Moore KR: Diagnostic Imaging: Spine. Philadelphia, Elsevier, 2005.

Harnsberger HR, Hudgins PA, Wiggins RH, Davidson HC: Diagnostic Imaging: Head and Neck. Philadelphia, Elsevier, 2005.

Castillo M: Neuroradiology: The Core Curriculum. Philadelphia, Lippincott Williams & Wilkins, 2002.

Gean AD: Imaging of Head Trauma. Philadelphia, Lippincott Williams & Wilkins, 1994.

6

Pediatric Imaging

There are anatomic conditions and pathologic processes that are unique to children and neonates. Some of these will be discussed in this chapter. This chapter is designed for the student who is taking a "mandatory" or required pediatric rotation. In this section you will read about commonly imaged abnormalities and a few not so commonly encountered abnormalities that should be recognized on x-ray examination in order to institute timely and effective treatment. Wonderful textbooks have been written to discuss in more detail the abnormalities presented here, as well as the many that are not included here. You are referred to the reading list for further tutelage. In the meantime, you should find that this chapter covers basic pediatric radiology.

Chest

How to Image

Imaging the chest in infants and children can be a challenge because of their "fidgety" nature. Sometimes this fidgety nature is due to illness, and other times it's genetic! In any case, when imaging the neonate, portable x-rays are obtained in the intensive care unit in a supine, anteroposterior (AP) projection. In slightly older children, a holder or restraint can be used during the examination. Obviously, it is difficult for the child to listen to commands such as "Hold your breath"! Therefore, the images are performed randomly when it comes to breath holding. In normal young children, the apex of the hemidiaphragm is located at the 8th or 9th posterior rib. If the diaphragms are lower than this, hyperinflation should be considered. A poor inspiratory effort is noted when there is tracheal buckling to the right. The lungs may mimic the appearance of pulmonary edema, pneumonia, and/or cardiomegaly. These findings should alert you to a poor inspiratory effort (Figure 6–1).

A major difference between the normal chest of an adult or older child versus that of a neonate or child younger than 2 years of age is the presence of the thymus. The thymus is routinely identified on chest films from birth to about 2 years of age. It is usually seen as a widening of the upper mediastinum. Occasionally, it does project into the lung ("sail sign"), and generally it points to the right. The

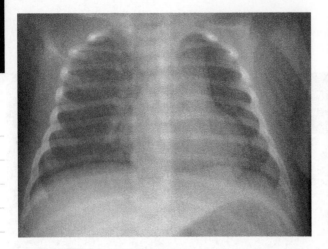

Figure 6–1   Frontal chest radiograph demonstrates normal inspiration and a normal cardiothymic contour with normal lung markings in this infant. The stomach bubble can be identified in the left upper quadrant.

thymus has a wavy border due to the indentations from the ribs. Parenchymal vessels can be identified through the thymus. Fluoroscopy will demonstrate that the thymus changes in size with respirations. This should eliminate any confusion that this density represents a pneumonia, because pneumonia does not do this (Figure 6–2). No air bronchograms are seen in the region of the thymus. On the lateral view, the thymus is anterior (anteriorly located mediastinal structure—see Chapter 2). It will regress by about 2 years of age, so there should be no density in the retrosternal space after age 2 (Key Point 6–1). The distribution of the vascularity and appearance of the hilum is otherwise similar in the child and the adult.

A not infrequently used examination is a combination of chest and abdominal imaging referred to as a "babygram." In very small babies, a single AP exposure can visualize pulmonary vascularity as well as abdominal gas patterns. However, if you are interested only in chest-related pathology, get only the chest film, and prevent unnecessary exposure to radiation.

Ultrasonography is a commonly utilized imaging technique in children that is employed to answer a wide variety of clinical questions, from evaluation of brain parenchyma in babies whose fontanelles are still open to evaluation of the genitourinary tract in patients with urinary tract infections or other suspected renal abnormalities. Cross-sectional imaging with magnetic resonance imaging (MRI) or computed tomography (CT) requires assistance with sedative medications. Depending on the age of the patient and his or her ability to cooperate, general endotracheal anesthesia may be necessary.

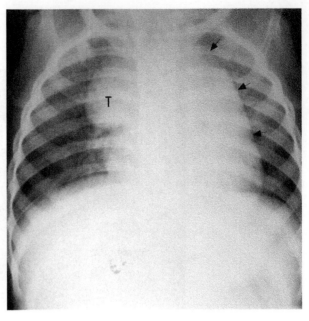

Figure 6–2   Thymus. Frontal chest x-ray in a 1-year-old demonstrating the appearance of the soft tissue density of the thymus (T) (*arrowheads*), which is causing the density in the upper portion of the chest. Parenchymal vessels can be seen through the thymus.

Key   Point 6–1
Radiographic Appearance of the Normal Thymus
Widened upper mediastinum Sail sign Wavy border Respiratory size variation No air bronchograms

The use of MRI in the newborn is usually in the evaluation of congenital abnormalities of the central nervous system or heart.

Lung Disease in the Neonate

Conditions leading to respiratory distress in the neonate are numerous. Some of these conditions need to be treated surgically—usually those associated with space-occupying lesions (cystic adenomatoid malformation, diaphragmatic hernia, pneumothorax). These entities will be mentioned a little later in this chapter. This discussion focuses on lung parenchymal abnormalities (**Table 6–1**).

Idiopathic respiratory distress syndrome is one of the most common causes of respiratory distress in premature infants. This abnormality can occasionally

Table 6–1 Lung Disease in the Neonate

Idiopathic respiratory distress syndrome (hyaline membrane disease)
Bronchopulmonary dysplasia
Wilson-Mikity syndrome
Meconium aspiration

occur in term infants of diabetic mothers. The abnormality is caused by a lack of the surfactant necessary to reduce surface tension of the alveoli, which causes the alveoli to remain collapsed. Respiratory distress is seen within the first few hours after birth. Radiographically, a fine, granular pattern with air bronchograms is present (Figure 6–3). On expiration, the lungs become opaque. With continued use of positive pressure-assisted ventilation and high oxygen concentrations, the lung parenchyma can be damaged, resulting in *bronchopulmonary dysplasia (BPD)*. Eventually this can lead to fibrosis. More severe cases result in an uneven pattern of aeration of alveoli. Areas of overdistention and areas of collapse give the appearance of variable-sized bubbles. The bubbles of BPD collapse on expiration, whereas the bubbles of *pulmonary interstitial emphysema (PIE—*air in the wall of the bronchus) do not collapse on expiration (Figures 6–4 and 6–5). Atelectasis is a common feature of BPD. This is most often imaged as streaky opacities emanating from the hila. PIE occurs in neonates with stiff lungs due to hyaline membrane disease. The interstitial air is seen as radiolucent

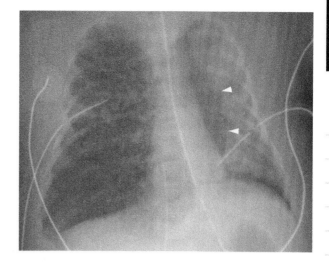

Figure 6–4 Pulmonary interstitial emphysema (PIE) and pneumothorax. Frontal chest x-ray demonstrates air density within the wall of the bronchus. This is best appreciated in the right lung. The entity has led to the development of a pneumothorax in the left lung, as indicated by the air density in the medial pleura of the left lung (*arrowheads*). An endotracheal tube, orogastric tube, and chest tube are also present.

lines when captured lengthwise and circular lines when imaged en face. The presence of PIE should alert the reviewer of the films to search for a pneumothorax or pneumomediastinum.

Meconium aspiration is a result of aspiration of meconium into the tracheobronchial tree after evacuation of meconium by the fetus into the amniotic fluid during intrauterine distress. The resulting subsegmental atelectasis and overdistention are a

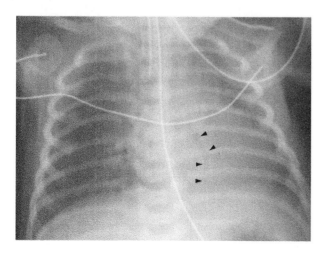

Figure 6–3 Hyaline membrane disease. Frontal chest x-ray in a premature infant demonstrates increased density in the lungs and an air bronchogram (*arrowheads*) superimposed over the cardiac silhouette. An endotracheal tube and an orogastric tube are also present.

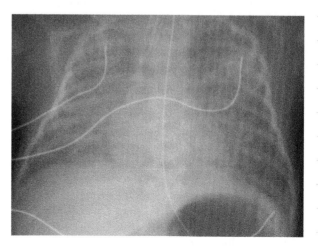

Figure 6–5 Bronchopulmonary dysplasia (BPD). Frontal chest x-ray showing marked peribronchial cuffing in this child who was born prematurely. The streaky opacities in the parenchyma are most prominent around the hila. An endotracheal tube and an orogastric tube are present.

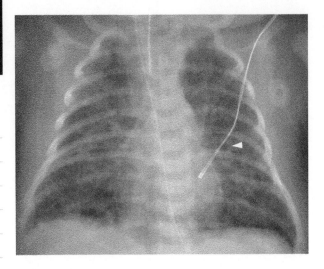

Figure 6–6   Meconium aspiration. Frontal chest x-ray demonstrates marked coarsening of the interstitium with peribronchial cuffing (*arrowhead*). This infant suffered meconium aspiration at birth. An endotracheal tube and an orogastric tube are present.

result of air trapping and obstruction of the small peripheral bronchioles. This creates a coarse, reticulonodular appearance of the lungs that is usually bilateral (Figure 6–6).

Lung Disease in the Non-neonate

Recognizing patterns of consolidation can be useful in trying to formulate a differential diagnosis. When alveoli are filled with a substance, *alveolar consolidation* occurs. Most often, the alveoli are filled with fluid from a bacterial pneumonia. The most common organism varies with the age of the child: *Haemophilus influenzae* is most common before 2 years of age, and *Streptococcus pneumoniae* is most common in older children. Primary tuberculosis should be considered if the infiltrate is accompanied by hilar lymphadenopathy (**Table 6–2**). A *round pneumonia* is, as its name describes, a round consolidation caused by a bacterial pneumonia (Figure 6–7). Viral and atypical pneumonias are not associated with round pneumonias. Round pneumonias should be followed-up after antibiotic therapy in order to exclude a mass.

Volume loss is a helpful clue as to the cause of an isolated consolidation noted on pediatric chest x-rays. If volume loss is present, the consolidation likely represents atelectasis that is seen in viral respiratory illness or atypical pneumonia. Atelectasis is not a typical imaging feature of bacterial pneumonia. In addition to being associated with infection, atelectasis can also be seen in acute asthma. The distinction between asthma and pneumonia can often be made with the clinical history. Some

Table 6–2 Focal Alveolar Consolidation
Bacterial pneumonia
<2 years of age
Haemophilus influenzae
>2 years of age
Streptococcus pneumoniae
Mycoplasma pneumoniae
Staphylococcus aureus
Nonbacterial infection
Tuberculosis
Actinomycosis
Pulmonary infarction
Pulmonary contusion

radiographic features that help distinguish the two entities are hyperinflation with flattening of the hemidiaphragms, prominent retrosternal "clear space," and segmental or lobar collapse in asthma. Effusions are not a finding of asthma, and their presence suggests another diagnosis. Clinically, a patient with an acute asthma flare is not usually febrile (**Key Point 6–2**). Multiple patchy lung consolidations can also be seen in the pediatric age

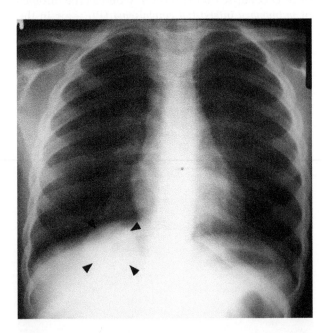

Figure 6–7   Round pneumonia. Frontal chest x-ray in this child with fever and abdominal pain demonstrates a round soft tissue density in the right lower lung (*arrowheads*). If this soft tissue density were originating in the liver (also a soft tissue density), it would not be visible as a separate structure on the x-ray. Because it is surrounded by the density of the lung (different from soft tissue), it can be localized to the lung. Round pneumonias are bacterial in origin. Remember that chest findings can present with abdominal pain.

Findings in Asthma Versus Bacterial Pneumonia

Asthma	Bacterial Pneumonia
Clinical	
Afebrile	Febrile
	Cough
	Chest pain
Radiographic	
Volume loss	No volume loss
Hyperinflation	
Prominent retrosternal "clear space"	
Segmental or lobar collapse	

Table 6–4 Causes of Bilateral Lung Hyperinflation

Diffuse peripheral obstruction

Viral bronchitis/bronchiolitis
Asthma
Cystic fibrosis
Immunologic deficiency diseases
Chronic aspiration
Graft-versus-host disease

Central obstruction

Extrinsic
   Vascular anomalies
   Mediastinal masses
Intrinsic
   Tracheal foreign body
   Tracheal neoplasm/granuloma

group in a wide variety of conditions, as listed in **Table 6–3**.

Bilateral lung hyperinflation is caused by airway obstruction due to a diffuse peripheral obstruction or a central obstruction. These processes are listed for you in **Table 6–4**. Two of these entities require additional mention. *Bronchiolitis* is of viral origin and represents a common cause of airway disease in children younger than 1 year old. Radiographically, peribronchial cuffing is noted in addition to hyperinflation. This is identified as a soft tissue density surrounding a bronchus. As you look at pediatric chest x-rays, you will notice that most children have some peribronchial cuffing. More than a couple of cuffs is abnormal. Bronchiolitis will demonstrate diffuse cuffing without a discrete infiltrate. The heart border may appear a bit shaggy, with increased lung markings emanating from the hila (Figure 6–8).

The other disease process that you should be comfortable diagnosing is *cystic fibrosis (CF)*. CF is caused by dysfunction of the exocrine glands, which produce thick mucus that accumulates in the lungs, leading to bronchitis and recurrent pneumonias. Radiographic findings include hyperinflation and bronchiectasis caused by irreversibly dilated bronchi with thickened walls. Parallel lines of increased density around the bronchi have been

Table 6–3 Multiple Patchy Lung Consolidations

Infection
   Staphylococcus aureus
   Mycoplasma
   Fungal
   Opportunistic organisms
Aspiration
   Hydrocarbon ingestion
   Near-drowning
Immune-mediated pneumonitis
   Milk allergy
   Hypersensitivity pneumonitis
Pulmonary hemorrhage
Pulmonary edema

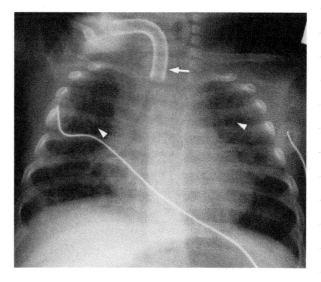

Figure 6–8 Bronchiolitis. Portable frontal chest x-ray in an infant demonstrating a tracheostomy tube (*arrow*) and the abnormal appearance of the bronchi through the lungs bilaterally (*arrowheads*).

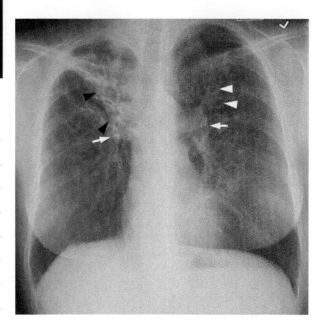

Figure 6–9 Cystic fibrosis (CF). Frontal chest x-ray in a female teenager demonstrates some of the characteristic findings of CF. Note the fibrosis in the right upper lobe (*black arrowheads*). The pulmonary arteries are also enlarged (*white arrows*). Peribronchial cuffing is present in the left upper lung (*white arrowheads*). The cardiac silhouette is also small.

referred to as having a "tram track" appearance. Mucoid impaction is another finding in CF. This appears as circular soft tissue densities in the periphery of the lung. Soft tissue density results from retained mucus in the bronchiectatic bronchioles. Atelectasis due to mucoid impaction is also a feature of this disease. The hila are enlarged in CF due to chronic colonization of organisms leading to adenopathy. Pulmonary arterial hypertension is also present. The mediastinum can also demonstrate a small cardiac silhouette. This is due to the negative intrathoracic pressure impeding venous return rather than large lung volumes (Figure 6–9). **Key Point 6–3** lists associated radiographic findings in CF. Children with CF are prone to a wide variety

---

Key Point 6–3

Radiographic Findings in Cystic Fibrosis

Hyperinflation
Bronchiectasis
"Tram tracking"
Mucoid impaction
Atelectasis
Enlarged hila
Small cardiac silhouette

Table 6–5 Causes of Unilateral Obstructive Emphysema

Bronchial foreign body
Mucous plug
Congenital lobar emphysema
Bronchial stenosis/atresia
Tuberculosis
Vascular abnormalities
Mediastinal masses

---

of gastrointestinal (GI) disorders in addition to pulmonary complications, including meconium ileus, intussusception, pancreatitis, jaundice, and vitamin deficiencies. CF should be suspected in a child with recurrent respiratory or GI symptoms.

Pulmonary aeration abnormalities can be unilateral as well. Hyperaeration can be caused by obstructive emphysema or compensatory hyperinflation. Evaluation of the pulmonary vasculature can sometimes help determine whether the hyperinflation is due to compensatory changes or obstructive changes. Obstructive emphysema will result in diminished size of the pulmonary vascularity because of hypoxia-induced arterial spasm. By contrast, vascularity to a lung exhibiting compensatory hyperaeration will appear normal or increased. If the frontal film does not clearly distinguish these two conditions, an inspiratory x-ray can be compared with an expiratory view. The lung that changes the least in volume between the two views is the abnormal lung. **Table 6–5** lists unilateral causes of obstructive emphysema.

Foreign Body Aspiration

No discussion of the pediatric chest x-ray or evaluation of the pediatric airway is complete without a discussion of foreign body aspiration. This must be considered in the differential diagnosis of a child presenting with difficulty breathing. Even diligent, watchful parents and caretakers can miss identifying a child who has put something in his or her mouth that either doesn't belong there in the first place or is too difficult to chew and gets aspirated instead of swallowed. Many children are like tiny vacuum cleaners, picking up almost anything that is not nailed down! Most aspirated foreign bodies are radiolucent (this includes plastic), which is an important reason you must think of this possibility from the clinical presentation.

As it happens, the peanut is the most commonly aspirated foreign body. Aspirated foreign bodies

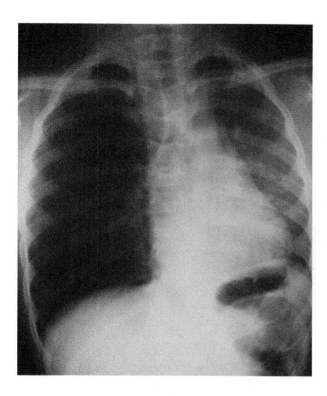

Figure 6–10 Air trapping. Frontal expiratory chest x-ray demonstrates lucent right lung with increased volume compared with the exhalation of the left lung. This finding is consistent with air trapping, and a foreign body must be a clinical concern.

lodge on the *right* side of the tracheobronchial tree more often than on the left. There are two possible lung findings. The first is that the object will become completely impacted and will not allow air to pass during inspiration or expiration. Air distally will become resorbed, and postobstructive atelectasis or a focal consolidation will be noted with associated volume loss.

The second possibility is that the object will incompletely obstruct the bronchus. The object then acts as a one way "ball-valve." The bronchus gets larger in diameter during inspiration, allowing air to pass around the lodged object. On expiration, however, air cannot escape around the object. Evaluation for foreign body with decubitus views is recommended in children who cannot cooperate for inspiratory and expiratory views. Decubitus views will help by demonstrating that the normal side (nonaspirated side) will have a change of volume in switching from dependent (down side) to nondependent (up side) status, whereas the abnormal side will have no such change in lung volume with this maneuver (Figure 6–10). Children who can cooperate with inspiratory and expiratory films will demonstrate air trapping in the lung with aspiration and reveal no change in lung volume in the affected lung between inspiration and expiration.

Epiglottitis is inflammation of the epiglottis affecting the pediatric and young adult population. Often the patient presents with drooling and severe throat pain with inability to swallow. Manipulation or evaluation of the throat should be prevented, because this can lead to complete airway obstruction. A lateral conventional x-ray of the neck demonstrates swelling of the epiglottis (Figure 6–11).

Another airway disease commonly encountered in children is croup or reactive airway disease. This is generally a clinical diagnosis associated with low-grade fever and difficulty breathing. Conventional x-ray studies reveals a "steeple sign" (Figure 6–12).

Masses in the Chest

Causes of pleural effusions are listed in **Table 6–6**. The evaluation of a pleural effusion in a child is much like that in an adult. Thickening along the lateral and apical portions of the lung are most often seen. Subpulmonic effusions demonstrate flattening of the diaphragms and laterally displaced curvature of the dome of the diaphragm. The most common cause of a massive pleural effusion in the neonate is a chylothorax. These are usually unilateral and more commonly right-sided. The cause is unknown, but the most likely explanation is a congenital defect or traumatic tear of the thoracic duct. Another relatively common cause of pleural fluid is iatrogenic, related to complications of indwelling catheters in thoracic vessels. Air in the pleural space is evaluated in the older child with a frontal and a lateral chest x-ray. Occasionally, inspiratory and expiratory films need to be performed. In the much younger child and in the neonate, cross-table lateral films are acquired in addition to the frontal chest x-ray (Figure 6–13). The nondependent air will rise to the top and be seen as a lucency in the anterior portion of the chest.

The most common pulmonary mass is in fact not a mass. It was mentioned previously: round pneumonia. Postinflammatory granulomas are the most common "true" masses and are usually seen after fungal or tuberculous infections. Another commonly encountered lung mass is a *bronchogenic cyst*. These cysts are lined with respiratory epithelium and filled with a tenacious liquid. They most often occur in a subcarinal location but occasionally can be found in the lung. If connected to the bronchial tree, they may be air-filled. *Esophageal duplication cysts* are developmental abnormalities resulting from abnormal division of the neurenteric complex during fetal development. Some of these cysts can be connected to the spinal canal (posterior mediastinal mass). The remainder of these cysts are middle mediastinal masses. Usually these are

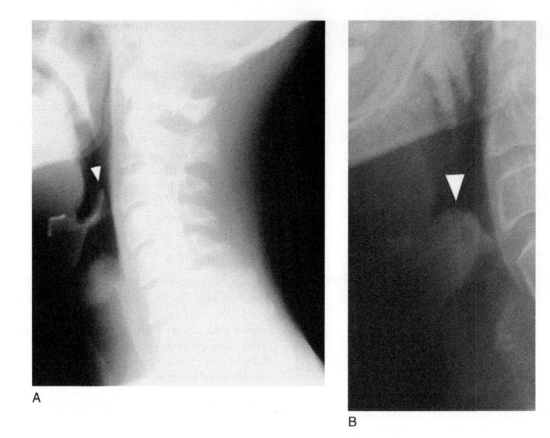

A

B

Figure 6–11   Epiglottitis. A, Lateral soft tissue of the neck demonstrating the normal appearance of the epiglottis (*arrowhead*). B, Lateral soft tissue of the neck in a young patient demonstrating swelling of the epiglottis (*arrowhead*). This is diagnostic of epiglottitis.

identified by their mass effect on the esophagus on contrast studies. These cysts do not communicate with the esophagus.

Not infrequently, a *pulmonary sequestration* can be identified. These are developmental bronchopulmonary foregut malformations that represent a mass of lung tissue that lacks a connection to the bronchial tree. Abnormal arteries from the descending aorta supply sequestrations. Usually, these are incidental unless they become infected. Recurrent pneumonias in the medial, basal portion of the lung (more commonly on the left) should prompt a search for abnormal vessels and a diagnosis of a sequestration. The sequestration can be enveloped by its own pleura (extralobar) or by the pleura of the adjacent normal lung (intralobar).

A rare congenital lesion of the lung that is typically unilateral and can affect any portion of the lung is *congenital cystic adenomatoid malformation (CCAM)*. It is characterized by abnormal lung tissue containing dysplastic adenomatous tissue within communicating cysts of variable size. The radiographic appearance can vary from a singular solid lesion with tiny cysts to multiple large, thin-walled cysts. In the newborn, the cysts are most often fluid-filled, and the lesion has the appearance of a solid mass. With time, the cysts fill with air and can enlarge to a degree that causes respiratory distress (Figure 6–14).

The mediastinum is arbitrarily divided into anterior, middle, and posterior portions, as it is in the adult. The differential diagnoses are the same, although some lesions are more common in the pediatric population. For instance, in the anterior mediastinum, the majority of lesions are tumors. The most common types are dermoids and teratomas. Remember that in children younger than 2 years of age, a normal thymus is also an anterior mass. A lesion not typically identified in adults is a *cystic hygroma*, a congenital malformation of lymphatic origin. Ultrasonography is a good way to evaluate this lesion.

Lymphadenopathy is the most common middle mediastinal mass. Massive lymph node enlargement is usually seen in lymphoma or leukemia. However, focal inflammatory lymph node enlargement is much more common than neoplastic disease.

Posterior mediastinal masses are mainly of neurogenic origin. Identification of bone erosion and rib space widening suggests such a lesion. The

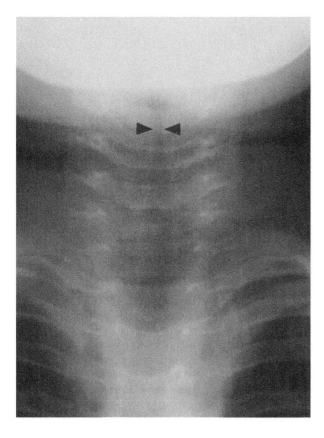

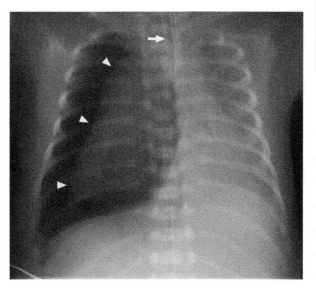

Figure 6–13   Tension pneumothorax. Frontal chest x-ray in a newborn demonstrates air in the pleural space (*arrowheads*) with a shift of the mediastinal structures away from the pneumothorax to the contralateral mediastinum. Although tension pneumothorax is a clinical diagnosis, it should be suspected based on the ominous findings on this x-ray. A central venous catheter is noted in the midline of the abdomen, and an endotracheal tube is present (*arrow*) with a shift to the left. A left lower lung opacification is also present. Note that the left hemidiaphragm is not visualized.

Figure 6–12   Croup. Frontal x-ray of the neck demonstrates tapered narrowing of the trachea (*arrowheads*) in a configuration resembling the "steeple" of a church. Although croup is a clinical diagnosis, occasionally an x-ray may be helpful to identify the characteristic appearance of the trachea.

mass is most often a neoplasm of *neuroblastoma-ganglioneuroma* origin. Thoracic neuroblastoma is not uncommon and has a more favorable prognosis than neuroblastoma that originates in the abdomen. Ganglioneuroma is the benign counterpart of neuroblastoma. The two lesions cannot be reliably distinguished from one another radiographically (Figure 6–15).

Congenital Heart Anomalies

Evaluation of cardiac abnormalities in the pediatric population is similar to that in adults. A variety of imaging modalities are available for diagnosing and evaluating congenital heart disease in children. Noninvasive modalities include echocardiography (ultrasound) and MRI. Nevertheless, evaluation always starts with a conventional x-ray. Assess the vascularity as either increased, decreased, or normal. *Active* and *passive* congestion were discussed in Chapter 2 and are reiterated for you here. *Active congestion* is defined as increased blood going through the pulmonary vasculature (left-to-right shunt, for example). *Passive congestion* is elevation of the pulmonary venous pressure, usually due to obstruction or dysfunction of the left side of the heart. Although it is not always possible to make a

Table 6–6   Causes of Pleural Effusions in Children

Unilateral

Pneumonia/empyema
Chylothorax
Iatrogenic
Trauma
Intra-abdominal inflammation
Intrathoracic neoplasm
Ruptured aneurysm of ductus arteriosus

Bilateral

Renal disease
Lymphoma
Neuroblastoma
Congestive heart failure
Collagen vascular diseases
Fluid overload

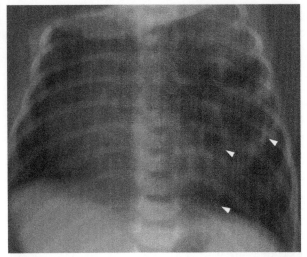

A

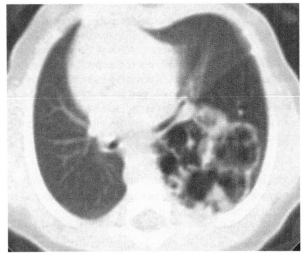

B

Figure 6–14   Congenital cystic adenomatoid malformation (CCAM). A, Frontal conventional x-ray demonstrating numerous round lucencies (*arrrowheads*) in the left hemithorax. The lucencies are a result of air filling the cysts in the CCAM. The left hemidiaphragm is visualized. Note the mass effect with shift of the mediastinal structures to the right hemithorax. B, Axial CT image in lung windows at the level of the carina shows the numerous air-filled cysts in the CCAM. This appearance should be distinguished from diaphragmatic hernia, in which the diaphragm would not be visualized. (Courtesy of Donald Frush, MD.)

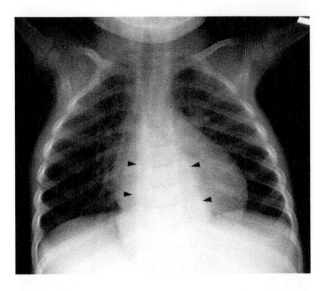

Figure 6–15   Neuroblastoma. Frontal chest x-ray demonstrates a soft tissue density along the paraspinous location (*arrowheads*). In a child of this age, a posterior mediastinal mass should be a consideration, and neuroblastoma is a leading candidate in the differential diagnosis. Extramedullary hematopoiesis can have a similar appearance, and the clinical history is imperative in excluding a hemoglobinopathy. (Courtesy of Elizabeth McGraw, MD.)

Table 6–7   Classification of Congenital Heart Abnormalities: Increased Vascularity (Active) without Cyanosis
Atrial septal defect
Ventricular septal defect
Patent ductus arteriosus
Aortic-pulmonary window
Ruptured aneurysm of sinus of Valsalva
Coronary artery fistula
Partial anomalous pulmonary venous return

Table 6–8   Classification of Congenital Heart Abnormalities: Increased Vascularity (Active) with Cyanosis
Total anomalous pulmonary venous return
Persistent truncus arteriosus
Complete endocardial cushion defect
Transposition of the great vessels
Single ventricle (without pulmonary stenosis)

specific diagnosis, the abnormality can often be placed in one of several groups listed in **Tables 6–7 through 6–12**. Examples of a few congenital anomalies follow. Cover the figure caption, and see how well you do categorizing the disease based on your organized approach (Figures 6–16 through 6–18).

Table 6–9   Classification of Congenital Heart Abnormalities: Increased Vascularity (Passive)

Total anomalous pulmonary venous return
Pulmonary vein atresia
Hypoplastic left heart syndrome
Cor triatriatum

Table 6–10   Classification of Congenital Heart Abnormalities: Decreased Vascularity

Tetralogy of Fallot
Pseudotruncus arteriosus
Hypoplastic right heart syndrome
Ebstein's anomaly
Uhl's anomaly
Tetralogy of Fallot
Single ventricle
Transposition of great vessels with pulmonary stenosis or atresia
Tricuspid or pulmonary insufficiency with right-to-left shunt

Table 6–11   Classification of Congenital Heart Abnormalities: Normal Vascularity (Left-Sided Lesions)

Coarctation of the aorta
Interrupted aortic arch
Hypoplastic left heart syndrome
Endocardial fibroelastosis
Cardiomyopathy
Aberrant left coronary artery
Mitral stenosis and insufficiency
Aortic stenosis and insufficiency
Cor triatriatum

Table 6–12   Classification of Congenital Heart Abnormalities: Normal Vascularity (Right-Sided Lesions)

Pulmonary stenosis or insufficiency
Tricuspid insufficiency

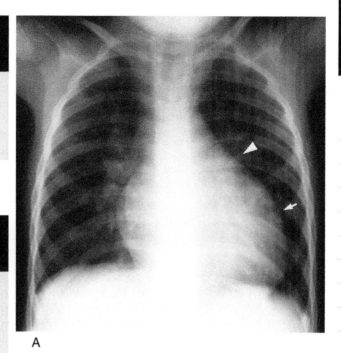

A

B

Figure 6–16   Patent ductus arteriosus (PDA). A, Frontal chest x-ray demonstrating enlargement of the region of the left atrium (*arrowhead*) and left ventricle (*arrow*). Hemodynamically, a shunt from the aorta to the pulmonary artery is present. The shunt functions in systole and diastole. The extra blood volume is circulated through the lungs and returned to the left atrium. It then passes to the left ventricle and finally out the aorta. Therefore, there is enlargement of all these structures. The right side of the heart is excluded from the hemodynamics of uncomplicated PDA. B, Lateral film demonstrates enlargement of the left ventricle. (*arrowhead*).

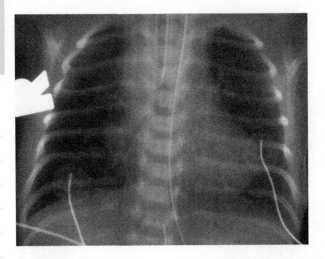

Figure 6–17   Tetralogy of Fallot. Note the "boot-shaped heart" with an upturn of the ventricle. The pulmonary vascularity is not very visible (particularly in the periphery of the lung). An endotracheal tube, an orogastric tube, and the tip of a central venous catheter (midline abdomen) are also present.

Lines and Tubes

A discussion of lines and tubes can also be found in Chapter 2. The lines and tubes unique to the pediatric population are umbilical lines. The endotracheal tube should be below the thoracic inlet and above the carina. The tube moves with chin movement. Often movement of the chin is the first maneuver that a clinician uses to manipulate placement of a tube that has been placed in too far or not far enough. Tubes that are too low usually descend into the right mainstem bronchus because of its more vertical orientation. This will lead to left lung atelectasis.

An umbilical artery catheter (UAC) and an umbilical vein catheter (UVC) are easily differentiated on x-ray. The UAC proceeds inferiorly from its insertion in the umbilicus into the pelvis, then turns and ascends into the aorta via a path through the umbilical and hypogastric (internal iliac) artery. The tip should be either at the L3–L4

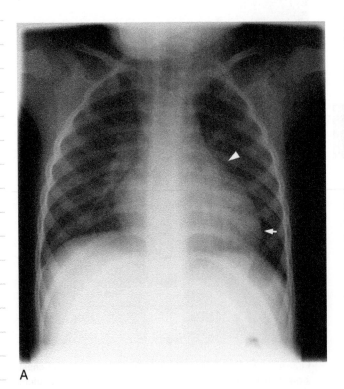

A

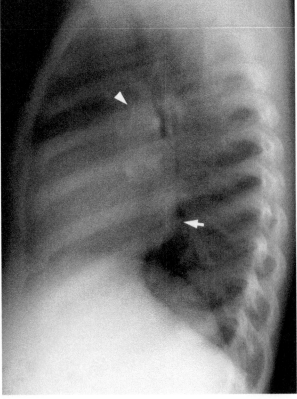

B

Figure 6–18   Ventriculoseptal defect (VSD). A, Frontal chest x-ray demonstrates increased pulmonary vascularity and moderate enlargement of the cardiac silhouette. Enlargement of the left atrium is present (*arrowhead*). The left ventricular dilation produces downward sagging of the cardiac apex (*arrow*). The enlarged pulmonary artery is hidden within the superior cardiac silhouette. B, Lateral chest x-ray demonstrates the enlarged left ventricle (*arrow*) and the enlarged pulmonary artery in the hilum (*arrowhead*). The hemodynamics depends on the size of the shunt. The more significant shunts lead to excessive pulmonary blood flow, active pulmonary vascular engorgement, and increased pulmonary venous return. Consequently, there is diastolic overloading and enlargement of the left ventricle (*arrowhead*).

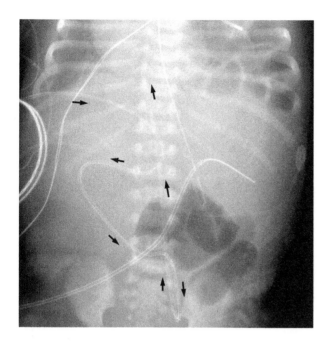

Figure 6–19 Umbilical artery catheter. Frontal abdominal film showing many lines and tubes going every which way. Unfortunately, this is what many x-rays show in the sick baby. It is helpful to try to remove any excess tubing from on top and under the baby before the x-ray is taken. However, this is not often possible when you are caring for a sick infant. Therefore, all lines and tubes should be evaluated from start to finish to determine their proper location. Umbilical artery catheter (*arrows*) begins external to the patient and then courses into the hypogastric artery and then along the aorta and finishes about T8. It appears shifted to the right. That is because there is bowel gas in the left chest! Can you deduce what is going on with this infant? An orogastric tube is also present, and there are numerous wires extraneous to the patient.

level or at T6–T10 (Figure 6–19). If the tip remains at the L1–L2 level, risk exists for thrombosis of the renal arteries, celiac axis, or superior mesenteric artery. Proximal migration is a problem if the catheter tip is too high in the thorax, with the possibility of extending into the great vessels to the head and neck or into the aortic arch.

The UVC proceeds superiorly from the umbilicus and courses posteriorly along the liver (best seen on lateral films) into the inferior vena cava (IVC) and right atrium. It passes from the umbilical vein into the left portal vein, ductus venosus, middle or left hepatic vein, and finally the IVC. The tip is ideally positioned at the junction of the IVC and right atrium (Figure 6–20). If the tip is too high, it may touch the atrioventricular node and cause an arrhythmia. It could also perforate the right atrium and lead to a pericardial effusion.

In infants, an orogastric tube is used instead of a nasogastric tube. The tip should terminate in a nondistended stomach.

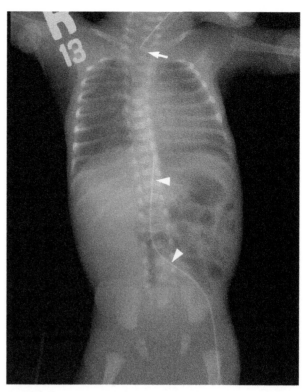

Figure 6–20 Umbilical vein catheter. Frontal image of the chest and abdomen in a newborn (babygram) reveals an umbilical venous catheter (*arrowheads*) and an endotracheal tube that is incorrectly positioned (too high) (*arrow*). (Courtesy of Elizabeth McGraw, MD.)

Abdomen

In the normal neonate, air should be seen in the stomach a couple of hours after birth, in the small bowel 6 hours later, and in the rectum in the first 24 hours. Healthy newborns don't need x-rays to evaluate gas progression. It is the infant who is not feeding or who has not passed meconium who warrants x-rays. A rule of thumb when evaluating the bowel in a newborn is that small and large bowel gas cannot be distinguished. When evaluating the gas distribution, assess proximal and distal bowel on a conventional x-ray (Figure 6–21).

A lesion that involves both the chest and the abdomen is a *congenital diaphragmatic hernia.* It causes respiratory distress in the neonatal period, and it carries a mortality rate greater than 50%. Clinical manifestations are a scaphoid abdomen and bowel sounds in the chest. Pulmonary hypoplasia exists due to the mass effect of the bowel in the chest. The hernias occur more commonly on the left and displace the heart and tracheal structures to the right (Figure 6–22). An orogastric tube may end in the right side of the chest if the stomach is involved with the herniation.

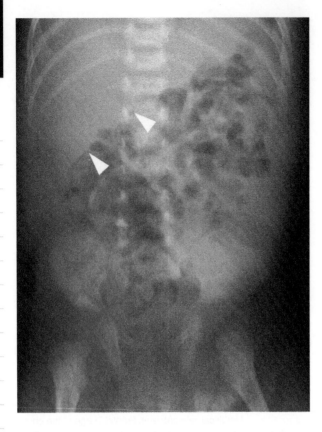

Figure 6–21   Normal kidneys, ureter, and bladder (KUB) view. Frontal x-ray of the abdomen in a newborn showing a normal bowel gas pattern. The soft tissue density in the right upper quadrant is the liver (*arrowheads*). (Courtesy of Elizabeth McGraw, MD.)

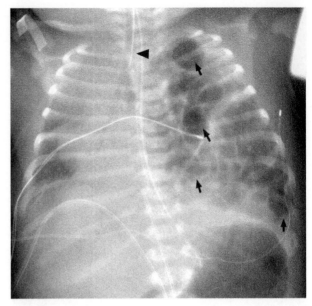

Figure 6–22   Congenital diaphragmatic hernia. Frontal chest x-ray of the patient in Figure 6–19 showing multiple air-filled, "cyst-like" structures in the left hemithorax. This is air-filled bowel (*arrows*). Note that the left hemidiaphragm is not visualized. The stomach bubble is distended. An endotracheal tube and an orogastric tube are present. Note the shift of the endotracheal tube to the right hemithorax (*arrowhead*).

Other congenital anomalies of the bowel can be seen in neonates. Tracheoesophageal fistula (TEF) may be suspected in an infant who has had in utero polyhydramnios. Clinically, there is excessive salivation and aspiration on feeding. In most cases of TEF, there is a blind-ending esophagus. The diagnosis can be confirmed by placing a soft feeding tube down the esophagus to the blind end and taking frontal and lateral x-rays. There is generally no need to provide contrast. Nearly 40% of infants with TEF have associated anomalies, such as the *VATER* syndrome (*v*ertebral anomalies, *a*nal atresia, *TEF*, *r*adial limb dysplasia).

Obstruction

A condition requiring surgery for repair that can be seen within the first 2 months of life is pyloric stenosis. There is a slight male predilection and a high incidence in a newborn whose sibling also had pyloric stenosis. Typically, these infants suffer nonbilious vomiting in the first month of life. A palpable "olive-shaped" mass to the right of the umbilicus is diagnostic. Conventional x-ray films will show a dilated, air-filled stomach. Ultrasonography demonstrates a donut-shaped, thickened pyloric muscle and is the study of choice to make this diagnosis.

Other causes of proximal obstruction include duodenal atresia and midgut volvulus. Conventional x-rays will show air in the bowel to the level of the obstruction. A "double bubble" is an x-ray finding that describes air in the stomach and proximal duodenum with no distal air. This appearance can be seen in duodenal atresia (Figure 6–23). Duodenal atresia is associated with Down syndrome. Annular pancreas and midgut volvulus less commonly cause a double bubble. Prenatal ultrasonography helps to disclose many of these abnormalities by demonstrating the presence of polyhydramnios.

Malrotation refers to any abnormality of rotation in which the ligament of Treitz (duodenal/jejunal junction) is not located to the left of the spine and at the same cephalocaudal level as the duodenal bulb. As you might remember from embryology (that class that you never thought was important but that keeps coming back to haunt you!), the small bowel first rotates 90 degrees outside of the body and then rotates an additional 180 degrees on returning to the body. The most significant complication of the malrotation is the *midgut volvulus*. A midgut volvulus occurs when the small bowel and proximal

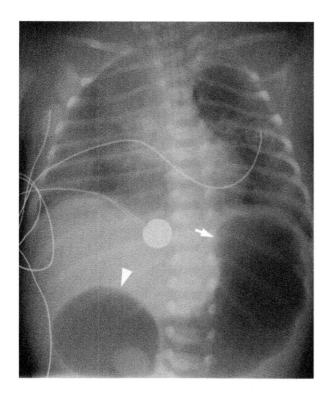

Figure 6–23   Duodenal atresia. Frontal chest and abdomen showing gaseous distention of the stomach (*arrow*) and of the first portion of the duodenum (*arrowhead*) in this patient with duodenal atresia. This has been referred to as the "double bubble." Note a low-lying endotracheal tube. The thymus is well demonstrated in this infant.

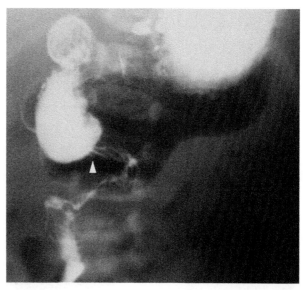

Figure 6–24   Midgut volvulus. Single frontal x-ray from an upper gastrointestinal series shows abnormal location of the duodenum and ligament of Treitz (*arrowhead*) in this infant with midgut volvulus. Slight distention of the proximal portion of the duodenum is also demonstrated.

colon rotate about the axis of the superior mesenteric artery. This can lead to arterial compromise and the development of gangrene if not thought of and diagnosed in a timely manner. The classic presentation of malrotation is bilious vomiting. Since the entire midgut can infarct, bilious vomiting in a newborn is an *emergency*!! Evaluation is made with a barium upper GI study to locate the ligament of Treitz (Figure 6–24).

If gas is not identified in the region of the rectum but is seen elsewhere in the bowel, a distal small bowel or colonic obstruction is possible. Two common explanations for this finding are *Hirschsprung's disease* and *meconium ileus*.

Meconium ileus is seen in half of patients with CF. Microcolon is seen on contrast studies in these patients, because the colon has been unused. Barium enema is performed with water-soluble contrast to draw fluid into the bowel, loosening the meconium. Reflux of contrast into the terminal ileum suggests that a colostomy is unnecessary.

Hirschsprung's disease is a condition in which the most distal bowel lacks neural ganglia. The proximal bowel is normal. Infants with this condition present because they have not passed stool. A transition

point is difficult to identify in the newborn after barium enema. A delayed film looking for a transition point or change in contrast is recommended as part of the evaluation. Older children generally demonstrate the transition point on barium enema (Figure 6–25). There is an association with Down syndrome.

Intussusception classically presents with "currant-jelly stool," a designation that is helpful only if the parents have ever had or seen currant jelly. Crampy abdominal pain is nonspecific but an important part of the presentation. Children with intussusception are often lethargic, which is important to remember. Lethargy often leads to a workup of sepsis, causing the diagnosis of intussusception to be delayed. The portion of the bowel that receives the intussuscepting bowel is the *intussuscipiens,* and the segment of intussuscepting bowel is referred to as the *intussusceptum.* Most of these occur in the ileocolic region. The conventional x-ray is most often normal, but since you now know what to look for, you can occasionally see an airless colon in the right lower quadrant or a soft tissue mass in this region. Children don't need a lead point mass for this telescoping to occur, whereas adults usually do. It is thought that intussusception occurs in children as a result of hypertrophied Peyer's patches in the terminal ileum. If the history is classic (particularly the currant jelly part), proceed immediately to Gastrografin enema for reduction. If this fails, surgery is necessary. Reduction should not be

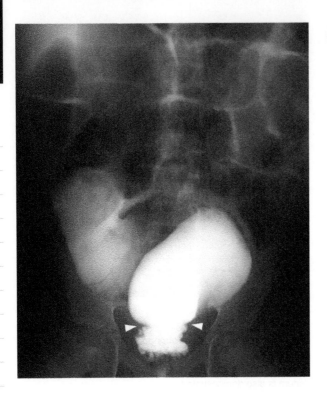

Figure 6–25 Hirschsprung's disease. Single anteroposterior film from a single-contrast barium enema demonstrates feature-less appearance of the distended rectum with transition point *(arrowheads)*.

attempted if there are clinical signs of peritonitis or shock.

Other relatively common lesions to consider when discussing bowel obstruction include incarcerated inguinal hernia and appendicitis. These generally occur in slightly older children (up to 3 years of age). The diagnosis of an incarcerated hernia is made on physical examination. The abdominal film should include the pelvis in order to see bowel below the level of the pubic ramus.

Appendicitis is not a diagnosis typically made on the basis of conventional radiography. However, in the appropriate clinical setting, visualization of a calcification in the right lower quadrant (appendicolith) indicates that no further studies are needed. Ultrasonography may show a thickened, noncompressible appendix, an appendicolith, or a complex fluid collection if a periappendiceal abscess has developed. Older children can be imaged with CT. Causes of obstruction based on age of presentation are summarized in **Table 6–13**. Evaluation of GI problems is outlined in **Table 6–14**.

Necrotizing Enterocolitis

Necrotizing enterocolitis (NEC) is the most common GI emergency in premature infants. The clinical presentation includes abdominal tenderness, rectal bleeding, and development of sepsis. Air within the bowel wall *(pneumatosis)* is the earliest radiographic finding. This produces a "bubbly" appearance of the bowel (Figure 6–26). An adynamic ileus is present, and therefore the small bowel dilates. A common complication is free air within the peritoneal cavity, indicating bowel perforation. Air in

---

Table 6–13   Common Causes of Gastrointestinal Tract Obstruction by Age

0–I Month

Congenital anomalies
    Atresia/stenosis
    Malrotation/volvulus
    Hirschsprung's disease
Meconium plug/small left colon syndrome
Meconium ileus

I–6 Months

Hernias

6–36 Months

Perforated appendix

36 Months and Older

Perforated appendix
Adhesions
Regional enteritis

Table 6–14   Radiographic Evaluation of Suspected Pediatric Gastrointestinal Problems

Condition	Imaging
Esophageal atresia or tracheoesophageal fistula (TEF)	Lateral x-ray with soft feeding tube
Gastroesophageal reflux (GER)	Barium swallow
Pyloric stenosis	Ultrasound
Duodenal atresia, stenosis, or midgut volvulus	Plain x-ray
Meconium ileus	Plain film, Gastrografin enema
Intussusception	Plain film, Gastrografin enema
Necrotizing enterocolitis (NEC)	Plain film
Hirschsprung's disease	Barium enema, Gastrografin enema
Meckel's diverticulum	Nuclear medicine

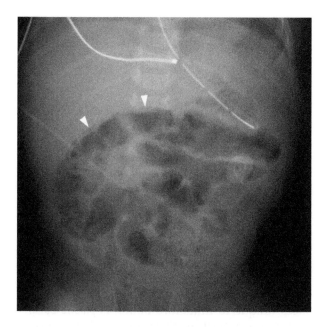

Figure 6–26 Pneumatosis, necrotizing enterocolitis. Frontal film of the abdomen demonstrates air in the bowel wall (*arrowheads*). No air is noted in the portal system (air superimposed over the liver). An orogastric tube is also present.

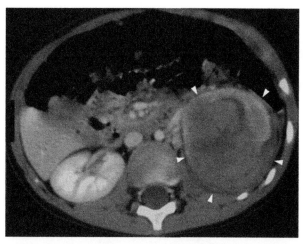

Figure 6–27 Wilms' tumor. Axial CT image after the administration of intravenous contrast at the level of the kidneys demonstrates a mass replacing the left kidney (*arrowheads*). This is characteristic of a Wilms' tumor in this young child.

the portal vein can also be identified. In children, unlike adults with portal venous gas, this does not portend a fatal outcome. In the setting of suspected NEC, cross-table lateral films are performed to assess for free air.

Meckel's Diverticulum

Meckel's diverticulum is the remnant of the omphalomesenteric duct. Clinical signs are more frequently related to painless lower GI bleeds. Meckel's diverticulum follows the "rule of 2's." It occurs in 2% of the population, usually presents before 2 years of age, and is usually located in the ileum within 2 feet of the ileocecal valve. The diverticulum may serve as the lead point of an intussusception. If the history is bleeding, a nuclear medicine study is the appropriate evaluation (see Chapter 8). Gastric mucosa is often present within the diverticulum. Technetium pertechnetate will avidly be taken up by normal and ectopic gastric mucosa. Barium enema is not helpful in making this diagnosis.

Abdominal Masses

The workup of a mass in the abdomen begins with a clinical history, a physical examination, and a conventional film of the abdomen. The differential diagnosis of an abdominal mass varies with the age of the child. Most masses in the abdomen arise from the kidneys, most commonly hydronephrosis. Other masses include GI duplication cysts and hemangioendotheliomas of the liver.

Hydronephrosis, Wilms' tumor, and neuroblastoma account for most flank masses. Neuroblastomas originate from neural tissue, and are seen along the course of the sympathetic chain. Calcifications are noted most of the time. This tumor is seen in children younger than 2 years of age. Neuroblastoma displaces the kidney when located in the adrenal gland. A Wilms' tumor deforms the kidney and distorts the collecting system (Figure 6–27). These tumors rarely calcify and occur in slightly older children than neuroblastoma.

Genitourinary Tract

The two common urinary problems in the pediatric age group are *hydronephrosis* and *ureterovesical reflux*. The most common cause of *hydronephrosis* is obstruction at the junction of the ureter and renal pelvis—the ureteropelvic junction (UPJ). Imaging with ultrasound provides information about the amount of dilatation of the collecting system, but not about the function of the kidney or the detail of the ureter. The best imaging study is an intravenous urogram. Follow-up studies can be performed with ultrasound or nuclear medicine to assess the degree of dilatation and function.

Reflux is most often due to maldevelopment of the flap valve created as the ureter courses obliquely through the bladder wall. This malfunctioning valve allows urine to reflux into the collecting system.

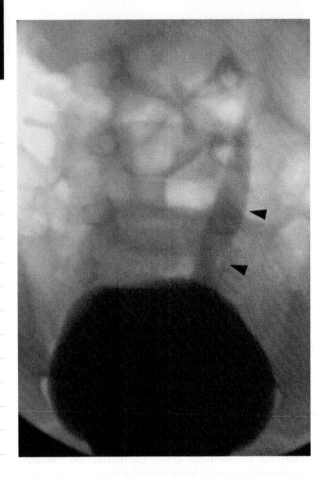

Figure 6–28 Voiding cystourethrogram (VCUG). Frontal film from a fluoroscopic examination after retrograde administration of contrast material. Contrast is demonstrated refluxed in the distal left ureter (*arrowheads*).

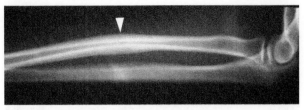

Figure 6–29 Plastic bowing deformity. Lateral x-ray of the forearm demonstrates volar bowing of the radius (*arrowhead*). Note the increase in periosteal reaction (thickened cortex) in the location of the bowing deformity.

Severe, long-standing reflux may lead to the development of infection. These abnormalities are therefore usually treated surgically when severe. Evaluation is performed with a voiding cystourethrogram (VCUG). Contrast is administered via a Foley catheter. The bladder is filled, and, while the child is voiding, the entirety of the collecting system is evaluated for reflux (Figure 6–28). This examination is associated with a high radiation dose to the gonads. Repeated examinations, if necessary, can be performed with nuclear cystograms that demonstrate function and allow for quantitative assessment of reflux with a lower radiation dose.

Musculoskeletal System

Fractures

The pediatric skeletal system differs from that of the adult by the presence of growth plates or *physes*. The bones are more flexible because pediatric bone is more porous. A child's bone can therefore tolerate a greater degree of deformity before fracturing completely. Children heal their fractures more quickly than adults do, except when the physis is involved.

Fractures in children have a variety of appearances unique to immature bones. A *plastic bowing deformity* is a fracture that causes a long bone to bend without breaking. The appearance is caused by microfractures on the concave side of the bone. Plastic bowing deformity is most commonly seen in the forearm. These fractures often require significant manipulation in the operating room to be reduced (Figure 6–29). *Buckle* or *torus fractures* occur at metaphyseal locations and resemble the torus or base of a pillar in architectural terms. Acute angulation of the cortex is noted, as opposed to the usual curved surface seen in this location (Figure 6–30). A *greenstick fracture* is a break in only one side of cortex. Think of the young limbs of a tree. When they are immature, they generally only break on one side of the branch and bend on the other. Fractures of this nature are treated by completing the fracture (after anesthesia) and then reducing it.

As mentioned earlier and in Chapter 4, in a skeletally immature patient, epiphyses are not fused to the remainder of the bone. The growth plates are open, and the physis is actively "maturing" by continuing to ossify. Injuries to this area can result in growth disturbances if not identified. The function of the *epiphysis* is to add to the length of the bone, while an *apophysis* is an ossification center that adds to the width of the bone. Tendons insert onto apophyses. Fractures through the growth plate can lead to unique complications if not identified. A classification scheme used for physeal fractures is the *Salter-Harris* classification (Figure 6–31). Type I is a fracture through the physis. This can be a difficult fracture to identify on conventional x-ray, but the physis should get wider compared with the contralateral extremity (Figure 6–32). Clinical suspicion is helpful. Conventional films may not be very revealing. An MRI is often very useful to see edema through the growth plate. A Salter-Harris

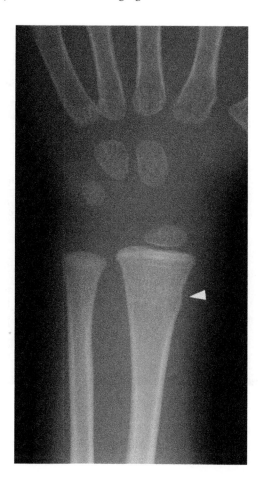

Figure 6–30   Torus fracture. Anteroposterior view of the wrist in a very young child demonstrates buckling of the cortex at the distal radius (*arrowhead*). This is a common result of a fall on an outstretched hand. Note the lack of ossification centers in the wrist. The nonvisualized carpal bones are still cartilage and have not ossified.

type II fracture involves the physis and the metaphysis (Figure 6–33). These are the most common type of physeal fractures. Type III fractures extend through the physis into the epiphysis. Type IV fractures traverse all three areas—the physis, epiphysis, and metaphysis (Figure 6–34). Type V fractures are considered crush injuries to the physis; they can be very difficult to identify on conventional radiography but are readily identified with MRI. MRI is an excellent means of evaluation when these types of injuries are suspected clinically. Narrowing of the physis with edema is noted. Marrow edema may be seen on either side of the physis.

A *toddler's fracture* is unique to this population. These are spiral, oblique fractures of the middle to distal tibia that may not be seen on AP or lateral views (Figure 6–35). Oblique imaging is often useful, and MRI is diagnostic when these injuries are occult by conventional imaging.

A *supracondylar fracture of the elbow* is the most common elbow fracture in children. These fractures occur from FOOSH (fall on outstretched hand) injuries. Analyzing the lateral elbow film for displaced fat pads is how the diagnosis is made. Evaluate the anterior humeral line and its relationship with the capitellum to identify the displaced supracondylar location (Figure 6–36). Identification of the displaced fat pads is essentially diagnostic. The child will be placed in a posterior splint and treated as though a fracture were present.

Avulsion fractures occur at tendon insertions. These types of injuries are much more common in children than in adults. Avulsion fractures usually result from sudden muscular pull during vigorous athletic activity (Figure 6–37).

The Salter-Harris Classification of Growth Plate Injuries

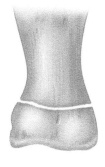
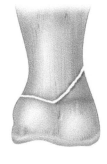
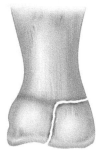
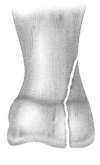
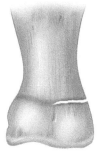

| I | II | III | IV | V |

Figure 6–31   Salter-Harris classification of physeal fractures. Type I is a slip or widening of the physis. Type II is a fracture through the metaphysis and physis. Type III is a fracture through the epiphysis and physis. Type IV is a fracture involving metaphysis, physis, and epiphysis. Type V is a crush injury to the physis. Type V is often delayed in diagnosis.

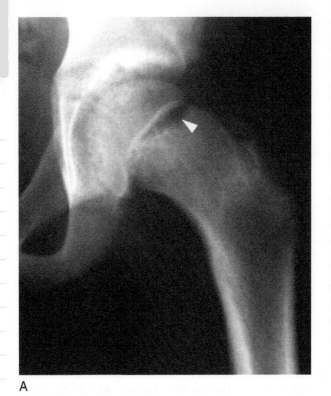

A

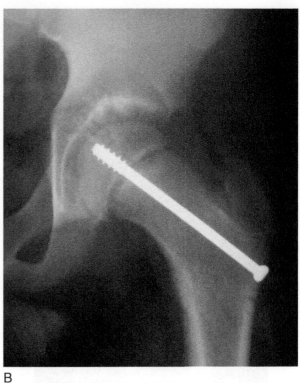

B

Figure 6–32 Slipped capital femoral epiphysis. A, Antero-posterior view of the left hip demonstrates widening of the physis (*arrowhead*) with abnormal relationship of the metaphysis and epiphysis. This is a Salter-Harris type I injury. B, After an intraosseous screw has been placed, the alignment of the physis as well as the relationship of the metaphysis and epiphysis has improved.

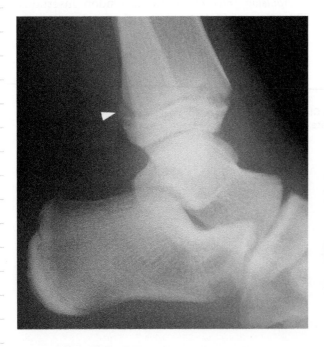

Figure 6–33 Salter Harris type II injury. Lateral x-ray of the ankle demonstrates a small fracture of the posterior portion of the tibial metaphysis (*arrowhead*).

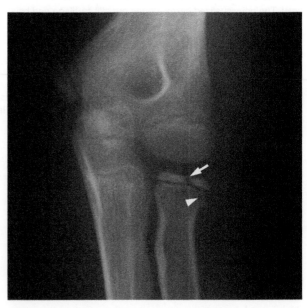

Figure 6–34 Salter-Harris type IV. Anteroposterior x-ray of the elbow demonstrates a linear lucency extending from the proximal metaphysis of the radius (*arrowhead*) through the physis into the epiphysis (*arrow*).

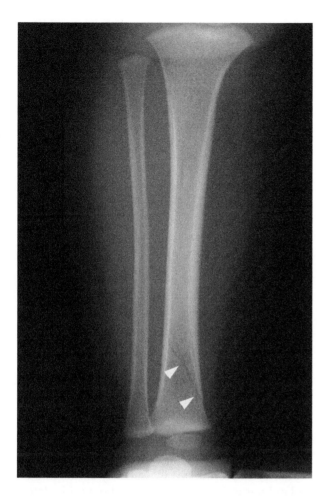

Figure 6–35 Toddler's fracture. Anteroposterior x-ray of the tibia demonstrates an oblique lucency in the distal tibia (*arrowheads*). This represents a nondisplaced, nondistracted fracture.

Infection

When you are seeing a child who cannot bear weight on an extremity because of a painful joint, you need to be concerned about a septic joint, particularly if the painful joint coincides with fever and leukocytosis. There are no imaging studies available to determine whether a joint is infected. An arthrocentesis is necessary to determine if pus is in the joint. Aspirated joint fluid is sent to the laboratory for cell count and culture. Bacterial infections can destroy a joint in short order. A delay in diagnosis can lead to marked cartilage loss, and ultimately to early joint destruction. Ultrasonography for evaluation of an effusion is less than 100% accurate and is therefore not recommended. MRI, although accurate in evaluating for the presence of an effusion, cannot determine whether an effusion is infected. *Toxic synovitis* is indistinguishable from septic arthritis by imaging. No organisms are

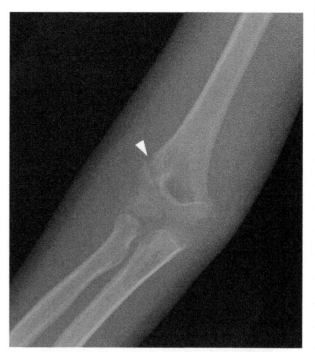

A

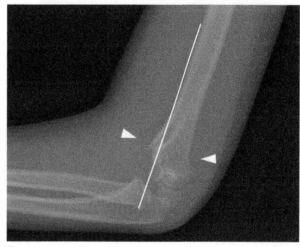

B

Figure 6–36 Supracondylar fracture. A, Anteroposterior conventional x-ray of the elbow in a child shows a lucency in the lateral supracondylar location (*arrowhead*). B, Lateral view of the elbow in a pediatric patient with a supracondylar fracture shows the utility of the "anterior humeral line." A vertical line drawn along the anterior aspect of the humerus should intersect the midportion of the capitellum when normal. In this case, the capitellum is posterior to the line, because the supracondylar location is displaced relative to the capitellum. The fat pads are present anteriorly and posteriorly (*arrowheads*) because of the joint effusion. (Courtesy of Elizabeth McGraw, MD.)

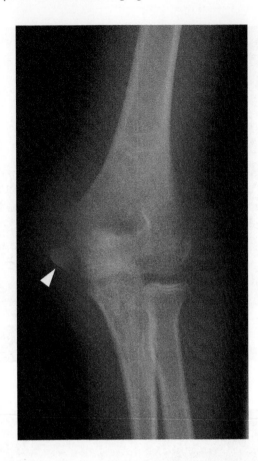

Figure 6–37 Avulsion injury. Anteroposterior x-ray of the elbow in a child, showing malposition of the medial epicondyle (*arrowhead*) with overlying soft tissue swelling. The common extensor tendon inserts onto this bone. This injury is referred to as "Little Leaguers' elbow." Note a small piece of bone avulsed with the medial epicondyle. This would be a Salter-Harris type II injury. This fracture was treated surgically with a pin. Occasionally, the ossification centers around the elbow can be confusing. When in doubt, examine the patient and correlate with the x-ray findings. If you are still not sure whether the bones are quite right, a comparison view with the other side can be helpful.

recovered in toxic synovitis, and the cell count is typically lower than in infection.

Osteomyelitis is discussed in Chapter 4. As a reminder, conventional x-rays are insensitive for the detection of osteomyelitis, whereas bone scan and MRI are much more sensitive, but not specific. A fluid collection may be identified with MRI, and a bone scan can be useful for determining multifocal involvement.

Neoplasms

Chapter 4 discussed the differential diagnosis for aggressive-appearing lesions in the pediatric patient population. A lesion unique to children is leukemia. Leukemia is a disorder of the marrow,

but it can affect any bone and demonstrate an aggressive-appearing lesion. Typical "metaphyseal lucent bands" are characteristic of leukemic infiltrates. Osteosarcoma can be lytic or sclerotic. The role of MRI is in determining skip lesions and involvement of neurovascular bundles. Ewing's sarcoma is a permeative process with poorly defined margins. In general, Ewing's sarcoma is more often diaphyseal in location, but this rule is often not helpful in distinguishing this tumor from other aggressive lesions. Langerhans histiocytosis (eosinophilic granuloma) is an abnormal proliferation of histiocytes that can involve any organ system but most commonly affects bone and has a variety of imaging appearances. The skull, ribs, and long bones seem to be the most commonly affected locations.

Congenital and Developmental Disorders

Commonly encountered congenital and developmental abnormalities include developmental dysplasia of the hip (congenital hip dislocation), tibia vara (Blount's disease), and clubfoot. Developmental dysplasia of the hip is due to a shallow acetabulum or a steep acetabular angle and ligamentous laxity. This abnormality is associated with a breech birth, and girls are more commonly affected than boys. In neonates, where the hip is primarily cartilaginous, no landmarks are available for radiographic determination of congenital dislocation of the hip. If strong clinical suspicion exists for hip dislocation in a neonate, ultrasonography is recommended. In children and older infants with more ossification of the hip joint, conventional films can be used to make this determination (Figure 6–38).

Blount's disease presents with marked depression, irregularity, and fragmentation of the medial metaphyseal tibial beak. This leads to the development of tibia vara and bowlegs (Figure 6–39). A third not infrequently encountered abnormality is that of *clubfoot* or *talipes equinovarus*. The ankle is in equinus position with both hindfoot and forefoot varus deformity.

Scoliosis is abnormal curvature of the vertebral column that can be divided into three subtypes: congenital, idiopathic, and neuromuscular. *Congenital scoliosis* occurs in association with vertebral anomalies and anomalies of other organs (e.g., VATER syndrome). Some possible vertebral body anomalies are hemivertebrae, butterfly vertebrae, and bony bar through the vertebral body. *Idiopathic scoliosis* is an S-shaped scoliosis with a primary and a secondary curve in the thoracic and lumbar spine (Figure 6–40). *Neuromuscular scoliosis* is associated with a C-shaped scoliosis. To evaluate scoliosis,

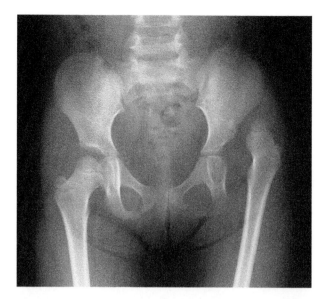

Figure 6–38   Developmental dysplasia of the hip (DDH). AP view of the pelvis demonstrates superior and lateral location of the femoral head with respect to the acetabulum. Note the under-development of the femoral head and acetabulum of the left side compared with the right. (Courtesy of Elizabeth McGraw, MD.)

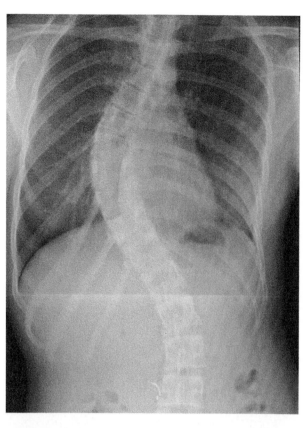

Figure 6–40   Scoliosis. Frontal view of the spine demonstrates an S-shaped scoliosis, which indicates an idiopathic form of scoliosis. However, a search for vertebral body anomalies as a cause is always indicated. Worth noting is that spine surgeons hang these films in an opposite manner from radiologists—as if the patient's back were to them. The curvilinear metallic density in the abdomen is a navel ring in this teenager.

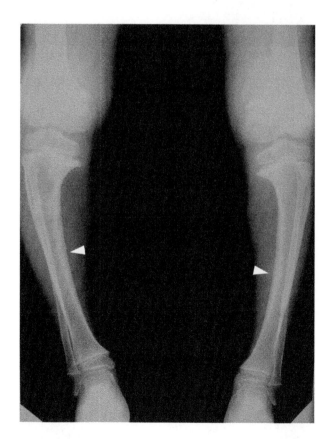

Figure 6–39   Blount's disease. Anteroposterior view of both lower legs demonstrates bowing of the tibia bilaterally. Note the increased sclerosis and irregularity of the medial portion of the tibial metaphysis bilaterally (*arrowheads*). This will lead to the development of tibia vara.

erect frontal and lateral films are necessary. Right and left bending films are also helpful to determine motion associated with the scoliosis. This combination of films helps the orthopaedic surgeon determine when surgical repair needs to be undertaken and which levels should be incorporated in the fusion.

Nonaccidental Trauma

Nonaccidental trauma (NAT) is said to affect 1,000,000 children per year in the United State. This statistic alone should give you pause. Children are an active bunch, and most of the time their injuries result from accidental trauma. However, it is important to recognize NAT. More than half of the children inflicted with NAT have detectable fractures. Imaging examinations are extremely important whenever child abuse is suspected, because they may supply evidence of multiple episodes of abuse,

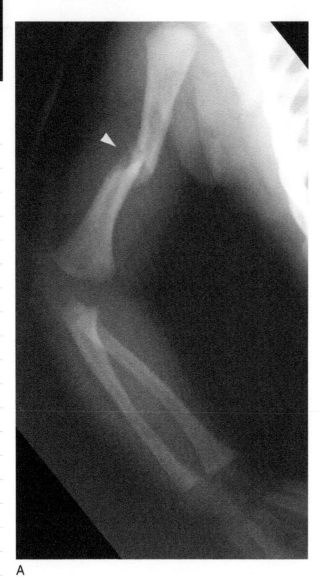

A

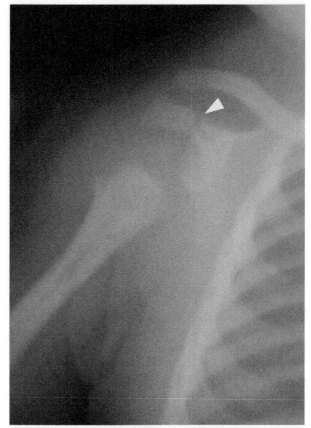

B

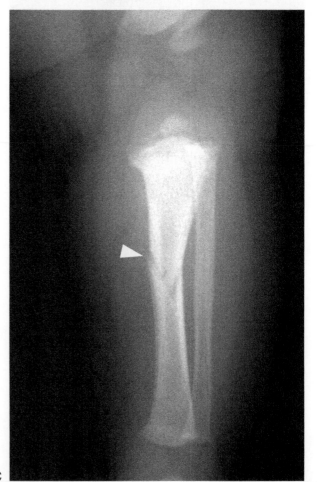

C

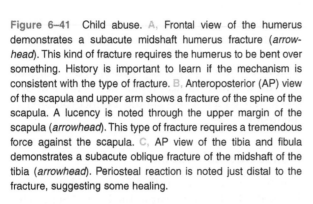

Figure 6–41 Child abuse. A, Frontal view of the humerus demonstrates a subacute midshaft humerus fracture (*arrowhead*). This kind of fracture requires the humerus to be bent over something. History is important to learn if the mechanism is consistent with the type of fracture. B, Anteroposterior (AP) view of the scapula and upper arm shows a fracture of the spine of the scapula. A lucency is noted through the upper margin of the scapula (*arrowhead*). This type of fracture requires a tremendous force against the scapula. C, AP view of the tibia and fibula demonstrates a subacute oblique fracture of the midshaft of the tibia (*arrowhead*). Periosteal reaction is noted just distal to the fracture, suggesting some healing.

whereas the clinical history and examination may provide evidence of only the most recent injury. If NAT is suspected, a skeletal survey should be requested. This series includes an AP and lateral view of the skull; lateral views of the spine; AP views of the chest, abdomen, and pelvis; and AP views of the long bones of the extremities, including the hands and the feet.

Highly specific x-ray fractures include those that involve the metaphysis of long bones (especially corner fractures), posterior ribs, scapulae, spinous processes, and sternum. Moderately specific x-ray findings include the presence of fractures at different stages of healing and in different locations, physeal fractures, and fractures of the bones of the hands, particularly in infants and young children (Figure 6–41). Complex skull fractures would also be suggestive of NAT.

Abdominal CT scans may show evidence of visceral injuries resulting from blunt blows or deceleration injuries, gastric rupture, or small-bowel perforation. Duodenal hematomas and mesenteric tears are also suspicious for child abuse. Splenic, hepatic, and renal lacerations can occur with motor vehicle crashes, but without that history, child abuse should be a consideration. CT or MRI examinations of the brain in NAT may show sub-galeal hematomas (superficial to the skull) and skull fractures. Facial injuries may be evident. Evidence of intracranial trauma such as subdural hematomas, cerebral contusions, or subarachnoid or intraventricular hemorrhages may also be seen.

Cerebral atrophy is a finding that can be seen as a result of previous injury to the brain.

Emergencies

There are many entities discussed above that require a timely response to radiographic findings. Free air, regardless of the location, should be correlated clinically and acted upon appropriately. Air in the interstitium of the bronchus or bowel wall should be correlated clinically to allow for appropriate timely intervention. Obstruction in the bowel or genitourinary system requires intervention for immediate relief. Causes of abdominal obstruction include congenital anomalies, hernias, intus-susception, and perforated appendix, to name just a few. A midgut volvulus is imperative to recognize due to the associated high mortality rate without surgical intervention. Bilious vomiting in an infant is therefore always considered an emergency. Neurologic emergencies are discussed in Chapter 5.

Suggested Reading List

Burton EM, Brody AS: Essentials of Pediatric Radiology. New York, Thieme, 1999.

Donnelly L: Diagnostic Imaging: Pediatrics. Philadelphia, WB Saunders, 2006.

Swischuk LE: Imaging of the Newborn, Infant and Young Child, 5th ed. Philadelphia, Lippincott, Williams & Wilkins, Philadelphia, PA, 2004.

Interventional Radiology

Interventional radiology is the subspecialty of radiology in which radiologists use imaging guidance to perform diagnostic and therapeutic procedures. Many radiologists enjoy this aspect of their job, because it provides immediate gratification by relieving patients of their presenting problem during the intervention. Procedures that were previously performed surgically are now being performed as outpatient procedures in interventional suites under conscious sedation, at a lower cost to the patient.

The focus of this chapter is to introduce basic techniques and indications so you will understand how this subspecialty of radiology contributes to patient care.

Techniques

Angiography is a technique of imaging blood vessels, usually by injecting contrast material via an intraluminal catheter. When imaging the peripheral vascular system, conventional angiography and intra-arterial digital subtraction angiography are preferred methods (Figure 7–1).

The technique used to introduce a catheter into a blood vessel is called the Seldinger technique. In this technique, a vessel is punctured with a needle (usually the femoral artery at the level of the femoral head), a guidewire is fed through the needle, the needle is removed over the guidewire (with the wire held in place by good radiology technique), a catheter is placed over the guidewire, and the guidewire is removed. Correct placement of the catheter tip is confirmed with a test injection of contrast material. Catheters and guidewires usually have floppy or curved ends to minimize possibility of damage to the walls of the vessels. Common indications for angiography are trauma (aortic transection, vascular injuries to the extremities, carotid or vertebral vascular injuries), bleeding (gastrointestinal and pelvic for embolization), claudication, renovascular hypertension (renal artery stenosis), pulmonary embolism (in the setting of an indeterminate ventilation/perfusion [V/Q] scan or for inferior vena cava [IVC] filter placement), and poorly functioning dialysis fistula (**Table 7–1**).

Potential complications of angiography are numerous and include those related to contrast administration, including allergic reactions and renal failure. Adequate hydration is key to minimizing the deleterious effects of iodinated contrast agents. Patients who have an elevated creatinine concentration (>2 mg/dL) are at greater risk of developing contrast-induced renal failure. Carbon

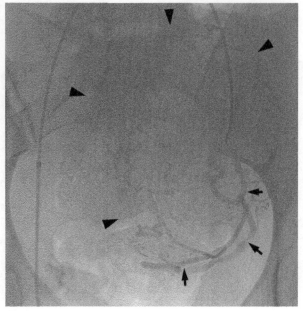

A

B

Figure 7–1 Conventional angiography (nonsubtracted and subtracted images). Fibroid (myomatous) uterus embolization. A, Nonsubtracted image from a cannulization for embolization of a myomatous uterus. Catheter is noted extending from the right femoral artery, through the right external and common iliac arteries to the bifurcation into the left iliac artery, and then selectively into a vessel that is feeding a very vascular fibroid uterus (arrowheads). The bones of the pelvis are seen on this image. Large arteries are seen wandering in the pelvis (arrows). B, The subtraction image shows only the abnormal vessels perfusing the abnormal uterus (arrowheads). The pelvic bones have been "subtracted." (Courtesy of Tony Smith, MD.)

dioxide gas is an alternative to contrast and is nontoxic and inexpensive. The disadvantage is that it is harder to visualize in smaller vessels. Non–contrast-related complications are those related to the puncture site, including the development of overt hemorrhage, hematoma, pseudoaneurysm, and arteriovenous fistula. Other vessel injuries that may occur as a result of vascular procedures include subintimal dissection, thrombosis, and distal embolization.

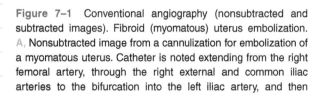

Table 7–1 Common Indications for Angiography

Trauma
   Aortic transection
   Vascular injuries to the extremities
   Carotid or vertebral vascular injuries
Hemorrhage
   Gastrointestinal and pelvic for embolization
Claudication
Renovascular hypertension
Pulmonary embolism
   Indeterminate ventilation/perfusion (V/Q) scan
   Inferior vena cava (IVC) filter placement
Poorly functioning dialysis fistula

Venography is not infrequently used for evaluation in the upper extremity, because ultrasound is technically more difficult to use due to the bone structure of the shoulder girdle. In the upper extremity, an antecubital vein is cannulated and contrast material is injected under fluoroscopic control. Venography of the lower extremity is still occasionally performed despite the advent of ultrasonography and magnetic resonance (MR) venography. A dorsal pedal vein is cannulated, and intravenous infusion of heparinized saline is begun. A tourniquet is applied above the ankle to force the contrast material into the deep system. Valsalva maneuver facilitates filling of the iliac system and IVC while the calf is massaged. The patient then relaxes, and the exposure is made while contrast material flows into the pelvis.

Computed tomography (CT) has limited use in the peripheral system but remains important in the evaluation of the abdominal aorta and the pelvic vessels. With the advent of flow-sensitive gradient echo techniques and cine acquisition, MR angiography has demonstrated its applicability for noninvasive imaging of the peripheral vascular system.

Ultrasonography is a good screening examination of larger vessels, and vascularity in the neck

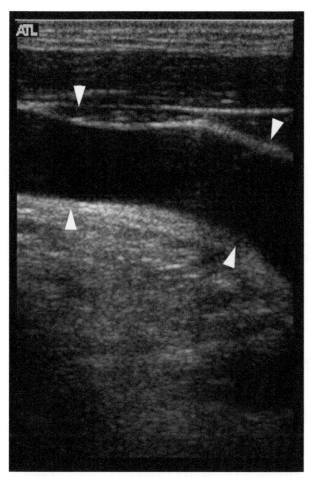

A

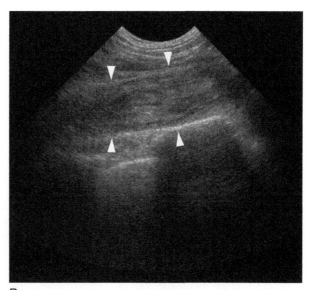

B

Figure 7–2   Ultrasound of normal leg veins and deep venous thrombosis. A. Longitudinal ultrasound image of normal patent leg veins (*arrowheads*). Normal vessels will demonstrate flow with Doppler imaging and will change capacity with respiration and Valsalva techniques. B. Longitudinal ultrasound image demonstrating echogenic material within the femoral vein (*arrowheads*). This is the appearance of thrombus in the vessel.

and extremities can be assessed with color Doppler and duplex ultrasound in a noninvasive fashion (Figure 7–2). The review of physics is beyond the scope of this introductory chapter. Refer to texts at the end of the chapter if you'd like to read more about the principles of color Doppler and duplex sonography. This is the technique employed in evaluating the lower extremity to exclude a deep venous thrombosis. The proximal deep veins of the lower extremity are examined from the inguinal ligament to the popliteal fossa. The vessels are evaluated in the transverse plane with compression and release every 1 cm to the level of the popliteal fossa. Compressibility of the vein and presence or absence of thrombus are assessed. Longitudinal views are used to assess the length of thrombus.

Commonly encountered vessels and disease processes will be noted in this chapter. There will not be a review of the entire vascular system.

Interventions

Angioplasty is a technique that uses special dilating catheters to open occluded or stenotic blood vessels. The combination of angioplasty with vascular stenting has greatly improved its results. Stents are mesh-like tubes that can be inserted through a catheter and expanded within a stenotic vessel in an attempt to restore adequate blood flow and prevent further stenosis. The main indications for stent placement include a residual pressure gradient of more than 10 mm Hg after angioplasty and dissection after angioplasty. In managing a dissection, the goal of stent placement is to appose the dissected flap against the wall to improve blood flow (Figure 7–3).

Embolization involves the deliberate occlusion of arteries, veins, or abnormal vascular spaces by the introduction of various materials through a selectively positioned catheter. Commonly used materials include Gelfoam, coils, wires, and balloons. Usual indications include acute bleeding, neovascularity from a vascular neoplasm, arteriovenous malformation, and intracranial aneurysm. Embolization procedures require diligent placement of the materials so that they do not end up in vessels other than those intended (Figure 7–4).

Patients suffering pelvic hemorrhage due to trauma receive a diagnostic pelvic angiogram with the catheter placed above the bifurcation of the aorta. Active hemorrhage is diagnosed by extravasation

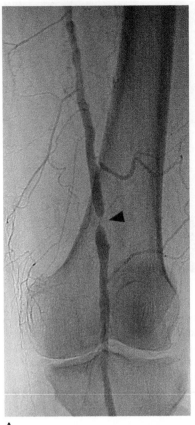

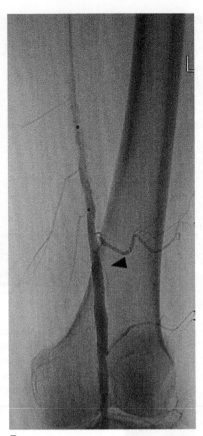

A

B

Figure 7–3 Peripheral vascular disease. A, Frontal image from a arteriogram performed for peripheral vascular disease. The common femoral artery and popliteal artery demonstrate opacification. Irregularities are noted along the femoral artery, but marked stenosis is identified at the popliteal artery (*arrowhead*). B, Contrast study done at the time of angioplasty to improve patency of the popliteal artery (*arrowhead*). Markers indicating the presence of the balloon are identified as small square foci just proximal to the arrowhead. If the patient's gradient were still abnormal after the angioplasty, a stent could be considered. The development of stents and interventional techniques has revolutionized the treatment of peripheral vascular disease.

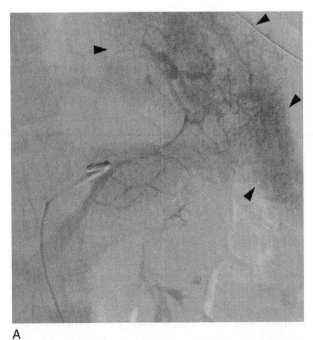

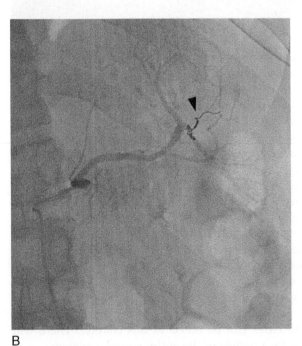

A

B

Figure 7–4 Splenic laceration. A, Single film from selected catheterization of the splenic artery shows pooling of contrast material outside the lumen of the vessel (*arrowheads*). B, After treatment with coils (*arrowhead*) and repeat injection, no pooling of contrast is noted.

contrast. The bleeding vessel may be embolized with Gelfoam or coils. Gelfoam recanalizes within 2 to 3 weeks, whereas coil embolization is permanent. A rich collateral blood supply exists in the pelvis, so ischemia resulting from an embolization procedure is unusual.

Gastrointestinal hemorrhage is evaluated with angiography after a diagnostic nuclear medicine tagged red cell study is performed (more about that in Chapter 8). Selective catheterization of the celiac, superior mesenteric, and inferior mesenteric arteries is performed. The choice of embolization depends on the cause and location of the bleeding. Vasoconstrictors (vasopressin) have been used in the past for gastrointestinal bleeds but are being replaced with embolization due to the improved choice of materials and ease with which embolization can be performed.

Interventional radiologists are often asked to place a venous access catheter for long-term administration of antibiotics or chemotherapy or for dialysis access. Commonly placed devices include peripherally inserted central catheters (PICC), permanent dialysis catheters, and triple-lumen catheters. The optimal placement for the tip of any of these catheters is at the junction of the superior vena cava and right atrium.

IVC filters are placed to prevent pulmonary embolism by trapping a clot from the lower extremities or pelvis before it embolizes to the lung. IVC filters are usually placed in patients in whom anticoagulation is not an option. These filters can be deployed via an internal jugular vein or femoral vein approach. Filters should be placed in the infrarenal IVC in order to reduce the risk of renal vein thrombosis (Figure 7–5).

Transjugular intrahepatic portosystemic shunts (TIPS) are placed in patients with portal hypertension who have intractable ascites or variceal hemorrhage. The purpose of this shunt is to decompress the portal venous system by shunting portal blood through the hepatic veins. Knowledge of the anatomy and the fact that this procedure can be performed via a right internal jugular vein approach decreases the morbidity for these patients. Before the advent of the TIPS procedure, surgery was required for these patients and the mortality in this group was high.

Great Vessels

Pulmonary arteriography is regarded as the gold standard in the diagnosis of pulmonary embolism. Many institutions now routinely perform CT for evaluation of pulmonary embolus (see Chapter 2). Pulmonary arteriography requires constant electro-

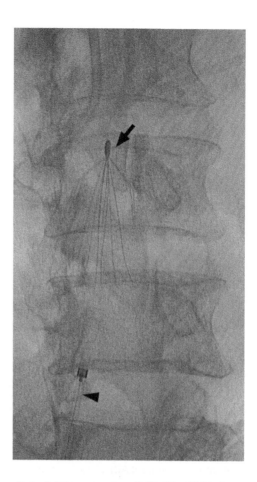

Figure 7–5   Inferior vena cava (IVC) filter. Single image from procedure to place IVC filter for prevention of pulmonary embolus. The right femoral vein was cannulated, and the sheath transporting the IVC filter can be seen (*arrowhead*). The IVC filter (*arrow*) is satisfactorily positioned.

cardiographic (ECG) monitoring because, in patients with left bundle branch block, conversion to complete heart block can occur during passage of the catheter through the right side of the heart.

The cause of death in most cases of aortic transection is exsanguination. The precise mechanism of injury is uncertain, but many investigators believe that it is sudden deceleration, which allows the mobile descending aorta to shear from the relatively fixed aortic arch. This is a reasonable explanation, since the most common site for aortic transection is just distal to the origin of the left subclavian artery. Injuries are clearly demonstrated with aortography. In particular, the left anterior oblique (LAO) view allows complete visualization of the aortic arch. Deformity in this location is diagnostic of an aortic injury (Figure 7–6). Keep in mind that the ductus bump, a normal anatomic variant in the arch, can be seen on the inferior surface of the aortic arch. It represents the site of attachment of the ductus arteriosus.

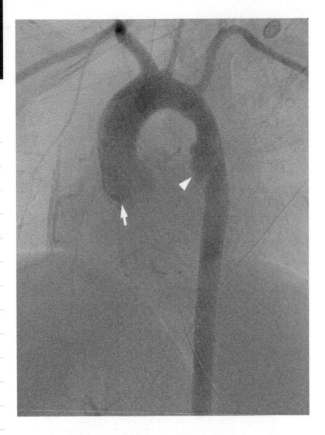

Figure 7–6 Pseudoaneurysm from aortic arch injury. Subtraction left anterior oblique (LAO) projection demonstrates a large pseudoaneurysm (*arrowhead*) from an injury to the aorta. This patient was injured in a motor vehicle crash. Remember that a widened mediastinum in the setting of trauma should prompt investigation for an aortic injury. Note the pigtail catheter at the root of the aorta (*arrow*).

Clinical symptoms of aortic arch injury are often obscured by other intra-abdominal or musculoskeletal injuries. Frontal chest x-ray signs of this injury include mediastinal widening, apical pleural density due to blood above the apical portion of the lung, and deviation of the trachea or nasogastric tube to the right (Key Point 7–1). The aortopulmonary window is usually opacified, and the arch is poorly defined.

Aneurysm, or dilatation of a vessel, can be a result of atherosclerosis, inflammation, trauma, or a congenital condition. Aneurysms located in the thoracic or the abdominal aorta are generally surgically repaired to avoid the complication of rupture. Sudden onset of chest pain in a patient with a known aneurysm should suggest rupture or ongoing dissection.

Evaluation of an aneurysm can easily be performed using CT scanning with a bolus of intravenous contrast material. Cross-sectional examination with CT allows visualization of the aneurysm as well as clot along the inner wall of the

---

Key Point 7–1

Frontal Chest X-ray Findings in Aortic Arch Injury

Mediastinal widening
Apical pleural density
Rightward deviation of trachea or nasogastric tube
Aortopulmonary window opacification
Poorly defined aortic arch

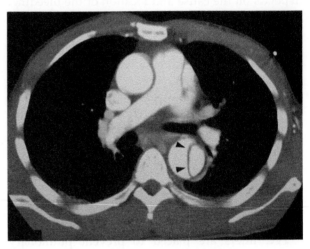

Figure 7–7 Aortic dissection. Axial image from CT after the administration of intravenous contrast material in the arterial phase at the level of the pulmonary arteries demonstrates a linear area of soft tissue attenuation in the lumen of the aorta (*arrowheads*). This is the appearance of a dissection. It is imperative to assess the proximal and distal aspects in order to determine management. Also, true and false lumens should be determined, and the origin of mesenteric and renal arteries should be assessed for involvement.

aneurysm. Arteriography is not the best way to evaluate an aneurysm. It does not allow for visualization of the clot. In addition, the catheter can release clot as it is being manipulated through the descending aorta, leading to embolism. Magnetic resonance imaging (MRI) can be used to evaluate aneurysms, but imaging times are longer than for CT and life support, if required by the patient, is difficult to manage in the magnet.

Aortic *dissection* is the result of an intimal tear causing separation of the layers of the wall of the aorta. Aortic dissection also commonly occurs in patients with atherosclerotic disease, particularly when associated with hypertension. Demonstration of an intimal flap by CT is diagnostic of dissection (Figure 7–7). Dissection of the thoracic aorta proximal to the left subclavian artery is a surgical

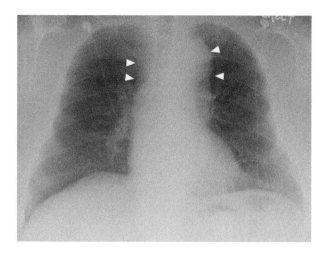

Figure 7–8   Aortic dissection. Frontal conventional x-ray demonstrating a widened mediastinum (*arrowheads*) in a patient who presented with chest pain and a dissection of the aorta.

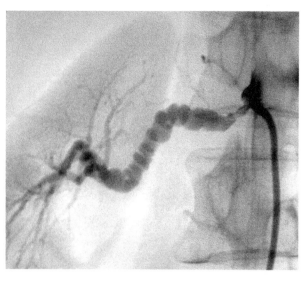

Figure 7–9   Renal fibromuscular dysplasia. Single film from selected renal artery catheterization demonstrating the stenosis and poststenotic dilation involving the right renal artery. This entity has been described as a "string of beads." It can lead to renal arterial occlusion, elevated blood pressure, and poor renal function. (Courtesy of Tony Smith, MD.)

emergency, whereas dissection of the descending thoracic aorta is usually managed nonoperatively by controlling the patient's hypertension.

Aortic dissection should be suspected on a chest x-ray if there is a double contour of the aortic arch, progressive serial enlargement of the aorta, or displacement of intimal calcification from the outer aortic margin (watch for rotation on the film). Additional findings on the chest x-ray include a dilated aorta with a widened mediastinum and cardiomegaly (Figure 7–8).

Peripheral Vessels

Evaluation of abdominal and pelvic vessels other than the aorta is best done by contrast angiography. The hepatic, renal, lumbar, and mesenteric arteries are well seen with arteriography. Atherosclerotic changes and areas of stenosis are clearly seen with this technique. Intervention can be performed, as described previously, as clinically necessary. Atherosclerotic disease can occur anywhere in the arterial system, but it commonly causes arterial occlusion in the lower extremities and carotid arteries. Other causes of peripheral arterial occlusion include thromboembolism (most commonly from the heart) and fibromuscular dysplasia (most often affecting the renal artery) (Figure 7–9). Vasculitis, such as temporal arteritis and collagen vascular disease, is readily diagnosed with arteriography.

Arteriography is also helpful in diagnosing entrapment syndromes such as thoracic outlet syndrome and popliteal entrapment syndrome. Thoracic outlet syndrome is evaluated with arteriography in provocative positions that reproduce the patient's symptoms. Most patients with arterial

involvement in this syndrome will have fusiform aneurysmal dilatation of the artery distal to the level of compression, representing poststenotic dilatation. Popliteal entrapment syndrome results from compression of the popliteal artery by an abnormal medial course of the popliteal artery in relation to the medial head of gastrocnemius, by an abnormal insertion of the medial gastrocnemius, or by the popliteus muscle. Unilateral calf claudication in a young male patient is the usual clinical presentation. Angiographic findings include medial deviation of the popliteal artery and stenosis. Other findings include popliteal artery thrombosis and aneurysm formation.

The popliteal artery also requires investigation in a patient who has sustained a knee dislocation. There is a high association of vascular injuries with knee dislocation, including thrombosis, intimal flap, and rupture. Physical examination is suspicious for a major vascular injury when pedal pulses are diminished or absent (Figure 7–10). MR arteriography can be performed in the acute setting with evaluation of the knee injury, but there should be no delay in the evaluation of this vessel. An overlooked popliteal artery injury can lead to occlusion and ultimately require amputation.

Other Procedures

Interventional radiologists can also play a role in feeding a patient. Percutaneous placement of

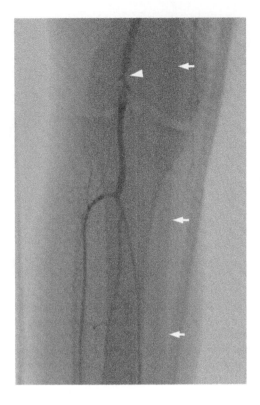

Figure 7–10 Popliteal artery injury. Frontal film from an arteriogram after a knee dislocation. The patency of the popliteal artery is the most critical factor to evaluate after a knee dislocation. This can be done with arteriography. Irregularity and narrowing of the popliteal artery is identified in this patient (*arrowhead*). This would be consistent with an intimal tear. Note that the patient is in a knee immobilizer (*arrows*) to maintain stability of the knee. (Courtesy of Tony Smith, MD.)

Table 7–2	Commonly Performed Nonvascular Procedures
Biopsy	
Abscess drainage	
Biliary drainage	
Gastrostomy tube placement	
Nephrostomy	
Stone extraction	
Foreign body retrieval	

gastrostomy and gastrojejunostomy tubes for enteral nutrition has gained widespread acceptance in management of patients who cannot eat for a variety of reasons. The Seldinger technique is used to access the stomach, and the tube is secured in place (**Table 7–2**).

Percutaneous nephrostomy is used to treat urinary obstruction caused by calculus, neoplasm, or stricture. Again, the Seldinger technique is

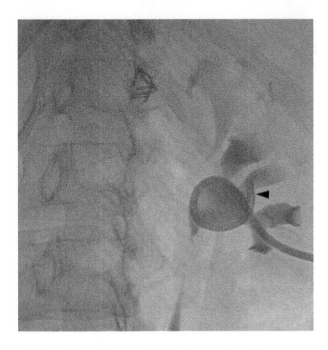

Figure 7–11 Percutaneous nephrostomy. Single image from percutaneous drainage of dilated collecting system. Drainage catheter is in place (*arrowhead*), and residual contrast material can be seen in the collecting system that has been decompressed by the drainage catheter. Surgical clips are incidentally noted adjacent to the spine on this image. (Courtesy of Tony Smith, MD.)

used for tube placement. A catheter is placed over the guidewire, allowing the renal collecting system to be decompressed. Through this access, ureteral stenting or stone removal may also be performed (Figure 7–11).

Obstructive jaundice may be further evaluated by percutaneous transhepatic cholangiography (PTC). A long needle is used to puncture the liver and identify bile ducts. The tract to the duct is dilated over a wire, and the obstructed area is traversed if possible. Stents can be placed to relieve strictures.

Percutaneous biopsies have prevented countless open surgical procedures performed solely to obtain tissue. These procedures are performed in most instances with CT guidance because of its superior depth control.

Abscesses and other fluid collections can be drained percutaneously using a modified Seldinger technique with CT guidance. A catheter is left in place in the fluid collection. Serial examinations can be performed with CT as necessary.

Emergencies

As discussed in this chapter, interventional radiology is often used to both diagnose and treat vascular abnormalities. In many cases, the diagnosis leads to emergent treatment. In severe occlusive disease with acute loss of distal pulses, angiography with vessel repair, stent placement, or angioplasty should be performed. In the setting of a motor vehicle crash and a patient with a widened mediastinum, suspicion for an injury to the aorta must exist. Aortography is used to locate the site of the injury. Similarly, embolization techniques can be used after identification of a damaged or leaky vessel.

Patients suffering from obstruction in nonvascular structures can have the obstruction relieved by the placement of a drainage catheter using the Seldinger technique. This includes obstruction in the renal collecting system and biliary tree.

Suggested Reading List

Kadir S: Teaching Atlas of Interventional Radiology, Diagnostic and Therapeutic Angiography. New York, Thieme, 1999.

Kessel D, Robertson I: Interventional Radiology, 2nd ed. Philadelphia, Churchill Livingstone, 2005.

Vedantham S, Gould J: Vascular and Interventional Imaging. Philadelphia, Mosby, 2004.

Nuclear Imaging

Chapter outline

Nuclear medicine is a subspecialty in radiology that uses radioactivity to help identify function and disease processes. A radioactive substrate is attached to a chemical that is taken up by the organ of interest. As the radioactive chemical decays, it gives off gamma rays. The gamma rays are detected by a gamma camera. Nuclear medicine studies provide physiologic information, but anatomic detail is lacking. Therefore, nuclear medicine studies should always be interpreted with corresponding radiographic images.

There are many types of nuclear medicine studies, and, in fact, there are therapeutic uses of nuclear medicine as well. In this introductory chapter, the examinations that you will most likely be ordering and need to understand are presented.

Technical Aspects

Radiopharmaceutical is the term applied to radioactive components attached to molecules that mimic a compound normally taken up by an organ of interest. The most common way to inject these pharmaceuticals is via a peripheral vein. The gamma camera uses a sodium iodide crystal to detect radiopharmaceutical decay. Emitted rays strike the crystal and produce light scintillations that are converted to digital signals. The resultant image is a "physiologic image" of the distribution of the radiopharmaceutical in the body (Figure 8–1). Very little ionizing radiation is associated with this technique. Because the gamma camera can change position, additional views can be obtained without additional injections of radiopharmaceutical. It is imperative to understand that the information provided is physiologic information, *not* anatomic information (Key Point 8–1). You can see how something works, but you won't necessarily see where it is or, for that matter, what it looks like. For that, you must remember to have the corresponding imaging studies (conventional films, computed tomograms [CT], magnetic resonance images [MRI]) available for proper and complete assessment. Nuclear medicine is very sensitive, but it is not very specific.

When describing a nuclear medicine study, the correct terminology to describe the tracer activity seen on the film (or monitor) is *increased* or *decreased radiotracer activity*. Terms such as "density," "echogenicity," and "signal intensity" are inappropriate.

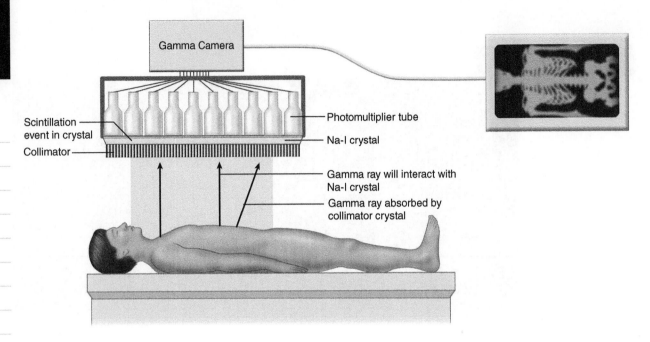

Scintillation event in crystal
Collimator
Photomultiplier tube
Na-I crystal
Gamma ray will interact with Na-I crystal
Gamma ray absorbed by collimator crystal
Gamma Camera

Figure 8–1 Schematic drawing of a setup in a nuclear medicine imaging area. The radioisotope is administered to the patient, and a gamma camera captures the gamma rays from the unstable nucleus of the atoms. The information is processed, and physiologic information is demonstrated.

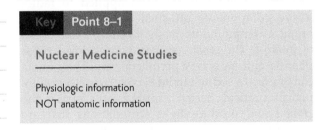

Key   Point 8–1

Nuclear Medicine Studies

Physiologic information
NOT anatomic information

By the way, do you remember which terms apply to which modalities?

Bone Scintigraphy

A number of disorders of the skeletal system can be assessed with bone scan imaging. The radiopharmaceutical used is technetium (Tc)-99m methylene diphosphonate. The mechanism of its function is not completely understood, but it adsorbs to the newly formed mineral phase of bone. New bone formation occurs in response to the presence of *almost* any skeletal pathology. Therefore, images will demonstrate increased activity localized to the site of bone abnormality.

After the radiopharmaceutical injection, the patient is required to hydrate and void as much as possible. The radiopharmaceutical is cleared through the kidneys and can concentrate in the bladder. Therefore, regular voiding is recommended. Imaging is usually performed 2 to 3 hours after injection unless a three-phase bone scan is being performed.

Increased activity will be seen where there is increased regional blood flow as well as increased osteogenic activity. Decreased tracer accumulation is seen in situations where there is decreased blood flow (infarction) or the skeleton is destroyed such that no matrix elements are present. Multiple myeloma, certain metastatic lesions, and some aggressive lytic lesions may not show activity on bone scan imaging for exactly this reason.

Before you can completely understand what is abnormal, you should know that there are some normal areas of increased activity. Growth centers in children—particularly the distal femur, proximal tibia, and proximal humerus—typically show increased radiotracer activity. One way to tell that the visualized activity is not pathologic is to note its symmetry. You can also expect to see activity in the kidneys, in the bladder, and at the intravenous injection site. What also affects the intensity of the image is the distance between the structure and the collimator (Figure 8–2).

Applications for bone scan imaging include evaluation for metastatic disease, trauma, stress fracture, insufficiency fracture, infection, and child abuse. Bone scan imaging is very sensitive for detecting metastatic lesions and will identify the focus before an abnormality can be seen on conventional x-ray films. The bone scan is not able to make a distinction between benign versus malignant processes. This is particularly true when a single lesion is identified on bone scan imaging.

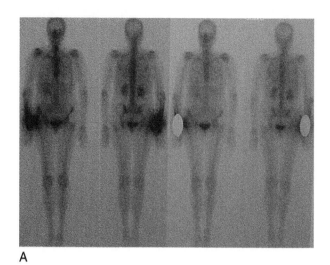

A

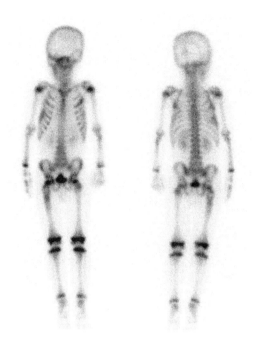

B

Figure 8–2   Whole-body bone scan. A, Bone scan in an adult. Anterior and posterior images with attenuation of counts. Note that the pair of images to the left demonstrate extravasation of radioactive tracer in the wrist. The second set of images, to the right, have a shield over the area. B, Bone scan in a skeletally immature individual. Note the increased activity (black) at the epiphyses. Subtle areas of increased activity are noted in the proximal femur and ribs in this child with lymphoma. (Courtesy of David Williams, MD.)

Multiple lesions are much more likely to be due to metastatic disease (Figure 8–3). Bone scan imaging is helpful in the setting of trauma, but it is largely being replaced by MRI for the evaluation of occult and insufficiency fractures. In patients with proven fractures, about 80% of bone scan images are positive 24 hours after the trauma and about 95% are positive at 72 hours. This doesn't quite reach the sensitivity and specificity of MRI. Bone scan imaging can show increased activity in a fracture site for up to 1 year after the trauma. In evaluating stress fractures, the bone scan will be positive 1 to 2 weeks before the conventional radiograph. Some clinicians prefer to order a bone scan for evaluation of stress fractures. Usually, a positive study leads to cross-sectional imaging with CT or MRI. Therefore, the patient has been subjected to the time and expense of two studies. Many clinicians prefer to order MRI for the evaluation of stress fractures, because the information is well visualized.

Bone scan imaging may not be as sensitive as conventional films in evaluating child abuse. Fractures more than 1 year old may not be appreciated. Therefore, a skeletal series should be obtained for nonaccidental trauma. A skeletal survey can demonstrate injuries at a variety of different stages of healing.

During your career, you will have many opportunities to see a patient who has a concern for osteomyelitis. A three-phase bone scan may be helpful in evaluating this pathologic process, especially when the patient has cellulitis on examination. During phase 1 or the flow portion, images are obtained in the first minute. Phase 2 is the blood pool phase, with images obtained 5 minutes after injection. Phase 3 is the delayed image, usually obtained 2 to 4 hours after injection (**Table 8–1**). Osteomyelitis can be suggested if there is progressive skeletal uptake and decreased soft tissue uptake. Cellulitis is suggested if persistent soft tissue uptake is noted without accumulation of skeletal activity.

Other uses of bone scan imaging are in the evaluation of metabolic bone disease (hyperparathyroidism, renal osteodystrophy), Paget's disease, and arthritis (any type) (Figure 8–4). In addition to uptake within bone, extraskeletal increased uptake can be seen in the kidneys. The kidneys should always be inspected on a bone scan image for evidence of renal masses, obstruction, displacement, and size. Dystrophic calcifications can also be identified and are not infrequently seen in the heart or skeletal muscle. Malignant pleural effusions may show increased activity, and some

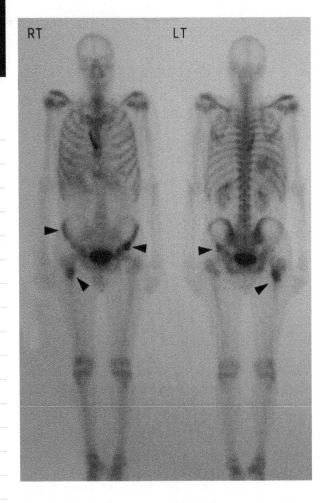

Figure 8–3 Bone scan in metastatic disease. Anterior and posterior projections demonstrate multiple foci of increased activity (*arrowheads*) in this patient with a known diagnosis of lung cancer. You can often tell which view you are looking at by assessing which bones you are seeing to better advantage. For instance, the image to the right demonstrates the scapula, a posteriorly located structure.

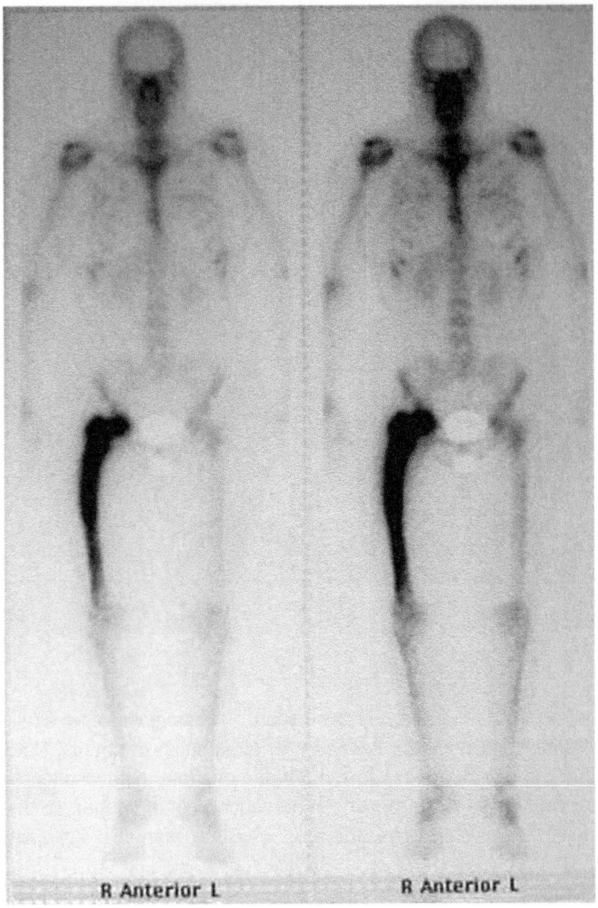

Figure 8–4 Bone scan in Paget's disease. Anterior and posterior projections from a whole-body bone scan demonstrate markedly increased activity of the femur. Note that the affected femur is slightly enlarged compared with the contralateral femur. The enlargement and marked activity are characteristic of Paget's disease.

Table 8–1 Three-Phase Bone Scan	
Phase	Time
Phase 1—Flow	1 minute
Phase 2—Blood pool	5 minutes
Phase 3—Delay	2–4 hours

extraskeletal tumors may demonstrate radiotracer activity. The activity in these locations must always be correlated with additional radiographic imaging.

Ventilation/Perfusion Scan

Pulmonary embolus (PE) is a common disorder associated with significant mortality rates. With proper detection and timely treatment, mortality can be significantly reduced. Establishing the diagnosis is not always easy. Mentioned in Chapter 2 are the evaluation of PE and the utility of CT to identify PE in patients who can tolerate the use of contrast material. The diagnosis is often difficult to make partly because the signs and symptoms are nonspecific. The classic triad of dyspnea, pleuritic chest pain, and hemoptysis are infrequently seen in clinical practice, and conventional chest x-ray and laboratory tests are also nonspecific. A conventional chest x-ray should be performed in all patients with suspected PE, both for comparison with the V/Q scan and to ensure that no other thoracic pathology is present to account for the patient's symptoms. A V/Q scan is one way to help suggest the diagnosis of PE.

The radiopharmaceuticals used in this study are xenon 133 gas or Tc99m diethylenetriaminepentaacetic acid (DTPA) aerosol to assess ventilation, and Tc99m macroaggregated albumin (MAA) administered intravenously to assess perfusion. Inhaling xenon gas allows the overall and regional dynamics of ventilation to be evaluated. The perfusion MAA particles are very tiny (<10–90 μm) and can become lodged in pulmonary capillaries. If xenon gas is used, the ventilation must be performed before the perfusion because of the lower energy of xenon compared with technetium. Patients are usually in a sitting position (for greater diaphragmatic excursion). Three phases of the xenon exchange occur. Wash-in/single-breath (inhalation) allows for the patient to take in and hold a maximal inspiration. This is followed by an equilibrium phase, during which the patient breathes air and xenon (steady-state breathing). Finally, during the wash-out phase, the patient

breathes room air and xenon is trapped abnormally (exhalation). The images are acquired from a posterior projection. The normal scan has homogeneous distribution of xenon with complete outlining of both lungs during the wash-in and equilibrium phases, and uniform wash-out of xenon (Figure 8–5).

Injection of radiopharmaceutical into a peripheral vein of a supine patient begins the perfusion portion. Images are obtained immediately, and multiple projections are acquired. The normal appearance of the perfusion scan is homogeneous tracer distribution. Normal defects are due to hilar and mediastinal structures as seen on the conventional chest x-ray.

The hallmark of PE is a perfusion defect corresponding to a bronchopulmonary segment that exhibits normal ventilation with no abnormality on conventional chest x-ray (Figure 8–6). It is not always this straightforward. Many processes can

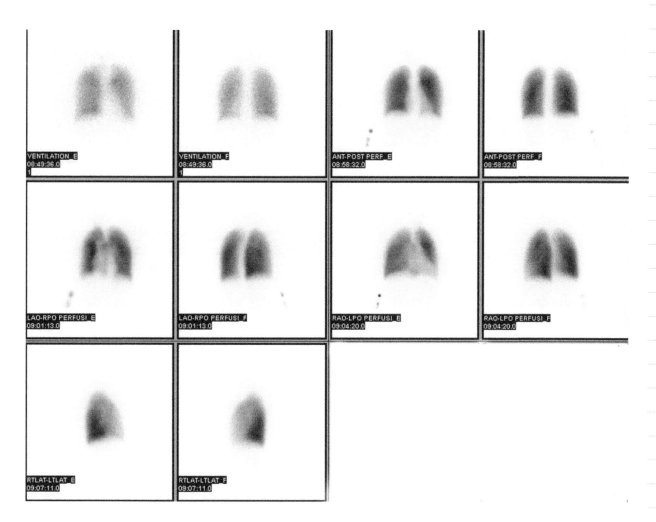

Figure 8–5   Normal ventilation/perfusion (V/Q) scan. Images show normal gas exchange with normal perfusion of the lungs.

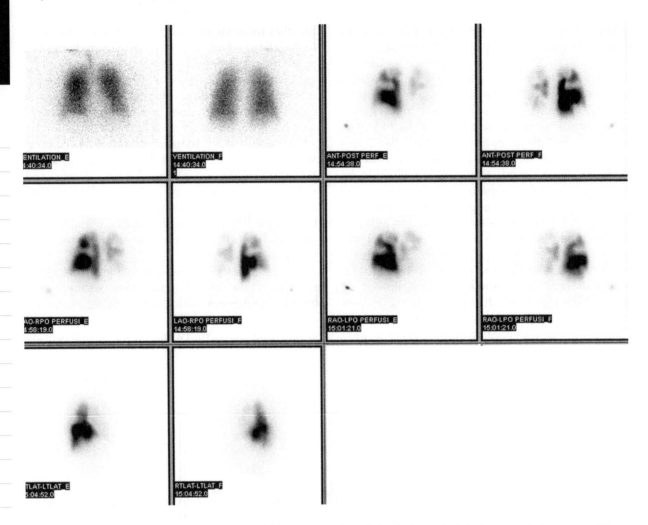

Figure 8–6 High-probability ventilation/perfusion (V/Q) scan. Normal ventilation is demonstrated. Marked perfusion abnormalities are demonstrated as areas of perfusion defects (decreased or no activity).

lead to a perfusion abnormality, so the chest x-ray needs to be assessed to see whether the non-perfused area corresponds to an abnormality on the chest x-ray. The more extensive the preexisting pulmonary abnormality, the harder it is to diagnose PE. A *V/Q mismatch* is suggested when there is normal ventilation and abnormal perfusion. **Table 8–2** lists the possible causes of V/Q mismatch.

A *V/Q match* is noted when there is abnormal ventilation and perfusion in the same area of equal size. **Table 8–3** lists possible explanations for a V/Q match. *Segmental defects* are wedge-shaped and pleural-based defects corresponding to a portion of lung supplied by a pulmonary arterial branch. Knowing the pulmonary anatomy can be helpful. Most nuclear medicine departments have this anatomy posted or a book nearby to look it up. These segmental defects are associated with a PE. A *nonsegmental* defect is not wedge-shaped, does not

Table 8–2 Causes of V/Q Mismatch
Acute pulmonary embolism (PE)
Chronic PE
Other emboli (drug abuse, iatrogenic)
Bronchogenic carcinoma
Adenopathy (obstructing vessels)
Hypoplasia of pulmonary artery
Swyer-James syndrome
Post-radiation
Vasculitis

correspond to a pulmonary segment, and it is not associated with PE. Some examples of abnormalities leading to nonsegmental defects are listed in **Table 8–4**. Defects are considered small if they

Table 8–3 Causes of V/Q Match
Chronic obstructive pulmonary disease
Bronchitis/bronchiectasis
Blebs/bullae
Congestive heart failure
Pulmonary edema
Pleural effusion
Asthma
Pulmonary trauma/hematoma
Inhalation injury
Mucous plug
Tumor

Table 8–4 Nonsegmental Defects
Pacemaker artifact
Tumor
Pleural effusion
Trauma
Hemorrhage
Bullae
Cardiomegaly
Mediastinal and hilar lymphadenopathy
Atelectasis
Aortic ectasia
Aneurysm

Table 8–5 Probability That a Pulmonary Embolism (PE) Has Occurred Based on Results of the Ventilation/Perfusion (V/Q) Scan (Modified PIOPED Criteria)*

High Probability (≥80% in the absence of conditions known to mimic PE)

Two or more large mismatched segmental perfusion defects or the arithmetic equivalent in moderate or large and moderate defects.[†]
Two large mismatched segmental perfusion defects, or the arithmetic equivalent[†], are borderline for "high probability." Individual readers may correctly interpret individual images with this pattern as "high probability." In general, it is recommended that more than this degree of mismatch should be present for the "high probability" category.

Intermediate Probability (20–79%)

One moderate to two large mismatched perfusion defects or the arithmetic equivalent in moderate or large and moderate defects.[†]
Single-matched V/Q defect with clear chest radiograph. Very extensive matched defects can be categorized as "low probability."
Single V/Q matches are borderline for "low probability" and should be categorized as "intermediate" in most circumstances by most readers, although individual readers may correctly interpret individual scintigrams with this pattern as "low probability."
Difficult to categorize as low or high or not described as low or high.

Low Probability (<20%)

Nonsegmental perfusion defects (e.g., cardiomegaly, enlarged aorta, enlarged hila, elevated diaphragm).
Any perfusion defect with a substantially larger chest radiographic abnormality.
Perfusion defects matched by ventilation abnormality provided (1) that there is a clear chest radiograph and (2) that there are some areas of normal perfusion in the lungs.
Any number of small perfusion defects with a normal chest radiograph.

Normal

No perfusion defects, or perfusion exactly outlines the shape of the lungs seen on the chest radiograph. (Note that hilar and aortic impressions may be seen and the chest radiograph and/or ventilation study may be abnormal.)

*Prospective Investigation of Pulmonary Embolism Diagnosis, Society of Nuclear Medicine, version 3.0, approved Feb 2004.
[†]A large segmental defect, >75% of a segment, equals 1 segmental equivalent; a moderate defect, 25–75% of a segment, equals 0.5 segmental equivalents; a small defect, <25% of a segment, is not counted.

account for less than 25% of the segment, moderate if they occupy 25% to 75% of the segment, and large if they represent more than 75% of the segment. Differential lung perfusion can be seen with prior pneumonectomy or lobectomy.

The results from the V/Q scan are used to estimate the probability that an acute PE has occurred. An entirely normal perfusion pattern indicates no chance of embolus, and other causes of the patient's symptoms should be entertained. A finding of

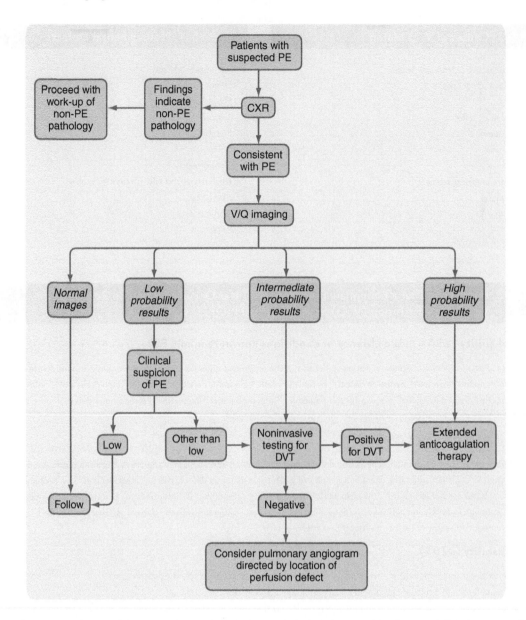

Figure 8–7   Pulmonary embolus (PE) workup. An algorithm for the workup of a PE as a quick reference. CXR, chest x-ray; DVT, deep venous thrombosis; V/P, ventilation/perfusion.

multiple (two or more) segmental perfusion defects with a normal ventilation study indicates a very high probability that the patient had a PE. As you can imagine, most cases lie somewhere in between (**Table 8–5**). If the diagnosis is uncertain, evaluation for deep venous thrombosis (DVT) is recommended. Most thromboemboli are a result of lower-extremity DVT. If the decision to perform pulmonary angiography is made, the perfusion study should act as a roadmap, guiding the interventional radiologist to the vessels that are most likely

affected. Figure 8–7 is an algorithm for the workup of suspected PE.

Hepatobiliary Scintigraphy

Patients with acute cholecystitis typically present with right upper quadrant pain and tenderness, fever, and an elevated white blood cell count. The diagnosis usually requires confirmation with ultrasonography or hepatobiliary scintigraphy. The radiopharmaceutical used is Tc-99m diisopropyl

Table 8–6 Causes of False-Positive Hepatobiliary Scintigraphy Results

Prolonged fasting (>48 hr)
Food within 2 hr
Chronic cholecystitis
Chronic alcohol abuse
Pancreatitis, hepatic insufficiency
Hyperalimentation
Severe illness

iminodiacetic acid (DISIDA), which is an analog of bilirubin. It is transported into hepatocytes, *not* conjugated, and excreted in its original form into the biliary tract. The patient must take nothing by mouth (NPO) for 4 hours (not longer than 24 hours) before the study. Prior to the study, the patient should use no opiates. Imaging is performed immediately after the injection in the anterior projection. One-minute images are obtained for 60 minutes. A right lateral view is obtained. Morphine can be given as well as cholecystokinin (CCK).

Certain conditions predispose to false-positive results. The most common is prolonged fasting. These patients will have lack of gallbladder visualization because the bilirubin derivative is blocked from uptake into the gallbladder due to viscous gallbladder contents in the fasting patient. On the flip side, if patients have eaten within 2 hours of the study, the gallbladder is likely to be contracted, which will limit the entry of radioactive bile into the gallbladder. Conditions that can lead to false-positive studies are listed in **Table 8–6**. Morphine can improve visualization of the gallbladder because it constricts the sphincter of Oddi, leading to a rise in pressure in the biliary system. This leads to improved gallbladder visualization and fewer false-positive results. The normal scan has prompt clearance of tracer by the liver (5 minutes), and the liver is homogeneous. The gallbladder, common bile duct, and small bowel are visualized by 60 minutes (Figure 8–8).

The test is extremely sensitive and specific, meaning that a normal study virtually excludes acute cholecystitis (Figure 8–9). The one exception is acalculous cholecystitis. In a small percentage of patients with acalculous cholecystitis, the gallbladder will be visualized.

Common bile duct obstruction can be detected with hepatobiliary scintigraphy within the first 24 hours of the disease, when ultrasound studies may be negative. Hepatic activity is identified without excretion. This study is also useful in distinguishing biliary atresia from neonatal jaundice, because small bowel is not visualized in a patient with biliary atresia. Additionally, bile leaks from trauma or surgery can be identified.

Gastrointestinal Bleeding

Evaluation of gastrointestinal (GI) bleeding is most often done with scintigraphy. The study helps to identify where the source is in the bowel by

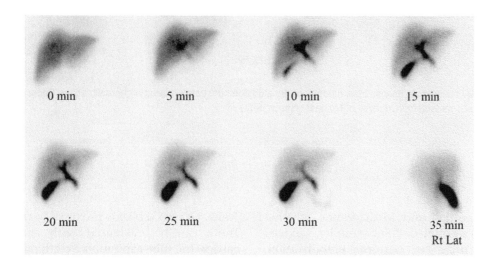

Figure 8–8   Normal hepatobiliary study. Filling of the ducts is noted in a timely fashion, and the tracer activity fills the gallbladder. (Courtesy of Michael Hanson, MD.)

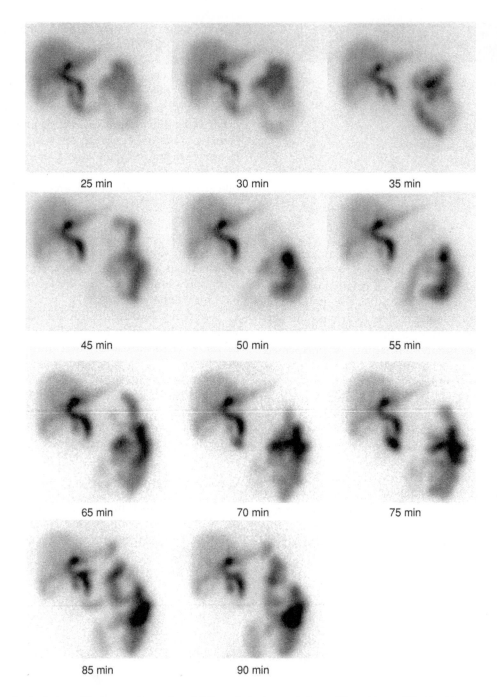

25 min   30 min   35 min

45 min   50 min   55 min

65 min   70 min   75 min

85 min   90 min

Figure 8–9   Acute cholecystitis. Images from a hepatobiliary study demonstrate no filling of the gallbladder. Tracer activity is seen in the small bowel and duct system. (Courtesy of Michael Hanson, MD.)

approximate location and to determine whether angiography is warranted. If angiography is indeed indicated in order to perform embolization, scintigraphy results can help guide initial vessel selection to shorten the study. This study is more useful for GI bleeds located distal to the ligament of Treitz. Upper GI bleeds proximal to the ligament of Treitz can be evaluated with endoscopy and nasogastric tube aspiration. Scintigraphy is used to evaluate patients with melena or bright red blood per rectum (BRBPR). It is not useful for a patient with guaiac-positive stools, in whom GI bleeding is

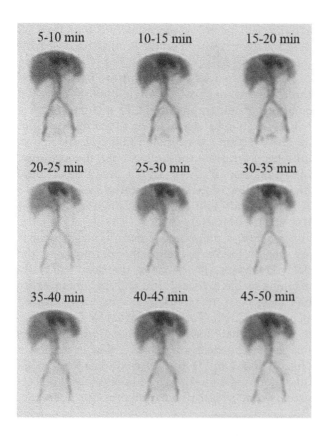

5-10 min   10-15 min   15-20 min

20-25 min   25-30 min   30-35 min

35-40 min   40-45 min   45-50 min

Figure 8–10   Normal tagged red blood cell study. There is no collection of tracer activity outside the normal pattern of vessels. (Courtesy of Michael Hanson, MD.)

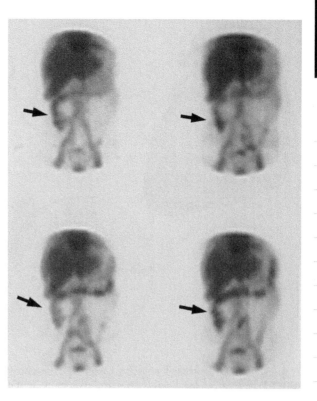

Figure 8–11   Abnormal tagged red blood cell study. Abnormal tracer activity is identified outside the vessels in the right upper quadrant (*arrows*). This was caused by a bleed affecting the cecum and ascending colon. (Courtesy of Michael Hanson, MD.)

not brisk enough to be detectable with scintigraphy. In this study, technetium is tagged to red blood cells (RBCs). Stannous pyrophosphate is injected and circulates for about 15 minutes. Technetium pertechnetate is injected to label the RBCs. This works because a stannous ion diffuses into the RBC, followed by pertechnetate. The stannous reduces the pertechnetate, which then binds to the beta chain of hemoglobin. The blood pool then is "labeled," and an area of active bleeding can be visualized. Continuous acquisition for 120 minutes in an anterior projection is performed. A normal scan is noted when all images are identical and show blood vessels, liver, spleen, stomach, kidneys, and bladder due to unreduced free pertechnetate (Figure 8–10).

Bleeding scans are more sensitive than angiography (hemorrhage rates of 0.1–0.4 mL/min versus 1.0 mL/min). Therefore, many angiographic studies are negative with positive bleeding scans. A positive diagnosis is made when active bleeding is identified as extravascular activity that increases and

Table 8–7	Pharmaceuticals Used for Myocardial Stress Testing
Dipyridamole	
Adenosine	
Dobutamine	

changes over time in the configuration of small or large bowel. Intraluminal blood can move antegrade or retrograde. Therefore, the bleeding site needs to be identified on the first images (Figure 8–11).

Tagged RBC studies are also used in evaluation of liver hemangiomas and in gated blood pool studies for cardiac evaluation.

Myocardial Perfusion Imaging

Continuing the discussion of gated blood pool imaging and its application to cardiac imaging, the

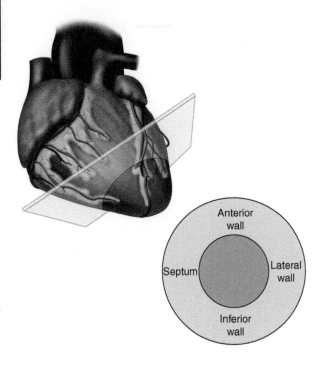

Figure 8–12 Single-photon emission computed tomography (SPECT) images of the heart. Schematic showing how the images of the myocardium are acquired with SPECT imaging.

ejection fraction (EF) of the heart can be estimated with this technique. This is done by counting the tracer activity at end-diastole (EDC) and end-systole (ESC) and using the equation, EF = (EDC − ESC)/EDC. Ventricular wall motion can also be assessed and categorized as hypokinetic, akinetic, or dyskinetic.

There are a couple of different radiopharmaceuticals that can be used to evaluate cardiac perfusion. Thallium (Tl) 201 acts as a potassium analog and accumulates in normally perfused myocardium. Tc-99m sestamibi provides a better quality image than Tl 201. A combination of the two studies can be performed, using Tl 201 for rest and Tc-99m sestamibi for exercise. Myocardial perfusion "stress" imaging can be performed with either exercise or a pharmaceutical (for patients who can't exercise). Pharmacologic agents include dipyridamole, adenosine, and dobutamine. Adenosine and dipyridamole are contraindicated in patients with asthma or severe bronchospasm (**Table 8–7**). The application of stress improves the sensitivity of myocardial perfusion imaging for detecting coronary artery disease. Arterioles distal to a normal vessel will increase the amount of myocardial perfusion after stress, leading to an increase in tracer activity. In a stenotic vessel, there will be little change in blood flow distal to the stenosis after stress, so the activity will be the same as before the stress. A defect is therefore seen on the immediate poststress images.

Perfusion images of the heart are performed in three dimensions using single-photon emission computed tomography (SPECT) imaging (Figure 8–12). This allows visualization of the myocardium in cross-section. A normal SPECT study shows uniform perfusion throughout the myocardium. Interpretation of these studies requires a little understanding of the different categories of disease. A *normal* study will show no change in images at rest versus after exercise (Figure 8–13). A *reversible* abnormality is diagnosed when perfusion defects are seen on the stress images that normalize on the delayed images. This area of the heart generally contains viable myocardium, and this abnormality has also been referred to as "exercise-induced ischemia" (Figure 8–14). A *nonreversible* abnormality is an area that does not change from the stress images to the delayed images. This is termed a "fixed" defect and is also referred to as myocardial infarction (Figure 8–15). These areas of fixed defects usually contain scar tissue from previous infarction.

PET/CT Imaging

This short section is meant to introduce the concept of positron emission tomography (PET)/CT to you. The idea of this imaging modality is to combine the information provided from nuclear medicine studies (physiologic information) with the cross-sectional imaging of CT (anatomic information). The isotope used in PET imaging is 18-fluorodeoxyglucose (18-FDG) (Figure 8–16). Foci of altered glucose metabolism (as occurs with a variety of disease processes) can be localized definitively to an anatomic structure, organ, or specific region within an organ. The impact of this technology on patient care is clear. It facilitates the diagnosis, identifies an optimal biopsy site, and monitors response to treatment.

Combined PET/CT scanners allow for images to be done in a timely fashion, and direct comparison of the imaging modalities can be made. Patients are injected with FDG radiopharmaceutical and placed on a CT scan-like unit. Images are acquired for PET and for CT. The CT images are performed without contrast. The implications for this technology are great, and it begs the question of what additional combined imaging techniques will come along in the future. Perhaps it will be one of you who pushes the envelope for this specialty by devising improved techniques and equipment and allowing for continued improvements in our ability to care for patients.

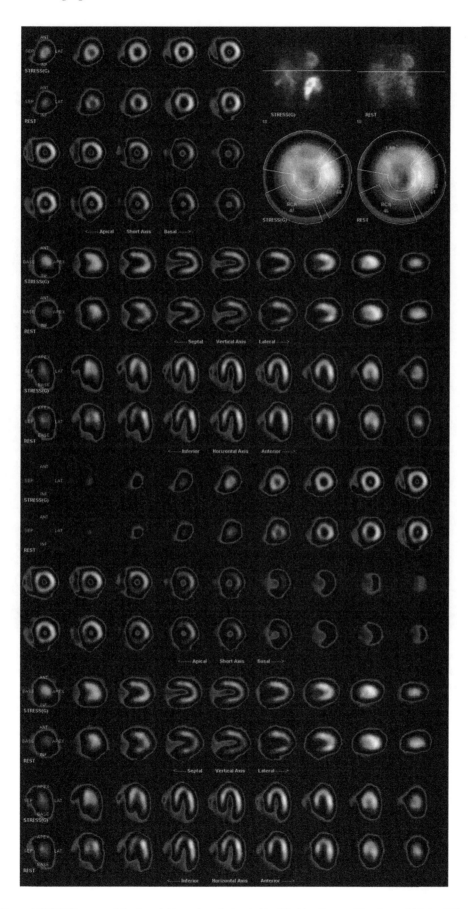

Figure 8–13   Normal SPECT images of the heart. Normal perfusion is identified in all axes. (Courtesy of Michael Hanson, MD.)

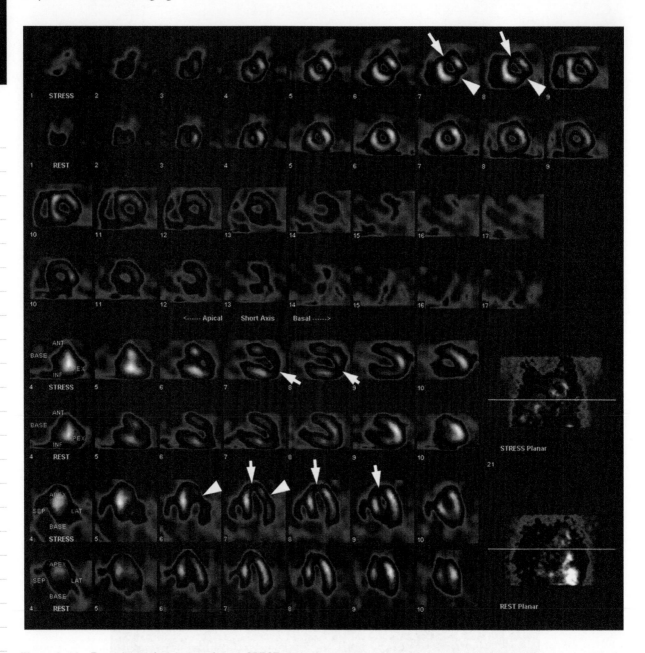

Figure 8–14 Reversible defect. Images from a SPECT study showing stress and rest. A reversible perfusion defect is noted in the distribution of the left anterior descending artery (*arrows*) and the lateral circumflex artery (*arrowheads*). With rest, the perfusion returns to normal. (Courtesy of Michael Hanson, MD.)

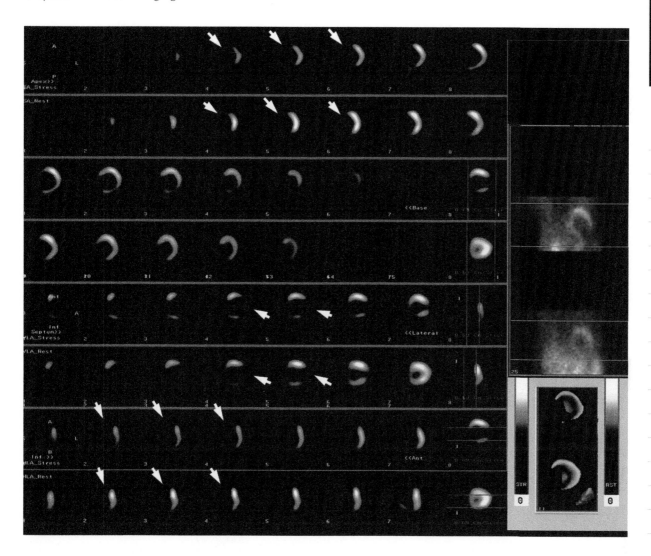

Figure 8–15   Irreversible (fixed) defect. Images from a SPECT study show a fixed defect in the distribution of the left anterior descending artery (*arrows*). This would indicate that the patient has sustained a myocardial infarction, and scar is now located in this area. (Courtesy of Michael Hanson, MD.)

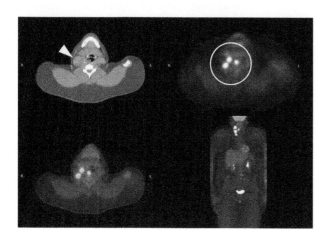

Figure 8–16   Positron emission tomography (PET)/CT. CT axial image through the region of the mandible shows asymmetry of the soft tissues of the neck. The right side of the neck is enlarged compared with the left (*arrowhead*). The corresponding fluorodeoxyglucose (FDG) PET image shows this area to have increased uptake (*circle*), compatible with disease in this patient with head and neck cancer. (Courtesy of David Williams, MD.)

Suggested Reading List

Donohoe KJ, Van den Abbeeale A: Teaching Atlas of Nuclear Medicine. New York, Thieme, 2000.

Mettler FA, Guiberteau MJ: Essentials of Nuclear Medicine Imaging, 4th ed. Philadelphia, WB Saunders, 1998.

Zeissman H, O'Malley JP, Thrall J: Nuclear Medicine: The Requisites, 3rd ed. Philadelphia, Mosby, 2006.

Breast Imaging

Mammographic images are not likely to be reviewed on call or in the middle of the night. Nevertheless, a chapter is devoted to breast imaging because many of you will need to be able to discuss the techniques available for imaging with your patients, and will have to order examinations based on the current guidelines. This information will be provided for you in this chapter.

Diagnostic Versus Screening Mammography

Breast imaging involves *screening studies* as well as *diagnostic studies*. The difference between the two studies is that the *screening* study is geared toward early detection of breast cancers. It is done on a routine basis in an asymptomatic female. The screening mammogram consists of two standard views: the craniocaudal (CC) and the mediolateral oblique (MLO). The radiologist interprets the examination but is not required to be present during the screening study (Key Point 9–1).

The *diagnostic study* is a specialized, tailored study designed to evaluate a specific breast complaint (such as a palpable lump) or to perform further workup or monitor an uncertain mammographic abnormality. The diagnostic examination is also performed in patients with implants and in patients with a history of breast cancer treated conservatively (minimal surgery). Special mammographic views are used including the true lateral view (90 degrees), magnification views, focal compression, and axillary views. Additional views and techniques are performed as the radiologist feels is necessary. The radiologist interprets and directs the diagnostic examination. The diagnostic

---

Key Point 9–1

Screening Mammogram

Indication
    Early detection of breast cancer
    Asymptomatic patient
Views
    Craniocaudal
    Mediolateral oblique
Radiologist
    Not present during image acquisition
    Interprets study

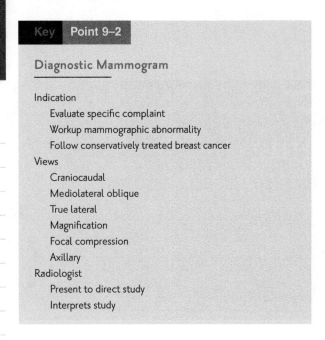

Key   Point 9–2

Diagnostic Mammogram

Indication
   Evaluate specific complaint
   Workup mammographic abnormality
   Follow conservatively treated breast cancer
Views
   Craniocaudal
   Mediolateral oblique
   True lateral
   Magnification
   Focal compression
   Axillary
Radiologist
   Present to direct study
   Interprets study

workup may require ultrasonography of the breast or breast magnetic resonance imaging (MRI) (Key Point 9–2).

Breast cancer survival is influenced by the size of the tumor and the lymph node status at the time of diagnosis. When the cancer is small and there is no axillary lymph node involvement, 5-year survival rates are greater than 95%. These cancers are rarely diagnosed by physical examination and are most often identified on screening examinations. When breast cancer becomes palpable with negative axillary lymph nodes, the 5-year survival rate

decreases to about 70%. In the setting of positive lymph nodes, the 5-year survival rate decreases to about 38%.

Techniques

Mammography requires high-contrast and high-spatial resolution for optimal imaging. Therefore, standard radiographic equipment is not satisfactory. Mammography is performed on special equipment dedicated to achieving high-contrast and high-spatial resolution. Mammographic units are equipped with compression paddles that are designed to squeeze the breast against the film holder. Good compression of the breast is essential to high-quality mammographic technique, because the compression spreads overlapping breast structures so that masses can be distinguished from summation shadows. Patient movement is minimized (who would want to move while the breast is being compressed in this device?) (Figure 9–1).

The MLO view depicts the greatest amount of breast tissue. The x-ray tube and holder are moved to an angle that parallels the orientation of the patient's pectoralis major muscle. For the CC view, the unit is placed in the vertical position so that the x-ray tube is perpendicular to the floor (Figure 9–2).

For the radiologist, the viewing conditions of the room need to be optimized. The room should be dark, and all ambient light should be blocked. A magnifying lens is always used for evaluation of breast tissue and allows for visualization of tiny microcalcifications.

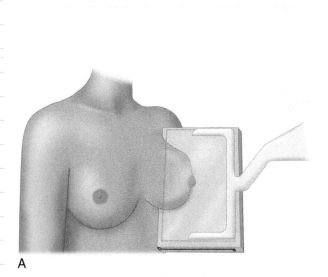

A

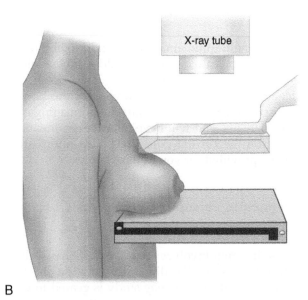

X-ray tube

B

Figure 9–1   Schematic diagram showing the normal setup to obtain mediolateral oblique (MLO) A and craniocaudal (CC) B compression views of the breast.

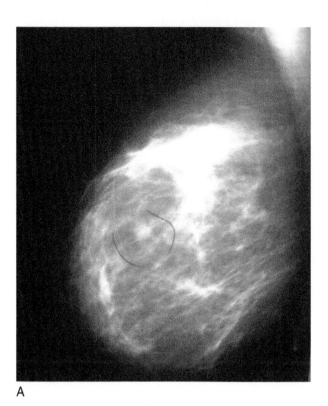

A

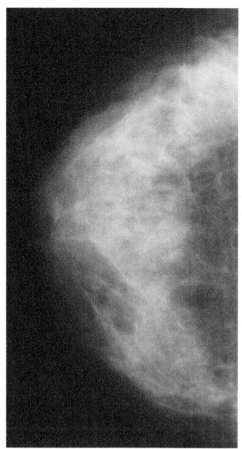

B

Figure 9–2 Mammographic views. A, Mediolateral oblique (MLO) view. Adequate chest wall and axilla is noted. A mass is noted on this image (*outlined*), which proved to be a fibroadenoma by biopsy. B, Craniocaudal (CC) view. Breast tissue has to be adequately compressed. One way to determine adequate compression is by noting crisp margins to breast parenchyma. Blurry margins suggest inadequate compression. Dense fibroglandular tissue (more white) is noted in a normal distribution.

Of all methods to image the breast, mammography provides the most information at a low cost. However, 10% of palpable cancers are not seen on mammograms. These false-negative studies may occur because of a poor-quality study (inadequate compression, incomplete coverage of breast tissue), error in interpretation (computer-automated systems are being developed to help in this regard—a controversial topic beyond the scope of this chapter), cancers hidden in dense breast tissue, and cancers that are difficult to detect because of their appearance (lobular carcinomas). Other modalities have been investigated for their potential in screening, but none can approach the sensitivity and specificity of mammography.

Ultrasound may help in differentiating cystic from solid masses. It is used as part of a diagnostic examination to evaluate a particular area of concern (palpable mass or mammographic finding). The entire breast is not evaluated with ultrasound. Since ultrasound does not involve radiation, it can be used to evaluate a problem in a young or pregnant female. MRI is most useful for evaluation of the integrity of breast implants. This technique is sensitive and specific for rupture of the implants (Figure 9–3). MRI is not useful as a screening technique because of the expense and time it takes to perform. However, it may be of help in localizing occult lesions. All of the studies mentioned thus far are noninvasive techniques (although the compression aspect is questionable!). Scintimammography is a relatively new nuclear medicine study that is still being investigated. This technique involves intravenous injection (which now makes this an invasive study) of a radiopharmaceutical (usually technetium-99m sestamibi). The radiopharmaceutical is taken up by the cancer cells. This technique may prove useful in patients with dense breasts and in those who are being followed after biopsy or lumpectomy. The radiopharmaceutical

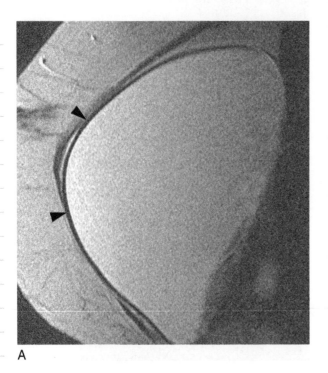

A

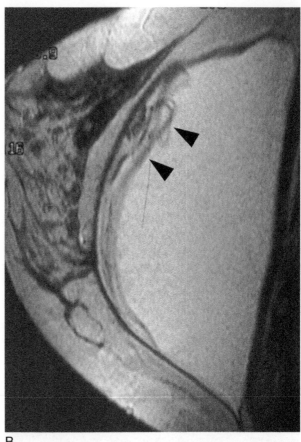

B

Figure 9–3   A, Breast implant. Sagittal T2-weighted image of a breast implant demonstrates well-defined low-signal "capsule" around the implant (*arrowheads*). B, Sagittal T2-weighted image of implant rupture demonstrates the "linguini" sign. Note the irregular lines of low signal (*arrowheads*). This is a finding of rupture of an implant by MRI. (Courtesy of Mary Scott Soo, MD.)

should be taken up by lymph nodes containing cancer cells. Increased uptake in the nodes has been referred to as the "sentinel node." The areas of increased activity can then get appropriately treated.

Screening Recommendations

Certain factors are known to increase a woman's risk of developing breast cancer. These include close family history of the disease (mother or sibling), precancerous breast lesions diagnosed at biopsy, first child born after age 30 years, nulliparity, and obesity. When adopting a screening policy, the physician must remember that all women are at risk for developing breast cancer. The American Cancer Society (ACS) estimates that one in every nine women will develop the disease. The majority of women will not have histories that place them at higher risk. The current recommendation from the ACS is that yearly screening should begin at age 40 years. This should be complemented by a

Table 9–1	American Cancer Society Guidelines for Breast Cancer Screening, 2006	
Age (yr)	Clinical Examination	Mammography
20–39	Every 3 yr	Not recommended
≥40	Annually	Annually

monthly self-examination and yearly physical examination. Younger patients with increased risk may be screened earlier than the average population (Table 9–1). Any breast mass, regardless of whether the patient has had a recent negative mammogram, requires immediate attention.

Anatomy

Normal breast tissue is composed mainly of lobules and ducts, connective tissue, and fat. Lobules are drained by ducts, which branch within lobes. The

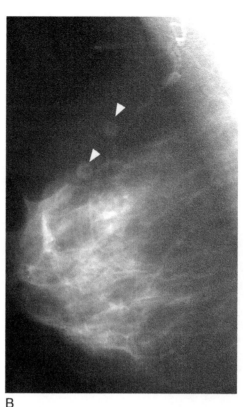

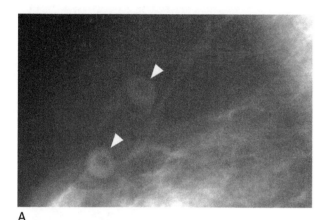

A

B

Figure 9–4   Normal lymph nodes. Mediolateral oblique (MLO) A and close-up B mammographic views show well-defined soft tissue densities with a lucent center (*arrowheads*). This is the appearance of normal lymph nodes. The lucent center is a fatty hilum seen in normal lymph nodes. (Courtesy of Jay Baker, MD.)

amount of glandular tissue is highly variable. Younger women tend to have more glandular tissue than older women. The breast is composed of a large amount of fat, which is lucent on mammograms (see Figure 9–2B). Lymph nodes are seen in the axilla and occasionally in the breast itself (Figure 9–4). There is a wide range of normal parenchymal density patterns related to variations in the ratio of fat to glandular tissue. Tissues that are lower in density (fat) are darker in the mammographic images. Tissues that are dense, such as fibroglandular tissue, are lighter (more white).

Abnormalities

Parenchymal density patterns vary for a variety of reasons (Table 9–2). Malignant masses are dense and may be hidden in normal dense background tissue. Breast tissue that contains a large amount of fat and little fibroglandular tissue allows for better identification of malignant masses and other dense abnormalities.

Classic signs of malignancy are spiculated masses or pleomorphic clusters of microcalcifications. Fewer than half of all cases of occult breast carcinoma present in these ways. The remainder

Table 9–2 Variations in Parenchymal Density
Weight changes
Hormonal changes
Pregnancy
Lactation
Menopause
Hormone replacement therapy
Genetic

of cases have more subtle or indirect signs of malignancy. False-negative and false-positive diagnoses must be balanced and minimized. Each time a woman is subjected to a surgical biopsy, financial and emotional costs as well as risks are incurred.

Masses

Once the radiologist has concluded that a mass is present, its size, margins, density, and location are assessed. The number of visible masses and their similarities and differences are noted. It is important that previous films be compared with the current study to look for new masses or an increase

Evaluation of Masses on Mammogram

Size
Margins
Density
Location
Number
Calcifications

Table 9–3 Lesions with Ill-Defined Margins

Breast cancer
Fat necrosis
Scar
Abscess
Hematoma

Table 9–4 Well-Circumscribed Masses

Cyst
Fibrosis
Fibroadenoma
Primary breast cancer
Metastatic disease
Lymphoma

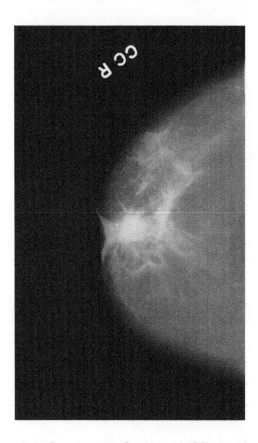

Figure 9–5 Breast cancer. Craniocaudal (CC) view demonstrates a mass with spiculated margins and associated microcalcifications. These findings are worrisome for malignancy. Two views are needed to localize the mass in the breast.

in the size of a mass (**Key Point 9–3**). Breast cancer is associated with ill-defined margins. Additional ill-defined masses include fat necrosis in an area that has been previously biopsied, scars, abscesses, and hematomas (Figure 9–5) (**Table 9–3**). Well-circumscribed margins can be seen with a number of abnormalities listed in **Table 9–4**. Architectural distortion is seen in some breast cancers. This process is also seen in scarring from previous surgery and in a sclerosing lesion known as a radial scar (Figure 9–6).

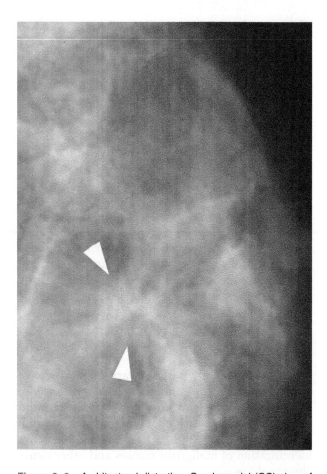

Figure 9–6 Architectural distortion. Craniocaudal (CC) view of the left breast shows an area in the retroareolar region which demonstrates increased density with a radial appearance of the breast tissue as the cancer tugs on the surrounding breast tissue (*arrowheads*). (Courtesy of Jay Baker, MD.)

Density

The density of a mammographically detected mass is an important characteristic. If the mass contains fat, for example, it is going to be a benign mass. There are a number of masses that contain fat density, including lipoma, oil cyst, and normal lymph nodes.

Location

Breast cancers can occur in any location, most often in the upper outer quadrant of the breast. Knowing the location of the intramammary lymph nodes is important in excluding these normally occurring structures as a pathologic process. Similarly, lesions located on the skin can erroneously be diagnosed as occurring within the breast. Identifying the air trapped around the lesion is key in not mistaking a skin lesion for an intramammary process.

Size

Cancers can be of any size. Size of the lesion is important in the follow-up step in the workup. Ultrasound is not as helpful in identifying lesions that are less than 5 mm in size.

Number of Masses

Many times multiple, well-defined round masses can be seen throughout one breast, or often in both breasts. These lesions most often represent cysts or adenomas. However, in a patient with a history of malignancy, these masses could represent metastatic disease. Benign and malignant lesions can coexist. The radiologist should evaluate these lesions using the criteria already described. A lesion with a different, suspicious morphology should prompt a biopsy.

Calcifications

When evaluating calcifications, the radiologist must note the features associated with the presence of this finding. These include form, distribution, size, and number.

Form Malignant calcifications are typically clustered and pleomorphic, with or without an associated soft tissue mass. These types of calcifications are seen in more than half of all mammographically discovered cancers (Figure 9–7). Benign calcifications may have a lucent center, may layer into a curvilinear or linear shape (milk of calcium), or may be tubular in orientation.

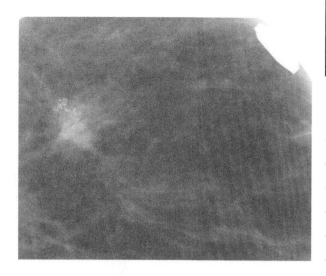

Figure 9–7. Worrisome microcalcifications. Magnification-compression views show a cluster of microcalcifications that are a variety of shapes and sizes. These are findings that are worrisome for carcinoma. Magnification-compression views are performed when an abnormality is found on the standard mediolateral oblique (MLO) and craniocaudal (CC) views.

Distribution Careful analysis with a magnifying glass is essential so that a morphologically dissimilar cluster is not overlooked. Such calcifications should be thoroughly examined with magnification views. Calcifications that are widely scattered (and bilateral) and morphologically similar are generally benign.

Size Malignant calcifications are generally less than 0.5 mm in size. Benign calcifications are often larger and similar in size when seen in clusters.

Number The greater the number of calcifications, the more likely it is that they are associated with malignant disease. Assessment with magnification views to determine morphology is imperative.

Implants

Various types of implants have been used in augmentation mammoplasty procedures. These implants can be filled with silicone gel or saline encased in silicone envelopes. Silicone is more radiopaque than saline (Figure 9–8). Screening mammography in a woman with implants requires the use of at least two extra views of the breast. Standard MLO and CC views are performed, and then the implants are displaced against the chest wall while the breast tissue is pulled anteriorly and vigorously compressed. Women with implants may present with complications related to the implant. These include abnormalities associated with the

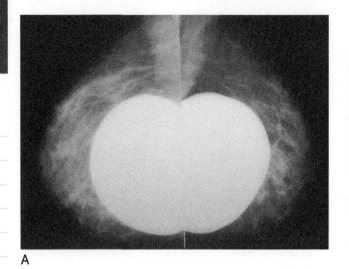

A

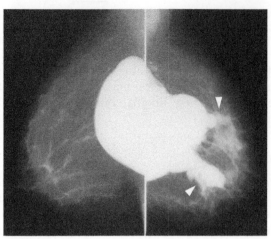

B

Figure 9–8. Mammographic appearance of silicone implants. A, MLO view of bilateral implants in this female. Note the well-defined contour of the implants. B, MLO view of a ruptured implant. Note the extravasation of silicone into the soft tissues (*arrowheads*) in this implant that ruptured. If you compare the two breasts, a contour abnormality of the breast with the ruptured implant can be seen. (Courtesy of Mary Scott Soo, MD.)

capsule, such as capsular contractures and herniations of the implant through rents in the capsule. The implant itself may rupture, and saline implants may deflate. Mammography is the first imaging method in patients older than 30 years of age with implants. MRI is useful in identifying ruptures and complications associated with implants (Figure 9–3).

In this brief overview, the salient points of radiographic examination and interpretation have been presented. For more in-depth reading on this topic, refer to any of the texts listed in the suggested reading list.

Suggested Reading List

Bassett LW, Jackson V, Fu K, Fu Y: Diagnosis of Diseases of the Breast, 2nd ed. Philadelphia, WB Saunders, 2005.

Cardenosa G: Breast Imaging (The Core Curriculum). Philadelphia, Lippincott Williams & Wilkins, 2004.

Ikeda D: Breast Imaging: The Requisites. Philadelphia, Mosby, 2005.

Index

Pages references followed by the letter *b* refer to boxes.
Pages references followed by the letter *f* refer to figures.
Pages references followed by the letter *t* refer to tables.

Printed and bound by CPI Group (UK) Ltd, Croydon, CR0 4YY

03/10/2024

01040345-0018